UNDOCTORED

WHY HEALTH CARE HAS FAILED YOU AND HOW YOU CAN BECOME SMARTER THAN YOUR DOCTOR

WILLIAM DAVIS, MD

#1 *New York Times* Bestselling Author of *Wheat Belly* and *Wheat Belly Total Health*

RODALE.

RODALE *wellness*

Live happy. Be healthy. Get inspired.

Sign up today to get exclusive access to our authors, exclusive bonuses,
and the most authoritative, useful, and cutting-edge information on health,
wellness, fitness, and living your life to the fullest.

Visit us online at RodaleWellness.com
Join us at RodaleWellness.com/Join

© 2017 by William Davis, MD

Rodale books may be purchased for business or promotional use or for special sales.
For information, please write to:
Trade Books/Special Markets Department, Rodale Inc., 733 Third Avenue, New York, NY 10017

Printed in the United States of America
Rodale Inc. makes every effort to use acid-free ∞, recycled paper ♻.

Book design by Amy King

Library of Congress Cataloging-in-Publication Data is on file with the publisher.

ISBN 978–1–62336–866–1   trade hardcover

Distributed to the trade by Macmillan

2   4   6   8   10   9   7   5   3   1   hardcover

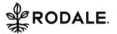

RODALE.

We inspire health, healing, happiness, and love in the world.
Starting with you.

Dedicated to all the readers who recognize that
health is something achieved through individual effort and has
almost nothing to do with doctors or the healthcare system.

Contents

Part III

Introduction

> I think the biggest innovations of the 21st century
> will be at the intersection of biology and technology.
> A new era is beginning.
>
> —Steve Jobs

Who doesn't love a gripping medical drama? Remember the George Clooney character on the TV series *ER,* pediatrician, womanizer, rebel-with-a-heart Dr. Doug Ross? Add characters like the cane-wielding Dr. Kerry Weaver and lovable nurse Abby Lockhart, and you've got the formula for a medical drama that addicted a generation of viewers, portraying health care as fast-paced and thrilling, flawed but well intentioned, and thoroughly human.

But that's TV—dramatized, idealized, sanitized. The private side of real health care is something altogether different. The bulk of what goes on in health care every day involves no drama, no urgency, no critical life or death decisions, no George Clooney winning smile, no surreptitious kisses in corners of the supply room. Having practiced medicine for over 25 years, I can tell you from personal experience that most health care involves routine, humdrum issues like blood pressure and bloating, bedsores and bladder infections, cost and copay and does not invite good-looking actors to play out drama as gripping as a case of itchy hemorrhoids.

Though as dull as dishwater, health care is big money. In 2014, we spent a total of $3 trillion nationally on health care ($9,523 per person), accounting for 17.5 percent of gross domestic product, compared to the 10 to 12 percent other developed countries spend with healthcare systems that match or exceed the United States in quality. Despite the dominance of glistening medical center images in the popular perception of health care, less than one-third of that total was spent in hospitals. The other two-thirds was spent on such uninspiring expenses as outpatient doctor visits, urinary catheters, and drugs for acid reflux.[1]

Many modern doctors hold themselves up as all-knowing, capable of managing every aspect of health, from delivery to death, from vaccination to senility. I know because I was guilty of this. The "I'm-the-doctor, you're-the-patient relationship" has been frozen in time since the days of Hippocrates. Despite the high-tech image, old-fashioned methods are still used to maintain paternalistic authority. Doctoring means wearing a white coat to impress ignorant, helpless patients, the appearance of authority designed to exploit the power of the placebo, long waiting room stays erected as barriers to the privilege of gaining the wisdom of presumed experts, while the monolithic world of medical billing remains impenetrable. All of it seems positively fossilized in an age of immediate information access, on-demand videos, drone deliveries, and the democratization of discussion via social media. Doctors hold themselves up as the gatekeepers of health information and regard the average person as ill-informed and inexperienced, a health simpleton who is powerless in administering any aspect of health. In what other industry can the provider of a service operate with such disregard for customer satisfaction? Imagine buying a car from a salesperson who used intimidation to raise prices, refused to answer questions, and brushed off your concerns as those of a naive automotive nonexpert; I doubt you'd drive off happily in a new hybrid convertible.

The information tide has shifted. Public ignorance in health may have been the rule in 1950, but rapid dissemination of information in our age has usurped this lopsided relationship, making the paternalistic doctor-patient relationship of the past as relevant as trepanation (drilling holes in the skull—yes, a real practice) to treat migraines. You have access to the same information as your doctor. And it doesn't involve leafing through dozens of thick volumes of the *Index Medicus* and then having to retrieve a study from dusty stacks of medical journals, like I did during my medical training. The newly leveled playing field of immediately accessible information means that a new clinical study read by your neurologist or gynecologist is available to you with a few mouse clicks. The cultlike, guarded monopoly over health information is long gone, replaced by immediate, widespread information readily accessible to everyone. The resources available to us have exploded. And they continue to increase at an exponential rate.

The growth in medical information means that the education your doctor received during medical school and training is dusty, moth-ridden, and obsolete. Information doubled every 50 years in 1950, every 7 years in 1980, and every 3.5 years in 2010. If current trends continue, it will double every 73 days by 2020.[2] And information growth is not just within medicine but also in other areas that impact human health, such as toxicology, due to the proliferation of industrial toxins in the environment that disrupt endocrine health and increase risk for cancer, or environmental science and urban planning, since city noise, smog, congestion, and stress all affect various aspects of health. No living human can keep up with the information load and hope to provide up-to-date health care, no matter how smart, how hardworking, how fancy their equipment, or how many operating rooms they have. Dealing with this boom in health information requires new tools to organize it all, put it to practical use, and extract maximum health benefit.

What if we combined the newly found informational freedom provided by Internet search capabilities with the human feedback tool of social media and the rise in direct-to-consumer testing that circumvents the doctor, then threw in a little benign guidance from sources that do not seek to profit from providing it? You might just be on your way to wielding considerable authority over your own health. When you apply the methods unique to the Information Age, unconcerned with ritual, intimidation, and profit, to your health, some pretty darned incredible things can happen: Weight melts away effortlessly, joint pain and skin rashes recede, acid reflux and irritable bowel syndrome symptoms reverse within days, fibromyalgia and ulcerative colitis begin a powerful retreat, prescription medications become superfluous—all by sharing in a growing collective information exchange.

The healthcare system is marvelous for developing the newest implantable defibrillator at a price tag of $36,000, even though a substantial portion of the people receiving such devices do not need them. But the system is miserable at delivering simple, self-managed nutritional solutions for heart disease.[3] The system is ready and willing to commit you to a life of taking drugs and injectable insulin for diabetes, dealing with the eventual heart disease, kidney failure, and peripheral neuropathy with more drugs and procedures, providing "education" designed by people who put commercial interests first, while no one provides the handful of inexpensive health strategies that have been shown to reduce, even fully reverse, type 2 diabetes. You can schedule a double mastectomy next week to avert breast cancer but spend years searching for credible advice on how to minimize exposure to xenoestrogens and organochlorine compounds and reduce inflammatory visceral fat, all of which cultivate cancer. If you are a middle-aged woman, a doctor has likely advised you to start a drug to treat osteoporosis and take it for life, but she likely never mentioned the proven-to-be-effective and inexpensive natural methods that can reverse bone thinning back to normal. In health care, success is measured by the number of surgeries performed and drugs prescribed and lives saved once disease shows itself, but it is almost never measured by the number of times the disease is prevented in the first place.

Unquestionably, there are situations in which doctoring and the healthcare system are needed. If you are bleeding, injured, or struggling to breathe with pneumonia, some old-fashioned suturing, bone setting, or antibiotics can still do the trick. Nobody around here is going to try to replace their own hip joint or treat a urinary tract infection with salves and tonics. There are also situations that are beyond our reach, such as childhood cancer, congenital defects, and lung disease from smoking cigarettes. There are even occasional healthcare professionals who, despite the biases of their education, understand their role as healers, not as cogs in this flawed, profit-seeking wheel. But I'm not talking about those situations. I'm talking about more common and costly (in total) health issues that plague modern humans, from constipation to migraine headaches, from eczema to erectile dysfunction, from acid reflux to plantar fasciitis, from acne to attention-deficit disorder. These are the problems that bore most doctors silly and are certainly never portrayed on TV medical dramas. Doctors are more eager to see exciting, better-paying problems like heart attacks, colon cancer, brain tumors, and kids swallowing peculiar objects. After all, in most hospital healthcare systems of the 21st century, physician pay is tied to hospital revenues, with a bigger end-of-quarter bonus, for example, for generating more MRI scans, surgical consults, organ transplants, and other big-ticket services—regardless of whether they are truly needed or not. (The Institute of Medicine reported that, in 2009 alone, $209 billion was spent on unnecessary medical services and $75 billion was lost to fraud, with many more hundreds of billions lost to inefficiencies, inflated pricing, and excessive administrative costs. The dollars spent on the unnecessary and the dishonest in health care nearly match the total dollars spent by the US military every year.)

But it's these less-than-interesting health issues for your doctor that are wonderfully and safely reduced, reversed, and—dare I say it—cured by a handful of simple strategies that you can implement on your own. You'll be spared the annoyances and dangers of the healthcare system, and because you are obviously not trying to profit financially, you will remove layers of unnecessary costs. You will also find personal health challenges far more fascinating to deal with since they involve you.

I got my first taste of the power of individually determined health 25 years ago when, despite being a faculty member at a teaching hospital and having been board certified in internal medicine and cardiology, I inadvertently gave myself type 2 diabetes with severe distortions of cholesterol values and triglycerides when I embraced a strict low-fat, vegetarian lifestyle dominated by vegetables and "healthy whole grains." I have since reversed all of these dietary disasters by following a few basic health strategies, not a single prescription drug involved. And it was easy.

Let's be absolutely clear: I propose that people can manage their own health safely and responsibly and attain results *superior* to those achieved through conventional health care—not less than, not on par with, but superior. Although you may find this proposal brash, if my experiences with thousands of people over the last decade are any indication, most people who adopt a handful of simple strategies gain health that is vastly superior to that obtained through conventional means with drugs and procedures, not to mention the awful message that passes for modern dietary advice. You will learn that the code has been cracked for an astounding and long list of health conditions. I propose that everyday people can achieve startling results without prescription drugs, without hospitals, without medical procedures by largely sidestepping the doctor, using tools that inform, measure, and support self-directed efforts. And it's relatively easy, inexpensive, safe, and even fun.

> **I propose that people can manage their own health safely and responsibly and attain results *superior* to those achieved through conventional health care—not less than, not on par with, but superior.**

This is something that was never before achievable and is part of the rapidly changing landscape of technology. Such an idea would have been impossible, or at least hazardous, just 10 years ago. Only now is it becoming a reality. Empowerment of the individual in health is really just one aspect of broader waves of change that include self-driving cars and the celebration of noncelebrities through reality TV and YouTube (surely you've seen "Evolution of Dance" and "Chewbacca Mom"). Computerized autopilot systems have been used to fly and land jetliners for years, technology has powered innovations in health care such as 3-D modeling of drugs and remotely operated robotic surgery, virtual nobodies show off impressive talents for national TV audiences, but modern innovations have not yet been fully exploited to empower the individual in health. Well, the time has come: The tools of technology, coupled with a critical mass of new information and crowd interactive potential, have reached levels that now allow the everyday person to take back personal control over health.

You may find the first four chapters of this book disturbing, even shocking, because that is where I dissect what modern health care has become, viewed over many years from the perspective of an insider. I don't do this just to point fingers or make you angry. I do this to reveal that what you thought was health care all along was really something different, a mere shadow of what health care should have been, built on outdated practices, cultlike adherence to rules, sometimes the pathological need to control people's lives, and profit. Only after I raise serious questions about modern health care do we dive into the much more interesting and engaging part of the conversation: how to begin living a life Undoctored. In the how-to part of the book, I share with you my 6-week program, complete with starting recipes, to get you confidently on your way to an Undoctored life, and I include steps to take to reduce or eliminate prescription medications.

Let me also be clear on what this book is not: It will not be a guidebook on how to self-diagnose various diseases, nor will it be a pharmacopoeia of over-the-counter treatments. You will see that the Undoctored process turns the health equation around 180 degrees by providing an approach that first restores head-to-toe health in unexpected ways, reversing numerous health distortions, many of which you are likely unaware that you had, as well as many overt health conditions. Only after this initial process do we veer off in directions that can involve exploring diagnoses and treatments. I will discuss how to distinguish good information from bad, biased advice designed to squeeze more money out of you from safe and unbiased guidance, and I will show you how adhering to a handful of basic ground rules can keep you on course.

Although the healthcare system is typically indifferent to real health outside of revenue-generating activities, never before has the volume of information and tools that could potentially be applied to health been greater. But the system is not equipped to provide such information—nor does it care to—and deliver it to you and your family. These are the roles that I want *Undoctored* to serve—a catalyst for change, a liberator from the bonds of helpless ignorance that allows conventional health care to thrive, a manifesto and map of the path to achieving something a lot better in health, as much of it as possible without a doctor.

Just as smartphones have transformed human communication—no one sent "selfies" back when Madonna sang "Vogue" or swiped through eligible men or ladies on Tinder—the information and tools of Undoctored, self-directed health will change the way we think about ourselves, how we achieve health, and our relationship to the healthcare system. They will release you from the stranglehold—yes, stranglehold—that conventional health care has had on people and replace it with health you create on your own, freeing you from the appointments, impersonality, neglect, and expense of what is presently passed off as health care. You haven't had leeches applied to your arms and legs to bleed you, but you have had to endure something only a bit better to the tune of nearly $10,000 per year, per person. Those days are now over if you simply follow along.

In the subsequent pages of this book, I will discuss why and how such wonderful self-directed strategies are not only possible but essential for you to succeed in health; leave your health up to the doctor and the healthcare system while you submit to their "care," and you are doomed to a life of following their rules for their gain. The power you hold reaches far and wide into multiple aspects of your and your family's health: Cholesterol can be reduced without medication, blood pressure controlled, prediabetic blood sugars squelched, just as I and thousands of others have. You can shed 30 pounds in a few weeks (since excess weight is a reflection of distorted health, not just a cosmetic issue), identify and correct thyroid problems, craft a program to prevent or reverse osteoporosis, and amplify energy—all using self-directed resources that are within your reach, many of which you already have. You can share your experiences with others, review the experiences of other like-minded people, and find new solutions to previously unsolvable problems, all without a doctor. And, as the tools and revelations of this new age unfold, that is just the start. Life and health by the end of your 6-week Undoctored program will be unrecognizably transformed, even to the point of drawing startled gasps from people around you.

Spiraling healthcare costs also make self-directed health not just the fascination of early adopters but a necessity, as the increasing costs of the healthcare status quo look like a bubble (and bubbles burst). Should the healthcare system collapse under the weight of its own unsustainable costs, the self-directed health movement will be catalyzed as individuals are forced to bear more costs through larger insurance deductibles, flex-spending, and medical savings accounts. As control over more of the healthcare dollar is returned to consumers, they will seek to spend more wisely and look for solutions that don't involve costly medical services. Cost savings will be realized as consumers take on more healthcare responsibility and avoid expensive doctors, prescriptions, and hospital services made unnecessary and counterproductive by our efforts.

As economically disastrous as spiraling healthcare costs are, you should also recognize that increasing costs are quietly celebrated by the healthcare industry, as they pocket the increased revenue. They have little incentive to fix this flawed healthcare system because your losses are their gains. Drug companies, medical device companies, doctors, hospital systems, health insurers—they all take their piece of this expanding pie, the pie that you and your family sacrifice to provide. Solutions to all the problems—cost, access, providing only as much care as is beneficial—are unlikely to come from within, so we provide the solutions that allow us to view health care as largely an option, not a necessity for the majority of health issues.

I predict that your Undoctored efforts will dramatically reduce your need for health care while helping you to feel better (and even look better) and sparing you from hundreds of health issues. They will, in effect, allow you to opt out of most aspects of health care. If you can't beat them—don't play the game, and win the game by playing by your own rules.

The ultimate cost savings emerge when you don't develop a disease in the first place or succeed in reversing chronic issues like acid reflux or high blood pressure on your own. The first year of not having acid reflux, for example, can save $2,000 in healthcare costs that year alone because you did not undergo the obligatory (and often unnecessary) endoscopy and were not prescribed the stomach acid–blocking medications that would have led to distortions of bowel flora and the associated bloating, constipation, intermittent bowel urgency, and inflammation, as well as loss of bone density and nutrient deficiencies, downstream health problems resulting from what is often regarded as a "benign" drug treatment. Instead, you institute simple measures that not only address the cause of the problem but also bring about other health benefits without causing unwanted side effects. And your approach costs, at most, a few dollars, or even results in saving money.

You are, in effect, failing to contribute to the physicians, nurses, dietitians, technicians, hospital executives, pharmacies, prescription management services, armies of salespeople, pharmaceutical executives, and medical device manufacturers that would have otherwise pocketed the money you would have been forced to spend. Multiply this cost savings by thousands, then millions, of people for just this one condition and you get a sense of what we could achieve if we persuaded the population to follow us and cut a path of health across hundreds of health conditions.

And we would also create a nation of healthy, slender, vibrant people who rely less on a bloated, profit-seeking healthcare system that costs more than any other system in the world. We would all come to view the healthcare system as nothing more than an acute and catastrophic service available when its services are needed—while we manage our own health safely, effectively, and inexpensively, doing it better than a system that places profit ahead of results.

I will explain how and why I chose to cultivate this daring path. In truth, I did not set out to develop a program that seized control over health or saved money. As with many things, it all happened through a series of fortuitous accidents, coupled with a desire for better answers, all unfolding on the cusp of an exciting and empowered Information Age. But, lo and behold, we (my development team and I) inadvertently created a system for dealing with a huge swath of health issues on our own—the first time in thousands of years that the traditional notion of doctor-patient relationship has been completely overhauled. And I think that Hippocrates would approve.

Along the way, I'll share some of the stories of people who have engaged in such an Undoctored process and achieved results that, just 20 years ago, would have been impossible, examples of people who seized the reins of health on their own and succeeded in some pretty big ways.

I will describe the basic requirements that virtually everyone should follow, practices that apply to everyone regardless of age: males; females; Democrats; Republicans; people who are tall, short, skinny, or overweight; those with gastrointestinal issues, autoimmune conditions, type 2 diabetes, or other diseases; and people who want to avoid such conditions in their lifetimes and just be healthy and function at their highest level. We will have to discuss the boundaries, where your Undoctored health efforts end and conventional health care picks up, including the role of your doctor in this new world.

I present the Undoctored discussion in three parts. In Part I, I go into detail on how and why the healthcare system, from doctors to agencies that pose as health advocates, fails in providing health or reliable health information. Recognizing unreliable or misleading health information is the first step in declaring yourself Undoctored. In Part II, I will take you full steam ahead into the world of Undoctoring, revealing the rationale and the essential tools needed to adopt this exciting life approach. In Part III, I discuss the foods, nutritional supplements, and other strategies of the Undoctored way of living in detail, laid out for you as a 6-week program, the amount of time required to have health and life transformed and be well on your way to freeing yourself from the bonds of the healthcare system.

Turn on the reading light, get cozy in your chair, grab the remote to switch off the medical drama airing on TV, and prepare to be enlightened and know that your future will be brighter and healthier, all because you decided that you've had enough of being a source of profit for the healthcare system while never really receiving health in return and that you are going to take back control over your health and fate, all Undoctored.

PART I

Talk to a toddler and you will quickly learn that she has not yet developed the ability to differentiate reality from imagination, right from wrong, denying, for instance, that she ate an entire chocolate bar while the evidence is smeared all over her face. It's not a matter of being good or bad; it's a matter of not knowing the difference yet.

At the start of your Undoctored journey, you may be like the chocolate-covered 3-year-old, unable to judge what is right, what is wrong, what is sheer fabrication and artifice in health care. It is therefore important that you first see health care for what it truly is before we get to the ideas and strategies that comprise your Undoctored experience. Knowing how to tell truth from fiction will take you from Undoctored toddlerhood to adulthood, an essential step before you reject many of the trappings of conventional health care and opt for ones you create on your own.

CHAPTER 1

Chimpanzees, Parasites, Travel Agents, and Stockbrokers

Chausiku . . . sits down in front of a shrub and pulls down several new growth branches about the diameter of my little finger. She places them all on her lap and removes the bark and leaves of the first branch to expose the succulent inner pith. She then bites off small portions and chews on each for several seconds at a time. By doing this, she makes a conspicuous sucking sound as she extracts and swallows the juice, spitting out most of the remaining fiber. This continues for 17 minutes, with short breaks as she consumes the pith of each branch in the same manner.

—Michael A. Huffman, PhD, primatologist at the
Primate Research Institute, Kyoto University, observing
the chimpanzee Chausiku in the jungles of Tanzania[1]

Dr. Huffman's description of the chimpanzee Chausiku documents an example of animal self-medication, unaided by human direction, no doctor's prescription or health insurance card in evidence. The chimp, weak and listless, clutching her back in pain, ingested the leaves of the plant *Vernonia amygdalina,* which purged an intestinal parasite. She recovered by the next morning. *Vernonia* leaves have since been found to contain over a dozen antiparasitic compounds.

Perhaps if chimpanzees can do it, humans can do it, too.

Undoctored: From the Cath Lab to Your Kitchen

You likely don't suffer from intestinal parasites like Chausiku. But you probably still have plenty wrong with you if you live in the modern age and have had interactions with the sorry excuse for health care that prevails today. If that seems needlessly harsh, stick with me: You will soon learn that you may have never learned to recognize genuine health in the first place and didn't even know that you were not receiving it.

It's not news that conventional health care has proven increasingly dissatisfying to the public. Doctors have been forced into a role of time-limited, crisis-driven interactions that leave little room for meaningful discussion. Just getting someone to look you in the eye seems a rarity. More than ever before, healthcare providers and hospital systems focus on the business of health care, hustling more people through revenue-generating hospital procedures. Ever see billboards posted by hospitals, staff in operating-room garb, informing you of the great "healthcare" services they provide, like coronary bypass surgery, heart rhythm ablation, laparoscopic surgery, or cancer radiation? And in settings where health care is publicly funded, such as in Canada and the UK, getting more than glancing attention generally requires a broken leg or open wound. In the modern system of health care, it is difficult or impossible to receive in-depth, personalized health insight, especially since the system regards such activities as inconsequential.

This situation is tragically and ethically wrong. It may have been right in 1950. But, in our modern Information Age, it is now needlessly wrong. You can fix it. You will not be able to fix the entire system, but you can fix it for you and your family and take health to an unprecedented new level. And you don't need a Mercedes-Benz with "MD" on the license plate to do it.

Let me tell you how I got the spark of this idea of empowering the individual that, over time, crystallized, gained scientific momentum, and made me tingle at its exhilarating potential. It did not begin as a flash of Archimedes-like insight that made me jump out of the tub, shout "Eureka," and run naked through the neighborhood. Nor did I set out to usurp the perverse economics of health care. As often happens, it was a sequence of misjudgments and blunders, with occasional flashes of enlightenment, that led me down this improbable path.

It started over 20 years ago. I was practicing as a successful interventional cardiologist, ballooning coronary artery blockages, inserting drilling devices and stents, aborting heart attacks. It was a time that invited creativity and daring, as methods and tools were evolving. It seemed that every week some new and exciting device was released, allowing us to improve procedural results. After performing 5,000 procedures, I, along with many of my colleagues, came to believe that "heart health" was delivered through the cardiac catheterization laboratory, the "cath lab," using an array of devices and drugs. Heart health was not obtained through an office visit, certainly not in your home. Diet? Let the dietitian take care of that!

Deep in this world, performing as many as 10 procedures per day, I received a call that my mother had died of sudden cardiac death. She had undergone her own balloon angioplasty procedure just a few months earlier.

Losing my mother without a chance to say goodbye was shattering. But it shook me further that she died of the disease I thought I knew something about. It made me question the view that the cath lab was a place to obtain heart health. Surely, there were better ways to identify, track, and control the disease that my colleagues and I so enthusiastically ballooned, drilled, and stented but resulted in my mother's death.

I began to search for better ways to recognize early coronary disease, preferably years before trouble erupted as heart attack or sudden cardiac death. Once I found a way to measure and track coronary atherosclerosis (the abnormal tissue, or plaque, of coronary disease responsible for heart attacks), it led to questions over whether we could stop, even reverse, its growth. (More on this later.)

Better questions eventually led to better answers. But the answers proved strikingly different than the usual "cut your cholesterol and saturated fat, eat more whole grains, and take a statin drug" advice that the rest of the world followed for heart health.[2] The search for these answers led to awareness of issues such as the incredibly disruptive effects of grains and sugars on lipoproteins (fat-carrying particles in the blood), the role of inflammation, the benefits of restoring vitamin D and omega-3 fatty acids, the huge impact of thyroid status on heart health, the importance of managing microorganisms inhabiting the bowel, and the astounding synergy that develops when you combine these apparently unconnected strategies. In an effort to increase awareness of benefits beyond such things as statin drugs (which barely worked, reflected in data I helped generate), I launched a Web site for heart health. The aim was simple: Cultivate discussions for people with coronary disease to learn about new ideas—period. I didn't say, "Dump your doctor" or "Manage heart disease yourself." I simply set out to provide better information, together with supportive discussions. Despite the complexity of some of the conversations, thousands of people embraced the approach.

Lo and behold, in addition to the 2,000 patients in my office having no heart attacks or hospital procedures over the years, likewise nobody in the online program (mostly high-risk people who'd undergone prior heart procedures or suffered heart attacks) was coming back needing stents or bypasses or having heart attacks. Heart disease came to a halt in people following a handful of simple strategies. And a growing number of them

FOOD, WEIGHT LOSS, AND SEX: THE LESSONS OF WHEAT BELLY

What captures the attention of most people and gets them to engage in a discussion or book? Not science. Certainly not heart disease. I'd say food, weight loss, sex, and money. If you're like most of us, you'd rather watch Carrie Bradshaw's love frolics on *Sex and the City* than explore quarks and dark matter on an episode of *Nova*.

If I wrote the finest book on heart health in history, it would receive a big yawn since it did not appeal to everyday interests. But what if the heart health message was delivered through conversations about food, weight loss, and sex that everyone wants to read?

This was the birth of the Wheat Belly book series. I called it Wheat Belly because abdominal fat is the signature pattern of weight gain from a diet based on wheat and grains. It is the outward expression of the deep visceral fat encircling the intestines and other abdominal organs that is inflammatory, disrupts hormones, keeps you from wearing a size four bikini, and yields the unsettling sight of middle-aged men with protuberant bellies spilling over Speedos. Wheat Belly conveyed the same lessons that I'd originally learned in the world of heart health, now repackaged to appeal to mainstream interests.

And it worked. Millions of Wheat Belly books and cookbooks have been sold in 44 countries; the Wheat Belly message has been featured on popular TV shows, from *The Colbert Report* to *The 700 Club*; and it now has its own public television special. It infuriated the grain industry, which then budgeted large sums of money to attack the message and its messenger. It spawned pushback from people who misperceived the Wheat Belly message as just another plug for a gluten-free diet.

Not only did the Wheat Belly message meet expectations in food, weight loss, and sex, it helped thousands of people recover from common health reversed the quantity of coronary atherosclerotic plaque in their arteries. A big part of the overall success of the program was due to the nutritional component. The diet proved enormously effective, resulting in weight loss and relief from gastrointestinal complaints, skin rashes, joint pain, and autoimmune diseases, as well as dramatically improving abnormalities leading to heart disease. This was, by the way, the birth of the nutritional approach discussed in my Wheat Belly book series, the books that revealed to the world just how aspects of health and control over weight can be regained by following a wheat-free, grain-free lifestyle. The success of the Wheat Belly message has not been driven by my charisma or good looks, but by the fact that it works: A multitude of health conditions melt in the face of

conditions, such as acid reflux and fibromyalgia, within *days* of starting; relieved lifelong sufferers of migraine headaches and binge eating disorder; and allowed people to get off prescription medications. People experienced reductions in appetite and increased energy and deeper sleep, and they felt and even looked different. (Take a look at the *Wheat Belly Blog*, for instance, or the Official Wheat Belly Facebook page, and you will see the "before" and "after" facial photos: facial edema gone, cheek/chin redness gone, around-the-eye puffiness gone revealing larger eyes, all developing within a few days to weeks. Some of the transformations are striking.) In short, Wheat Belly works. This wacky-named collection of ideas that originated with efforts at heart health, subsequently embraced by millions while driving the grain industry crazy, simply works. It worked in showing that food choices entirely contrary to conventional wisdom yielded impressive weight loss, made you feel and look sexier while restoring a healthy hormonal status, and reversed a long list of health conditions.

And with more people reading the books and following their advice, newer lessons emerged as larger numbers of people provided feedback. It became clear that efforts at health could not end with a shift in food choices, as crucial as they were. There were nutritional deficiencies remaining, for instance, some caused by wheat and grains, others not, that needed correction, such as magnesium and iodine deficiencies. People needed guidance on how to get off medications, as many doctors proved unhelpful or incapable of dealing with people who no longer had diabetes, for example, but were still taking insulin and diabetes drugs. (Doctors struggle to deal with healthy people who no longer need drugs.)

But the Wheat Belly experience provided a starting point for the concepts that are further advanced in *Undoctored*. And, yes, we will be discussing food, achieving weight loss, and talking about the sexier aspects of this lifestyle, all while reversing or preventing hundreds of health conditions with little or no doctoring involved.

removing foods that "official" agencies tell us to eat more of, a real-world experience backed by a substantial body of existing evidence. (For those of you unfamiliar with the Wheat Belly message, I will discuss some of the science and rationale behind this approach and why it yields such extravagant and unexpected benefits. For those of you already familiar, I will expand on ideas presented in the Wheat Belly books and take you even further down the path to self-directed health.)

In other words, my efforts to create a source for better information on heart health yielded solutions to an unexpectedly broad panel of health conditions, with participants succeeding on their own, unimpeded by their doctors, in the comfort of their kitchens and living rooms. From that unexpected and fortuitous start, Undoctored insights and health tools emerged.

DIY Heart Care?

While I never set out to create a do-it-yourself-at-home heart disease management program, that is how it turned out—to my great surprise. It made for some interesting stories, like Perry, who, after surviving a heart attack and receiving a stent, was told by his doctor to cut fat intake, eat more whole grains, exercise, take aspirin and a beta-blocker drug, and reduce cholesterol with a statin drug. After educating himself with the resources from my online program, Perry returned to his doctor and declared, "I'm not ready to just go along with 'reducing cholesterol' for heart disease risk. My goal is to gain as much control over coronary disease as possible, so I'd like to address issues I believe may be important. I'd like to have my lipoproteins analyzed; I'd like to obtain levels of omega-3 fatty acids and 25-hydroxy vitamin D; and I'd like a thyroid assessment. I believe that I should also have an assessment of inflammation and my blood sugar status measured with fasting glucose, insulin, and hemoglobin A1c." (All of this, by the way, I discuss later.)

Perry's doctor was speechless. Rather than reveal his ignorance or appear to have neglected crucial aspects of his patient's health, he advised Perry that none of this was necessary, and then sent him on his way. But Perry was determined to get these questions answered, having engaged in online discussions with people who had successfully obtained such information and enjoyed dramatically improved heart health. So Perry found a way to obtain the testing on his own. Within a couple of weeks, he returned to our online community and shared his information.

Within moments, he received feedback to help understand the values.

He also compiled information on nutritional supplement choices, how and where to get supplements such as iodine and vitamin D, and even how to find the best sources, quality, and prices. Engaging in this process, self-directed but collaborative, he witnessed marked transformations in his health. Not only did he never again—over several years—redevelop heart symptoms or require any additional trips back to the cath lab (which is uncommon in the conventional experience, where multiple repeat trips, what I call the heart disease "revolving door," are the norm), but he also lost weight, reversed a prediabetic sugar profile, improved cholesterol values without drugs, got rid of acid reflux symptoms he'd endured for many years, dropped his blood pressure to normal, and enjoyed better mood, energy, and sleep. In short, his life and health were better, all achieved without his doctor—in spite of his doctor.

Slender, energetic, on no drugs except the aspirin for his stent, Perry returned to his doctor for a routine follow-up 1 year later. Holding the basic laboratory assessment he ordered for Perry in front of him, his doctor admitted, "Well, I don't know how you're doing it, but these values look like a 20-year-old substituted his blood for yours. They're unbelievable. Your blood sugars are normal, your triglycerides are incredible, and you've doubled your HDL cholesterol. What medications are you taking to do this?" "No medications," Perry replied. "I'm following a program to reverse heart disease, but it means doing some things that are different from standard approaches." His doctor closed the meeting with the signature response of doctors: "Well, I don't understand what you are doing, but just keep doing it."

Yes, Perry knew more about how to control heart disease than his doctor, more than his cardiologist, though neither would admit it. Perry's goal was to achieve heart health, while the doctors' goals were to avert catastrophe with drugs and procedures. The cardiologist knew how to insert a stent to open a blocked artery or implant a defibrillator to abort sudden cardiac death. But could they provide information that empowered Perry in all aspects of health from head to toe, while also dramatically reducing, even eliminating, coronary disease risk and avoiding the need for procedures? As you now know, that is not what conventional health care does, nor is it interested in doing so, as it would take too much time, involve economically unproductive discussions, and potentially cut off a hugely profitable procedural revenue stream.

Having managed to inadvertently create a largely do-it-yourself program for coronary health, among the toughest of all areas of health to tackle, I had to wonder: If it can be done with heart disease, why not expand this to other areas of health, such as bone health, weight loss, hormonal health, and others? Provide access to unbiased information and a community of people with similar concerns engaged in collaborative discussions, share health data, and then stand back and watch what happens. I also decided that, as revolutionary as it sounded, people needed to hear about these concepts in a world where their local healthcare system boasts about high-tech surgical suites and a growing organ transplant program but does nothing for genuine health.

Skeptical? Well, it's already under way, whether you join in or not. You can recognize a crude and rudimentary form of self-directed health in its primitive predecessor, "wellness," the eat-a-balanced-diet, don't smoke, exercise break, check-your-blood-pressure, and know-your-cholesterol practices followed at workplaces to reduce healthcare costs. Home testing, such as do-it-yourself pregnancy tests, has been around for decades. You've likely had your blood pressure checked at those automatic blood pressure devices at the drugstore. And who knows how long chimpanzees have successfully purged intestinal parasites? But the concept is evolving rapidly from these humble beginnings. And it's going to grow, coming to homes and workplaces near you. Access to better information combined with crowdsourced collaboration and tools are going to trigger a 9.5 Richter scale health earthquake that will topple the status quo, leaving an entirely new model of health to emerge from the rubble.

And I invite you to be part of a community that shares and collaborates through the Undoctored experience: Engage in the Wild, Naked, and Unwashed program that I will introduce soon and that forms the core of your Undoctored effort, and then share your data and results on the Undoctored Web site, anonymously, of course. As the community grows, the cumulative data grow, and I will report back to you exactly what we have accomplished: how much blood sugar and blood pressure have dropped, how much weight people have lost, how many health conditions have reversed, how many medications people have been able to stop, etc., all accomplished on our own. As our crowdsourced experience grows and I tabulate the results and report them back, we will get smarter and more capable at taking the reins back over health in even greater ways.

Who's Smarter: You or Your Doctor?

Undoctored will do for health what Lady Gaga has done for the idea of wardrobe restraint. But even more than the evolution in popular entertainment from girl-next-door Doris Day to the provocative Lady Gaga, technology has irrevocably altered the landscape of life. It will, in effect, make you smarter than your doctor.

The explosion of technology has generated tidal waves of disruptive innovation these past 30 years: e-mail displacing regular mail; digital data replacing cassette tapes and encyclopedias; cell phones making hard-wired telephones antiquated curiosities, all since the Information Age burst on the scene. Airline schedules, previously inaccessible to the public, are now viewable 24-7 by anyone, allowing consumers to book a cross-country flight within seconds, leaving travel agents idle and in search of something else to do. Investing in the stock market 40 years ago meant relying on a stockbroker who charged fees for every transaction, not uncommonly "churning" your account with unwise trades to generate commissions, all because he had access to the tools of the trade that you did not. Today, you can analyze the financial health of a company, compare it to its peers, rank the performance of mutual funds, and make investments with a few mouse clicks on your computer, while stockbrokers are left staring idly at the ticker tape. The same disruptive innovations that swept through the travel industry and stock market are now sweeping through health care. Perhaps you occasionally need a travel agent to assist in booking a Mediterranean cruise or the input of a stockbroker about a new exchange-traded fund, and you could sometimes benefit from some unbiased guidance on navigating the flood of new health information coming your way, but given the attitudes of most doctors, that sort of guidance is unlikely to come from your primary care physician or other healthcare personnel.

But raw information by itself is not enough. What if we combined information with the wisdom of crowds? Crowd behavior can lead to mass panic and hysteria, yes, but with the proper "lens," collective wisdom can be focused on answering questions. By sharing experiences through tools such as social media and online interactions that support, affirm, and collate human experience, collective wisdom can be harnessed to lead us through the tangle of complex health questions. Data, such as that provided by the Web site health project PatientsLikeMe (patientslikeme.com), for example, are yielding answers to health problems by gathering the experiences of tens of thousands of participants—everyday people, not doctors or scientists. There's only so much wisdom one person can acquire. But harness the knowledge, life experiences, and insights of thousands of people, all working to answer the same questions, and something wonderful happens.

This is not a phenomenon experienced by you, all on your own; it is a shared experience—and the more we share, the greater the potential gain. A survey conducted by PatientsLikeMe revealed that 84 percent of people would be willing to share personal health data if that information could be helpful to the health of others, completely contrary to modern notions of health privacy.[3] The power of crowdsourcing is still in its infancy, but it is just a matter of time before the potential of this phenomenon is harnessed with Google-like efficiency.

Self-directed health is also already at work on a large scale in the nutritional supplement industry, a $30 billion confirmation that people are looking for self-managed health solutions. Though we may dispute the wisdom of some of it, nutritional supplements have exploded, and the public has embraced them. In the United States, lax regulation imposed by the Dietary Supplement Health and Education Act of 1994 has allowed the definition of *nutritional supplement* to be stretched widely. And, as a result, obviously non-nutritional (though still potentially interesting) products like the hormones pregnenolone, dehydroepiandrosterone (DHEA), and melatonin can be sold on the same shelf as vitamin C. We have access to powerful choices—such as probiotics that restore healthy bowel flora and vitamin D that can reduce or reverse dozens of health conditions—that are, in my experience, more beneficial for health than any prescription drug available. Likewise, in publicly funded healthcare systems, despite regulatory agencies that pooh-pooh nutritional supplements as folly, an astounding choice in such products is still available. The international, borderless nature of the Internet has also made virtually every nutritional supplement out there available to the worldwide public.

Though still in its infancy, direct-to-consumer medical imaging is another facet of emerging self-directed health. Today, it is possible to diagnose coronary disease (CT heart scan), measure bone density for osteoporosis (DEXA, ultrasound, or bone densitometry), or quantify the severity of carotid atherosclerosis (ultrasound) with tests available directly to the consumer, without a doctor's involvement.

Direct-to-consumer laboratory testing is now a reality with a mind-boggling number of self-directed tests now available, from advanced markers for heart disease, to genetic cancer and blood clotting risk markers, to hormonal assessments. An analysis of personal genetic markers is obtainable today for less than $200 with just a sample of saliva, and an assessment of bowel flora microorganisms performed via the newest technology is just a small stool sample away, also for about the cost of a nice dinner for two.

We can only imagine the journey that technology will take us on with

KAY IS **UNDOCTORED**

Decatur, Illinois

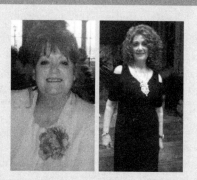

As a former Weight Watchers instructor for 10 years, I thought I knew how to eat right until what I was eating was making me sick. I struggled with years of bloating, cramping, nausea, diarrhea, vomiting, irritable bowel syndrome, and diverticulosis, and I was diagnosed as prediabetic in 2014.

In 1981, I started having weight issues—gaining, losing, gaining, losing, gaining, and losing. I lost eight teeth to gum disease at the age of 35. I lost 1½ inches in my height according to a bone density test; I've always been 5 feet 8 inches, but now I'm 5 feet 6½ inches. I was devastated by that, and all the doctor said was that it was age (little did I know it was from using omeprazole for 11 years). I have a bulging disk and have had steroid shots, pain patches, but none of that worked for me. I have arthritis on my whole left side and osteoarthritis took my left hip, and I had a left hip replacement July 2016.

At the age of 53, my doctor did an arthroscopic surgery on my left knee and told me I would probably have to have my knee replaced in 10 years. In 2005, I had a colonoscopy and was diagnosed with diverticulosis. Being so overweight caused my back to hurt constantly.

I viewed Dr. William Davis on *The Dr. Oz Show* in September 2014, in which he shared the effects that you would have from eating wheat, grains, white flour, and white sugar. It upset me to find out that they had changed wheat and its genetics and it is now an appetite stimulant and a poison to my health. I was ready and willing because I wanted my life and my health back.

I don't experience pain, nausea, cramping, bloating, vomiting, or diarrhea from eating all the wrong foods now because I'm eating the right foods and taking a probiotic and vitamin D. Now I understood why I always had bloating, cramping, and pain all my teenage and early years of my life.

My BMI at the beginning was 35.5, obese. Now it's 23.33, normal. I have not let any of these health issues stop me from losing and maintaining a 70-pound weight loss and 36 inches. The weight off of my back has helped immensely. Don't ever think you're too old, because I'm 64 and have four grown daughters, nine grandkids, and two great-grandkids. I'm keeping off 70 pounds and 36 inches for 14 months!

exciting innovations such as voice-reading software that diagnoses and tracks progression or regression of parkinsonism or identifies voice patterns that suggest depression. You can now diagnose sleep disorders in the comfort of your own bed, assess mood by chemical changes in the skin (then enhance mood with scent therapy), and reduce blood pressure using biofeed-back facilitated by your smartphone. (I will fold in discussions on how to put some of these new technologies to use along the way.)

Combine the leveled information playing field with the multitude of health tools that have appeared on the scene and the prospect of self-directed health care has arrived. Someone just needs to show you how to get it. Self-directed health is a phenomenon that will stretch far and wide into human health. It will encompass preventive practices, diagnostic testing, smartphone apps, and therapeutic strategies. It puts the astounding and unexpected wisdom of crowds to work, providing you with a depth and breadth of collective information and experience that far exceed that of any one person, no matter how much of an expert. You may not have a freshly starched white coat or smartly dressed drug sales reps calling on you, but you have the advantages of information, innovation, self-motivation, and collaboration in this new age. Over time, it will dramatically shift the land-scape of health care, change the economics of payment, and revolutionize the health of millions for the better. Disruptive innovation defines the mod-ern age, and it's coming to health care. It's coming to your home. And the healthcare system cannot stop it.

The answer to the question "Who's smarter: You or your doctor?" is a resounding *you*. Yes, the doctor knows more about conventional healthcare issues in her specialty delivered through drugs and procedures. But you have the collective power of thousands of people and technology and access to tools that were never before available, and you are going to focus your efforts on genuine health. After all, there is only one person genuinely capa-ble of knowing how well you feel: you. Put it all together and you are capa-ble of accomplishing some impressive things.

Let me paint you an example.

Undoctored Health in Action

"Looking over your medical record, Nancy, I'm a bit concerned about your risk for osteoporosis and hip fracture. It looks like your mom had a hip fracture at age 67. Is that right?"

"Yes, she did," Nancy responded, "and her life was never quite the same for the 5 years she lived after that."

"You're 53 years old. Bone thinning develops over many years. Let's get you scheduled for a bone scan."

Two weeks later:

> "Your Z-score is -1.5. This means that your bone density is below normal and you've got a mild form of bone thinning called osteopenia. Here: This is a prescription for alendronate, what used to be called Fosamax."
>
> "Aren't there side effects with that drug? A friend of mine said that her mom had a leg fracture from it."
>
> "Well, yes, of course. All prescription drugs have potential side effects. They're uncommon, but they can happen, and we can't predict when and where. Besides leg fracture, there's something called jaw osteonecrosis in which the jawbone dies and has to be surgically replaced. But would you rather run the risk of a hip fracture?"
>
> "Before we make the jump to drugs, aren't there natural things I could do first?"
>
> (Big sigh.) "You can take calcium, but that only helps a bit. You've got to make a choice: Take the drug or risk a hip fracture."
>
> "I think I'm going to explore some natural remedies on my own first."

Nancy's dialogue with her doctor is fictional but based on thousands of similar encounters. Identify a problem, prescribe a drug. Natural remedies? "They don't work." "I don't know anything about that." "None of that is proven." "I only practice evidence-based medicine," even though the "evidence" is generated by industries and committees that profit from the message.

Each of Nancy's fictitious interactions was no more than 10 minutes long. If she is like most people, unless she develops an acute illness, she will have one or two such interactions over the course of a year. She's got less than 30 minutes per year to compress all of her health counseling into the allotted time—30 minutes per year to discuss bone health, nutrition, blood sugar issues, cholesterol issues, blood pressure, female issues, genetic questions, sleep issues, joint questions, skin questions, emotional and mood struggles, and all the rest of her concerns, all while the doctor writes in his chart or types on his tablet, barely looking at her face-to-face. Perhaps she has developed some chronic gastrointestinal complaints, too, and a rash on her elbows and struggles with headaches. Regardless, she's going to have to

(continued on page 18)

WHAT HEALTH CONDITIONS ARE ADDRESSED BY THE UNDOCTORED APPROACH?

Here is a list of conditions that can be impacted by the Undoctored program laid out on these pages. Most of these conditions will respond favorably and dramatically just by adhering to the basic strategies of the program, while others will require additional efforts discussed later in the book.

It's a pretty impressive list that includes autoimmune conditions, metabolic diseases, and risk for dementia and cancer. Of course, this is not to say that a well-established case of dementia or cancer will reverse, but that the factors that lead health in those directions are at least partially, if not entirely, reversed by the Undoctored strategies.

Acanthosis nigricans

Acid reflux

Acne

Addison's disease

Allergies

Alopecia areata

Ankylosing spondylitis

Antiphospholipid antibody syndrome

Anxiety

Asthma

Autoimmune hemolytic anemia

Autoimmune hepatitis

Autoimmune inner ear disease

Autoimmune lymphoproliferative syndrome

Autoimmune pancreatitis

Autoimmune thrombocytopenic purpura

Barrett's esophagus

Behcet's disease

Bile stasis

Binge eating disorder

Bipolar illness (manic phase primarily)

Bulimia

Bullous pemphigoid

Cardiomyopathy (dilated or congestive)

Celiac disease

Cerebellar ataxia

Chronic fatigue syndrome

Chronic inflammatory demyelinating polyneuropathy

Cold agglutinin disease

Constipation, obstipation

Coronary disease, angina

CREST syndrome

Crohn's disease

Cutaneous vasculitis

Dandruff

Depression

Dermatitis herpetiformis

Dermatomyositis, polymyositis dermatomyositis

Diabetes, type 2

Discoid lupus

Dysbiosis

Eczema

Esophagitis, esophageal spasm

Essential mixed cryoglobulinemia

Fatigue

Fatty liver

Fibromyalgia

Food protein–induced enterocolitis syndrome

Gallstones, bile stasis

Gastroparesis

Gluten encephalopathy

Graves' disease

Hair loss, nonimmune

Hashimoto's thyroiditis

Heartburn

Hypertension

Hypertriglyceridemia

Hypochlorhydria

Ichthyosiform dermatoses

Idiopathic thrombocytopenic purpura

IgA nephropathy

Insulin-dependent diabetes (type I)

Iron deficiency anemia

Irritable bowel syndrome

Juvenile arthritis

Ménière's disease

Metabolic syndrome

Migraine headache

Mixed connective tissue disease

Multiple sclerosis

Myasthenia gravis

Myocarditis

Nonalcoholic fatty liver disease

Obesity, overweight

Pemphigus vulgaris

Peripheral neuropathy

Pernicious anemia

Plantar fasciitis

Polyarteritis nodosa

Polychondritis

Polyglandular syndromes (nongenetic)

Polymyalgia rheumatica

Prediabetes

Primary agammaglobulinemia

Primary biliary cirrhosis

Psoriasis

Pyodema gangrenosum

Raynaud's phenomenon

Reiter's syndrome

Rheumatoid arthritis

Sarcoidosis

Schizophrenia, paranoid (paranoia, auditory hallucinations)

Scleroderma

Seborrhea

Seizures, primarily temporal lobe

Sicca syndrome

Sjögren's syndrome

(continued)

WHAT HEALTH CONDITIONS ARE ADDRESSED BY THE UNDOCTORED APPROACH? *(CONT.)*

Small intestinal bacterial overgrowth

Systemic lupus erythematosus

Takayasu's arteritis

Temporal arteritis

Ulcerative colitis

Uveitis

Vasculitis

Vitiligo

Wegener's granulomatosis, granulomatosis with polyangitis

The degree of response can vary depending on the individual and the condition. For example, the response of ulcerative colitis and hypertriglyceridemia (high triglyceride blood levels) can be complete, conditions that can wonderfully revert back to normal with Undoctored efforts. On the other hand, type 1 diabetes does not revert back to normal because the pancreas that produces insulin will not regenerate after incurring damage; however, improved blood sugars and reduced hemoglobin A1c (HbA1c), a long-term measure of blood sugar control, will develop, along with reduced potential for other autoimmune conditions that are a substantial problem in people with type 1 diabetes. Likewise, the autoimmune process in primary biliary cirrhosis can be halted, but the liver damage will not reverse. Thankfully, situations like this are the exception, rather than the rule; most chronic health conditions can be reversed, or at least minimized.

And I will be tracking the results of the Undoctored approach on undoctoredhealth.com. Over time, you will be able to view the collective experience of thousands of people following this approach, all working toward the same goal: to take back control over health by applying simple, inexpensive, commonsense strategies and avoid the healthcare system.

WHAT CONDITIONS ARE NOT ADDRESSED BY THE UNDOCTORED APPROACH?

I've already pointed out that acute injury, such as a broken leg or a concussion, and infections, such as pneumonia or a bladder infection, are not

confine her healthcare interaction to those few minutes, perhaps receiving one or more prescriptions or imaging procedures for each. That's how modern health care works: Provide the minimum interaction; address a few, perhaps no more than one, problems; and then prescribe a drug or procedure. Imagine you had to care for your car by the same formula, having to be content with the 10 or so minutes your mechanic was permitted to maintain and repair your car; you'd have to start taking the bus.

Let's pick up again with Nancy. Upon learning of her osteopenia and amenable to our Undoctored efforts (though your ability to recover from such conditions is improved by them). The list of conditions successfully addressed by the Undoctored strategies are indeed wide and varied, but there are other conditions that will not be improved by these efforts. These include:

Genetic disorders. As the world of genetics continues to yield health insights that will empower us in our Undoctored world, there will also be conditions that remain inaccessible, such as Tay-Sachs disease or hemochromatosis.

Organ damage due to prior disease or life habits. Cirrhosis of the liver or chronic obstructive pulmonary disease, COPD, from decades of cigarette smoking will not be addressed by Undoctored efforts. Cerebral palsy from birth trauma is another.

Congenital and structural/anatomic disorders. This consists of a long list of very difficult disorders that even conventional medical care often struggles with, such as congenital heart defects, brain aneurysms, and scoliosis.

Chronic diseases that can be addressed via Undoctored efforts but are too far advanced. Kidney failure, dementia, established cancers, and pancreatic injury are among the conditions that might have been prevented by introducing Undoctored efforts earlier, but not once they are established and/or advanced.

Neurodegenerative diseases. Parkinson's disease, established dementia, and Lou Gehrig's disease (amyotrophic lateral sclerosis) are among the nervous system degenerative diseases that will not respond to our efforts (although many such conditions can be avoided in the first place through Undoctored strategies).

Psychiatric illnesses. While conditions such as depression and anxiety can respond partially or totally with Undoctored strategies, responses will vary. The same goes for the behavioral excesses of schizophrenia (paranoia, auditory hallucinations), the learning impairment and behavioral outbursts in attention deficit hyperactivity disorder (ADHD) and autism spectrum disorder, and the mania of bipolar illness. There are also conditions that will not respond, such as some forms of schizophrenia, personality disorders, or the effects of childhood abuse or post-traumatic stress disorder.

long-term risk for osteoporotic fractures, she started searching for solutions. Not only did she discover that there are indeed safe and effective natural ways to deal with osteopenia, she also learned that some strategies have even been examined in clinical trials, pitted head-to-head with prescription drugs and shown to perform as well as, if not better, at little cost and without side effects. (She also discovered how out-of-date and ineffective, even dangerous, her doctor's advice to take calcium was.) She found that there are online communities in which she could discuss health questions with other people with similar health interests. During one such interaction at the start of her effort, a woman living in another part of the country who shared an interest in restoring bone health commented to Nancy, "Don't sweat it, Nancy. I was in your shoes a little over a year ago. I followed a program for bone health: I took vitamin D, vitamin K_2, and magnesium; I made sure that I included leafy green vegetables at least once or twice per day; and I added strength training for a few minutes twice per week. I started with osteoporosis. My most recent bone density test showed that I reversed it completely; it's now normal. My doctor didn't know what to make of it, and I told her to stick her drugs you-know-where! So hang in there and be sure to share your questions and concerns with us here."

That is what *Undoctored* is all about. *Undoctored* fills the gaps of health knowledge not provided during brief medical interactions and reveals the often astonishing amount of credible, safe scientific information that allows you to actively participate, and often take over completely, various aspects of your health. You don't have to fire your doctor; these efforts *supplement* the information and advice you obtain (or don't obtain) in the doctor's office.

Our fictional woman, Nancy, returned to her doctor 1 year later after undergoing a repeat bone scan. The doctor opened her chart expecting to scold her for her foolhardy and careless attitude and worsened bone thinning (although, he had to admit, she sure looked healthier, including having lost the extra 30 pounds of weight she'd been carrying). Instead, he was speechless. After a pause, he said, "I don't know how you did it, but your bone density is now normal, the density of a healthy 30-year-old woman. Your blood sugar is perfect, cholesterol numbers all in order. Just continue doing what you're doing." He closed the chart and walked out.

Yes: "Just continue what you are doing," not "Please tell me what you did so that I might learn something new," or "Where did you learn about such strategies? I knew nothing about this!" That response defines what modern health care has become: You don't need drugs or procedures; you therefore don't need health care.

You don't want that kind of health care. It's reassuring to know that the doctor and hospital are there in case you tumble down the stairs or need to be helicoptered to the trauma unit after a head-on collision. But why not follow day-to-day health advice of the sort that improves bone density naturally, keeps you slender, maintains blood pressure in the normal range, normalizes insulin response, keeps bowels operating happily, and can even reverse conditions such as autoimmune joint pain, type 2 diabetes, or skin rashes, while costing next to nothing? That is the kind of health care you want.

Nancy conducted her own Undoctored health effort to correct her reduced bone density. She experienced no ill effects from the strategies she adopted, it was inexpensive, and, while she focused on bone health, she obtained health benefits across a wider spectrum because genuine health develops as a body wide process. Her simple efforts to improve bone health helped reduce her risk for heart disease, diabetes, dementia, and numerous other health conditions, while feeling and looking better—all Undoctored, all self-directed, all safe. It confused the doctor, but Nancy knew exactly what she was doing.

Potholes, Detours, and Drunk Drivers?

Primum non nocere. That's Latin for "First, do no harm." It is a doctrine followed by doctors—in an ideal world. If we take a reality check, though, it is far from what happens in day-to-day health care.

In the real world, the system plays fast and loose with your health and safety, since its primary goal is no longer health but profit. But when you are the captain of your fate, you have no interest in profit, only health.

Nonetheless, critics will warn that there is the potential for danger in this Wild West of personal health exploration, turning to Dr. Google, health apps, and nonprofessionals—even crowds of anonymous people, for heaven's sake!—for answers. They fear that we will misdiagnose, misinterpret, and fail to recognize various conditions; choose the wrong tests; and institute the wrong treatments. Healthcare insiders view the medical system as a sleek 12-lane highway with traffic flowing smoothly; to them, your self-directed version of health will be congested and chaotic with unwarned lane changes, fender benders, and 10-car pileups. Unnecessary or unwise treatments will be instituted, chaos unleashed, hell and eternal damnation just around the bend.

I disagree. Surely, increased freedom necessitates increased responsibility. Boundaries need to be established, guidelines provided, feedback made available. First of all, we do not abandon common sense: accidentally slice open your finger with a kitchen knife, go straight to the emergency room or urgent care—no question. If you have a child with brain injury incurred at birth, now with cerebral palsy, this lifestyle will have no impact on brain function. But I predict that self-directed health will improve health enormously outside of such situations and that you can observe improvements as they unfold. My experience—and the experience of the many thousands of people who have followed such a plan—is that people do better by taking the reins of health themselves. We may have to endure a few outbreaks of informational acne and social awkwardness as we progress from health adolescence to adulthood, but we will get there, just as adults survived their teenage years.

My experience has also been that when people begin to realize just how much they are capable of when directing their own health, a spark of interest ignites and a fascination with learning more emerges, very different from the conventional health interaction that begins and ends with ignorance and acquiescence to the healthcare professional. If a health condition is present, there is nobody more motivated to understand and correct the causes than you. We can harness that desire. We apply the synergies of collaboration and crowd wisdom, we track measures, and we receive and provide feedback, all taking us closer and closer to the desired health answers.

But we have to be aware of the potential for being misdirected. The same tools that enlighten can also mislead. Take, for example, the proliferation of "colon cleanse" products with graphic photographs of piles of disgusting goo purportedly purged from intestines of people taking this or that formula. Claims include curing cancer, dementia, and diabetes, all by drinking a magical formula or administering enemas. While we embrace tools and insights that empower us in health, we also have to exert a healthy skepticism over any product or process that has no validation, makes too-good-to-be-true claims, or comes with hard-sell tactics, a high price tag, and piles of goo. I will include a discussion on the basic rules of engagement needed to safely process information in this new age.

There will also be opposition to some aspects of an Undoctored health experience. Genetic testing, in particular, has drawn fire from conventional medicine. This is reflected in a 2011 letter sent to the FDA by the American Medical Association (AMA): "We urge the [FDA Molecular and Clinical Genetics] Panel to offer clear findings and recommendations that genetic testing, except under the most limited circumstances, should be carried out under the personal supervision of a qualified health care professional, and provide individuals interested in obtaining genetic testing access to qualified health care professionals for further information." In other words, the AMA wants to bar individuals from obtaining access to their own genetic information except under the supervision of a health professional. No surprise: The AMA wants to safeguard the role of the physician, despite the fact that 74 percent of them admit that they have no idea what the various genes even mean.[4] There is indeed value to FDA oversight of genetic testing to ensure, for instance, the

RUTH IS UNDOCTORED

Royal Oak, Michigan

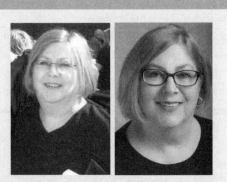

My ever-present asthma wheeze was gone in a day or two, never to return. There is no more sinus gunk either. My constant eczema vanished after about a week grain-free. I lost 20 pounds in about 6 weeks, and my fasting blood sugar dropped 15 points.

I am free of the uncontrollable cravings I once had and find it easy to refrain when faced with food offerings at dinner parties or lunch meetings.

After 8 weeks grain-free, my periodontist said my gums were the best he had seen them in 25 years; the hygienist said my tissues looked normal and healthy.

A few weeks ago, I knelt down to talk to a seated employee and then stood back up without assistance and realized I hadn't been able to do that in years.

Best of all has been the change in mood. The low-level depression that has dogged my heels for years is gone. It feels as if a cloud cover has lifted and I have access to a baseline sense of well-being.

accuracy of testing. Imagine BRCA testing for breast cancer by a genetic testing lab, for example, that proved inaccurate, an error that prompts some women to wrongly undergo bilateral mastectomy. Accuracy in testing, as well as in any correlations made with disease conditions, needs to be assured. But that oversight falls under the authority of the FDA, not your doctor.

And let's be absolutely clear on something: Conventional health care is not perfect, has not always gotten things right, and frequently violates the rule of "first, do no harm." We don't have to dig very deeply to uncover astounding blunders committed in medicine. For example, the drug diethylstilbestrol, or DES, was prescribed for 30 years to reduce miscarriage and premature labor but induced vaginal cancers and reproductive deformities in offspring, and thalidomide, which was prescribed for morning sickness, caused limb mutations in thousands of newborns. The popular surgical procedure called extracranial-intracranial (EC-IC) bypass, used to treat stroke, was performed at high volume in hospitals until 1985, when it was shown to be a sham. And the widely prescribed anti-inflammatory drugs Vioxx and Celebrex caused heart attack and cardiovascular death in over

100,000 people. The list of systematic and widespread blunders made in medicine involving millions of people would fill an entire book. No, conventional medical care has not always gotten it right and has not always been good for the health of the patient. So we are not replacing something that is flawless, scientific, and effective. We are trying to improve on something that is deeply flawed, largely unvalidated, often misguided by less-than-perfect motivations, and limited by the knowledge and experience of single individual practitioners.

The AMA may raise objections, naysayers may criticize, but this movement will grow, even if you choose not to participate. And it will do so widely and rapidly. The growth of self-empowerment in health can no more be squashed than a social medium like Facebook or Twitter can be stamped out—even though countries like China try. It's going to be tough for critics, terrified of the Pandora's box we are opening, to envision exactly what I am talking about and where this will take us. But, as travel agents and stockbrokers have learned, it is indeed going to happen.

Become an Unpatient

To break free of the shackles of the healthcare system, you are going to have to stage a quiet but determined revolt. It is going to create some interesting and unexpected surprises along your journey. For instance, after you've come to understand the ideas presented here, adopted the strategies, and engaged in online discussions, you'll see your doctor again for whatever reason, perhaps just to say hello. In just a few minutes, you will be struck with the realization that, of the two people in the room, you know more about your health than the doctor ever will. Your doctor knows more about drugs, medical procedures, and navigating the tangle of modern hospitals. But you will know more about healthy nutrition, the purposeful use of nutritional supplements, how to interpret basic lab values from the perspective of ideal health, and how to build a solid foundation of health applying real information.

You will learn that the nurse knows how to take blood pressure but doesn't know how to reduce it herself. The phlebotomist can draw your blood but has no idea how to put the values it yields into the service of health. You will recognize that the dietitian is not an expert in healthy eating but delivers a message friendly to breakfast cereal and soft drink makers. You will laugh when you see advertisements for the healthcare system and realize that they are all part of the broad deception of healthcare marketing for profit. Best of all, you will derive a new sense of confidence in yourself as the real arbiter of health.

Part of our uprising is to do away with the common label of traditional doctor-patient relationships and never regard ourselves as "patients" in following this Undoctored pathway. As we innovate and collaborate without the doctor and gain considerable advantage in health, the notion of "patient" completely loses relevance. We, like the doctor and others in health care, are all people. After all, the word *patient* originates from the Latin word for suffer (*patior*); we're simply not playing that game. Not only are we Undoctored, we are Unpatients. And the doctor is not director, but advisor, suffering no longer required.

But before you get to the point of engaging in Chausiku-like self-administered health, let's talk more about some of the problems in the current healthcare system, as I'd like to drive home the point that we are not rejecting an altruistic, efficiently run system. We are rejecting a predatory, self-serving, perversely overpriced hodgepodge that deserves to be cut back to its essentials. And you can personally advance that process by opting out of health care as much as possible and regaining health on your own.

Chapter Summary:
Your Next Steps to Becoming Undoctored

Undoctored is not about diagnosing your own illness or prescribing your own medication. It is about taking back control over health by taking advantage of new informational and interactive tools at our disposal. By doing so, not only can we push aside a lot of the aggravation, unnecessary expense, and hazards from what is passed off to us as "health care," but we gain health that is dramatically superior to what most doctors provide.

CHAPTER 2

Who Took the "Health" out of Health Care?

I think we're heading towards a world of what I call
"technological socialism." Where technology—not the
government or the state—will begin to take care of us.
Technology will provide our healthcare for free.
The best education in the world—for free.

—Peter Diamandis, MD,
Founder of the XPRIZE Foundation and Singularity University

Hamburger contains no ham, Grape-Nuts don't have grapes or nuts, and health does not come from health care.

Undoctored wouldn't be necessary if the healthcare system lived up to its name and provided actual "health"—but it does not. It does nothing of the sort, no more than pouring a glass of moonshine gives you a piece of the moon. Modern health care shares similarities with the prison system. Prisons provide incarceration but generally do a lousy job of rehabilitation or preventing crime, and the healthcare system delivers products and procedures to deal with illness, while maximizing financial return to its insiders, but does not provide health.

That concept is so important that I'd like to say it again, rephrased: *Health care is the system created to deliver the greatest revenue-generating products and procedures to address illness, but not provide health.* Prison time comes with its own unique hazards and tattoos, while health care likewise yields its own collection of infections, scars, errors, side effects, and unanticipated consequences as part of its imperfect effort to address illness. But unlike prison, the healthcare system puts on the pretense of being a system that provides health. We all recognize that prison is not a nice place to be, but imagine prisons calling themselves "good behavior systems." We would all laugh, of course, at such a gross misrepresentation, yet we tolerate this charade when it comes to the healthcare system.

The pretense reaches absurd heights in healthcare advertisements that portray doctors and nurses as healthcare personnel devoted to your welfare, and hospitals as friendly places, using buzzwords like "miracles," "healing," "extraordinary," "compassionate," and "personalized." An ad for the Baylor Health Care System in Dallas boasts, "For some people healthcare is a job. For us, it's our calling." Florida's Jackson Health claims, "Miracles made daily." In Milwaukee, where I live, there are billboards claiming that doctors are your "guardian angels." The Lake Wobegon effect, where "all the women are strong, all the men are good looking, and all the children are above average," doesn't come close to the hyperbole of health care, where every hospital is number one, internationally recognized, and staffed by benevolent and wise world experts.

If health care truly provided health, then your primary care doctor would counsel you on correcting common nutritional deficiencies, and an annual physical would not end at just looking for disease with a chest x-ray and a rectal exam. Seeing a rheumatologist would involve advice on how to preserve joint health and correct environmental and nutritional factors that create inflammation. A visit to an oncologist would include a review of day-to-day exposures to household carcinogens and dietary strategies that reduce the likelihood of cancer in your lifetime. A visit to a neurologist would mean having an extended discussion about the nutritional and life strategies you can follow to minimize lifetime risk of dementia. Of course, modern health care almost never involves such interactions, certainly no angels or miracles in sight.

And it's not because the doctors are not doing their jobs; they are doing the jobs they were taught to do. The medicine they were taught involved drugs, scalpels, catheters, monitors, imaging procedures—all the accoutrements of intervening or "fixing" a problem. Ironically, some doctors have knowledge that could indeed empower their patients in health, but they don't feel that this is part of their role. Doctors in procedural specialties, in

(continued on page 30)

HEALTHCARE MYTHBUSTERS

While not as dramatic as a TV *MythBusters* episode blasting a school bus into the air with a jet engine, we can still bust a few widely held myths surrounding modern medical care. This will help you get past any reluctance or fear that the medical system is holy and exalted and cannot be bested by everyday people.

MYTH #1: HEALTH CARE IS ABOUT HEALING

That may have been true many years ago and may still be alive in hospital advertising slogans. But the ethic of healing is largely lost from modern health care, now subverted into the pursuit of increased fees and revenues, the expansion of healthcare systems, the growing dominance of the pharmaceutical industry, and other factors, none of which place healing first. Health care is no more about healing than gambling on horse races is about preparing for retirement. In the doctor's mind, handing you a prescription for insulin may be her version of "healing," but you know better: There is no healing that can come from handing out pharmaceutical Band-Aids while ignoring the causes of a health problem. Don't bet on horses to grow your retirement account; don't count on doctors for healing.

MYTH #2: DOCTORS ARE ALL-KNOWING

Doctors can know a lot about a limited menu of issues, but any individual doctor can master only so much information. This is especially true today, as the amount of health information has grown far beyond the capacity of any single human being. Given the rapid rate at which medical information is increasing, the education your doctor received in medical school is obsolete by the time he finishes his internship, and the training he received in his internship is obsolete by the time he completes his residency, with the cycle continuing and accelerating every year. If you want to test a doctor's knowledge, ask an orthopedist about the bone health benefits of vitamin K_2, or an oncologist about the emerging science behind ketogenic diets and tumor shrinkage, or a gastroenterologist about the importance of prebiotic fibers for healthy bowel flora. You will most likely encounter complete ignorance or indifference, or your question will be dismissed as unimportant, irrelevant, or a waste of time, even though each of these questions relates to crucial aspects of health in each of the respective specialties, with the science already available to back it up.

The medical model of one doctor, one answer is woefully outdated. You will see, however, that as we fold in the expanding wisdom of the "crowd" collected via new technology, we can harness the information that comes to us from widely disparate sources at faster and faster rates. But it is unlikely to be delivered to you through your doctor.

MYTH #3: HEALTHCARE COSTS ARE HIGH
BECAUSE HIGH QUALITY COSTS MONEY

You will be learning later on in *Undoctored* that because the healthcare system operates with misguided motivations and imperfect methods, the more health care a population receives, the less healthy they become—actually, the more deaths experienced, death being the ultimate example of poor health. Yet the healthcare system is designed to be increasingly costly; it is expensive because it is designed to be that way.

As the Undoctored experience unfolds in this book, you will find that genuine health is inexpensive and within reach of nearly everyone—because you take charge of your health without the need for layer upon layer of skyrocketing fees, revenues, and profits. The potential cost savings are breathtaking because if you are healthy, you don't need the healthcare system.

MYTH #4: IT TAKES YEARS OF EDUCATION AND TRAINING TO DEAL WITH HEALTH ISSUES

This used to be true—until the Information Age came upon us and broke all the rules. We used to think that a shelf packed with encyclopedias was the perfect example of collective human wisdom; now, it is a relic of a time gone by, a static and unchanging behemoth in a world of rapid change and expanding knowledge. Though unnecessarily flattering, your doctor is, in many ways, the *Encyclopaedia Britannica* of health: largely static, trying to manage an unwieldy amount of information, struggling to keep up with information that changes every week. It's not entirely your doctor's fault; it is part of the disruptive Information Age.

We are therefore not going to try and memorize the contents of medical textbooks. We will take advantage of the new health tools coming our way, handily exceeding the knowledge of any one doctor.

MYTH #5: HOSPITALS ARE HAVENS OF CARING AND HEALING, OPERATED BY PEOPLE LOOKING OUT FOR YOUR HEALTH AND SAFETY

Health care is a business. If you donate money to a hospital, it would be like donating money to Wal-Mart: You'd be donating to a thriving business that does not need your money, though your contribution helps defray the cost of paying the CEO his multimillion-dollar annual salary and perks. (With rare exceptions: There are a few hospitals that do indeed operate as charities, but they are rare exceptions.) And contrary to the claims of high-paid hospital CEOs, salary has no relationship to quality of care.[1] Even though most hospitals enjoy "nonprofit" tax status, it does not mean that well-positioned insiders cannot profit handsomely.

The system is rigged for profit. This is why it is so difficult to understand the mind-numbing process of hospital billing, why hospitals spend billions of dollars every year on advertising, why your orthopedist drives a Maserati. Last I checked, these are not the emblems of charitable operations.

You are trying to avoid being pulled into the grips of an aggressive, profit-seeking system that views you as an opportunity to generate revenue, even willing to bend the rules to do so, exposing you to the dangers of modern health care: errors, infection by resistant bacteria, drug overprescription, deplorable food.

particular, such as surgery, cardiology, ophthalmology, and gastroenterology, would "waste" time that could have been spent charging higher fees for performing gallbladder surgery, heart catheterizations, eye injections for macular degeneration, and colonoscopies. If it doesn't involve a prescription, an injection, sedation, a bowel prep, a trip to the hospital, and big fees, health issues such as nutrition and correcting nutritional deficiencies are typically pooh-poohed as meaningless or ineffective by the medical community, or at least not part of their role.

The unspoken secret is that providers prefer treatment over prevention, expensive over inexpensive, patent-protectable over non-patent-protectable, billable procedure over nonbillable procedure, BMW over Toyota Prius. Spiraling healthcare costs are the expected result because greater revenues are built into the basic principles that drive the system. The endless year-over-year increase in your health insurance premiums should therefore come as no surprise because this system is designed to take more and more of your money.

Health care is a business, a big business (the biggest business of all in the United States), a business that seeks to continually grow its revenues and profits. With 1 in 10 Americans employed in the gargantuan healthcare industry, as much as 20 percent of workers in some metropolitan areas, health care also represents a huge wealth transfer from those not in health care to those in health care (many of them multinational corporations based outside the United States). It adds up to the largest wealth transfer in the history of mankind. You can stop blaming the burgeoning price of the educational system or the skyrocketing costs of military campaigns worldwide for increasing burdens on consumers—it's what is being passed off to us as health care.

The push to grow health care even bigger is all around us. Direct-to-consumer drug advertising is designed to get you to ask your doctor whether you should take a drug, even if it costs tens of thousands of dollars per year and comes with the risk of liver failure and suicide. There is a continual push to "medicalize" human life: Shyness is now "social anxiety disorder" to justify "treatment" with antidepressant medication; binging in the middle of the night is now "sleep-related eating disorder" to justify treatment with seizure medication and antidepressants; obesity, declared a disease by the FDA, justifies insurance payment for gastric bypass and lap-band. Don't be surprised if, sometime soon, bad dreams, between-meal hunger, and excessive love of your cat are labeled "diseases" warranting treatment.

The spotlight shines on new drugs and medical technologies. Hospital ads boast about the newest robotic surgery and high-tech imaging procedures. It all seems wonderful—until you stop to realize that these are the

RICK IS UNDOCTORED

Forth Worth, Texas

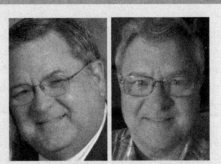

I began (nutrition, supplements, and pre- and probiotics) on the recommendation of a friend who had great success correcting a range of medical conditions over 2 years, while losing 40 pounds.

On day one, I was a miserable 277 pounds (a lifetime high) and had diabetes with fasting blood sugars in the 140 to 160 range, chest pressure, gum disease with receding gums, brain fog, low energy, insatiable carb cravings and appetite, and, worst of all, joint pain, especially in my lower back and knees, that made walking and standing very difficult. My doctor declared, "On our next visit, I'll discuss how to live with diabetes."

I experienced "wheat flu" during the first week, caused by withdrawal from wheat-opiate addiction. Like a bad case of flu, I was in bed for 3 days with high temperatures and alternating chills and fever. At the end of that first week, I lost 14 pounds (263), all joint pain, and carb cravings.

By day 18, I lost 27 pounds (250). Blood sugar dropped into the 120s. Energy returned, and no more joint pain. I was able to play racquetball again—that was a great joy. Chest pain disappeared, as did the brain fog. At the end of the first month, I had lost 6 inches from my belly, dropping from 54 inches to 48 inches.

In the fourth month, I had a semiannual dental exam, and my dentist declared my gum disease much improved: Gums were healthy and growing again. I told him what had happened with my lifestyle. "Whatever you are doing, keep it up."

By the end of the 12th month, I lost 45 pounds (232). Waist was 44 inches.

I am now in my 18th month. All the initial benefits continued. I weighed in at 234 this morning. Despite a long weight plateau, health benefits continue. Fasting blood sugar is 100 to 110. The greatest change has been joint pain. I love racquetball, and before I had so much joint pain I couldn't play racquetball; I could barely walk. I could hardly get out of the chair. Now I'm much more athletic; I'm working in the yard, playing racquetball, walking, standing. I have mobility and flexibility and strength. Friends say I look 10 years younger. Strangers don't believe I'm nearly 70.

I have directly experienced the body transformations, and I have seen them in countless others. I await the day that the medical profession yields to the overwhelming evidence that low-fat, high-carb eating produces the very diseases they claim to battle.

technologies created to deal with the results of neglected health, the alchemy of converting neglect into revenue. Neglect the real causes of osteoporosis, for example, and you are going to require an expensive course of prescription drugs or a new hip prosthesis. Neglect the real causes of diabetes, and you are going to need diabetes drugs, insulin, cataract and retinal surgery, coronary bypass, an implantable defibrillator, and dialysis. Neglect the real causes of autoimmune conditions, and you are going to need oral drugs to suppress the immune response, injectable biological agents, biopsies, and organ transplants. Neglect the real causes of obesity, and you will need drugs for weight loss, drugs to treat high blood sugar and high blood pressure, a CPAP device for sleep apnea, gastric bypass or lap-band for weight loss, and knee and hip surgery and prostheses to deal with weight-bearing destruction of joints.

In other words, neglect the cause, profit from the treatment. It is the unspoken but defining mantra of modern health care. Health is not part of the equation.

Recent efforts at healthcare reform are small steps in the right direction by expanding access. The Obamacare initiative, for example, which aims to insure everyone in the United States, has made health insurance premiums affordable through government subsidies and has eliminated some unfair insurance practices, such as exclusions for "preexisting conditions." Medicare and, to a lesser degree, private health insurers have also introduced initiatives to cap reimbursement. Some states have taken a further step by introducing tort reform to reduce defensive medicine— excessive and unnecessary testing and procedures performed by doctors to avoid lawsuits.

But such efforts only dance around an essential and driving flaw in the healthcare system. Let's put aside the cost inflation introduced by such factors as performing unnecessary procedures, fraud, and inefficiency; those are indeed problems, but problems that are increasingly under scrutiny and are largely solvable. But there is an aspect to the healthcare system that has nothing to do with dishonesty or sloppiness.

The Creed of Greed

Despite efforts at healthcare reform, almost nothing has been achieved to address the issue of healthcare costs. It's not for lack of trying, but every time any administration tries to tackle this issue, armies of lobbyists converge on Washington to protect the interests of Big Pharma, the medical device industry, the hospital industry, and the dozens of other special interests that all stand to lose plenty of money. Whenever the federal government, for instance, tries to cap charges for drugs prescribed to Medicare recipients, PhRMA, the Pharmaceutical Manufacturers Association, wields its considerable clout to squash it, unrelenting until it succeeds. Congressmen and senators listen to health lobbyists since they are near the top in donations to politicians. Some call this lobbying; others call it bribery.

Say you manufacture socks. You make nice wool socks, as do several other manufacturers. It costs you $2 to make a pair of socks, which you then sell to the public for $4. One year there is an increase in the cost of wool. You compensate for increased costs by raising the price for a pair of socks to $4.25—a reasonable increase based on your increased costs. Another sock manufacturer, however, purchased wool from another source, allowing the company to charge $3.75; they will have a competitive advantage. These are the simple rules of a competitive marketplace that everyone understands.

But such competitive rules do not apply to health care. Let's take the pharmaceutical industry. Unlike socks being sold in a competitive marketplace, drug companies can charge anything they like, even when it makes no sense whatsoever; prices are not based on supply and demand, not on competitor's prices, not on cost of materials, not on affordability or any sense of fairness. It would be as if a new pair of socks doesn't cost $4, but $400—pay up or you go sockless. Prices are set on whims that do not follow any sense of right or wrong, availability, or costs of doing business but are motivated by greed, a desire to maximize profit.

Take the drugs Harvoni and Sovaldi, for example, both from the company Gilead Sciences for treatment of hepatitis C, that carry price tags of $84,000 to $94,000 for 120 tablets, or around $750 per pill. To treat the two and a half million people medically appropriate for this drug treatment in the United States, the total bill would exceed $300 billion. (Worldwide, 160 to 180 million people have been infected with hepatitis C.) Treating even 10 percent of Americans with the condition would yield a huge financial payoff to the company, far beyond any justification for funding research and development and fair compensation for risks taken. That's just one drug. Yet the cost of manufacturing these drugs is small, around $68 to $136 for the entire 12-week course, one-thousandth of the retail price, meaning our $4 pair of socks would cost $4,000 if socks followed the lead of the drug industry.[2]

The biopharmaceutical company Celgene understands that the rules of drug pricing are largely unwritten. Despite its biotech heritage, it did something not-so-biotech with the drug thalidomide. You may remember thalidomide from headlines in the 1960s; it was a drug prescribed to pregnant mothers for morning sickness that was withdrawn from the market when 10,000 infants were born with *phocomelia*, underdevelopment or absence of arms and legs, nearly half dying after birth. Despite this scarred history, Celgene rehabilitated thalidomide as a cancer treatment for multiple myeloma, shown to prolong survival by 6 months.[3] Originally, the drug was inexpensive, as were most prescription drugs in the middle of the 20th century. It was even sold as an over-the-counter drug for a few years. Prior to FDA approval for treating multiple myeloma, a 50 milligram tablet of thalidomide cost $6, even though you could buy a tablet in Brazil in that year for seven cents, reflecting its low cost of production.[4] By 2013, thalidomide cost $197 per tablet—a thirty-two-fold increase in its original price—or $5,900 per month.[5]

Celgene did not develop this nearly 70-year-old drug, nor did it bear the cost of development. The company simply acquired the rights, performed a small clinical trial that revealed modest benefits, negotiated with the FDA, and then jacked the price up to anyone who wanted to squeeze out a few more months of life. (Because of the awful history of thalidomide, the FDA imposed severe restrictions on how the drug is prescribed, giving Celgene a virtual monopoly.) In other words, the oft-repeated argument that drug companies charge high prices to recover research and developments costs simply does not apply; the price is high because they like it high.

Celgene is not alone. Celgene executives justified the high cost of the drug by claiming that it is still cheaper than other drugs used for similar purposes. (Imagine using this argument in any other industry. Say your real estate agent proposes to charge you a 25 percent commission for the sale of your home, a usurious rate. When you object, she claims that other agents charge 30 percent, so you should be happy.)

The arbitrary and cavalier nature of drug pricing was recently epitomized by the shenanigans of Martin Shkreli, CEO of Turing Pharmaceuticals, when he raised the price of the drug Daraprim, for treatment of the fungal infection toxoplasmosis, from $13.50 to $750 per tablet, a 5,500 percent increase, overnight, an increase that the Infectious Diseases Society of America estimated raised the annual cost (treatment with this antibiotic, unlike most others, is long term) to $634,500 per patient.[6] Similar to the situation with thalidomide, the drug is off-patent and generic, and Turing did not develop the drug or file the FDA application, so he had no development costs to recover. The market of around 10,000 patients is too small for many companies to want to bother getting into, leaving Turing a virtual monopoly. Outrage over the increase prompted Shkreli to remark at a Forbes summit in New York, "I probably would have raised the price higher. My investors expect me to maximize profits."

Here's another twist on the pharmaceutical game: Take an agent already in the public domain and classified as a nutritional supplement, perform a clinical trial to treat some condition, and then declare that this new agent is a drug. This is how prescription fish oil, Lovaza (called Omacor in Europe), got its start, when the drug company Reliant spotted the opportunity. It's been known for decades that supplements of omega-3 fatty acids from fish oil reduce the level of triglycerides in the bloodstream, a risk for cardiovascular disease and other conditions. A clinical trial of the "drug" was performed, demonstrating its effectiveness for reducing triglyceride levels, just as over-the-counter fish oil does. The FDA approved Lovaza for treatment of hypertriglyceridemia, or high triglyceride blood levels. Pharmaceutical giant GlaxoSmithKline purchased the rights from Reliant and has since built the Lovaza franchise into a $1 billion-per-year business. Marketing for Lovaza uses clever wording like, "Lovaza is the only FDA-approved medication made from omega-3 fish oil. It's purified. It's concentrated. And you can't get it at a health food store." The wording is meant to persuade doctors and the public that Lovaza is somehow different from its low-cost competitors: purer, more concentrated, so powerful you can't get it on your own. Doctors, being as poorly informed about nutritional supplements as they are, jumped on the prescription form.

Lovaza costs about $60 per capsule per month. Most people take four capsules per day: $240 per month, or $2,880 per year, to obtain 3,360 milligrams of EPA and DHA omega-3 fatty acids per day.

What if I instead went to Costco and bought its high-potency fish oil? This version is in the same common ethyl ester form as Lovaza. The Costco form of omega-3 fatty acids costs $14.99 for 180 capsules, or $2.50 per capsule per month; each capsule contains 684 milligrams EPA + DHA. I would therefore have to take five capsules per day to obtain the same 3,360 milligrams EPA and DHA per day as with Lovaza. This would cost me 5 x $2.50 = $12.50 per month, or $150 per year to achieve the same effect, or 95 percent less than the cost of the prescription form. High-grade fish oil that is pure (contains essentially no contaminants such as mercury) and has a similar or greater omega-3 fatty acid content than the prescription form is widely available over the counter at a fraction of the price of Lovaza. You can even purchase another form of fish oil, the triglyceride

OF HORSES AND WOMEN

This one little tale about hormonal health of human females, pregnant horses, and drug patents paints a microcosm of the bigger healthcare picture. It is an example of how when money becomes the primary goal, health may not be served.

For years, physicians prescribed estrogen hormone replacement for women experiencing menopause, believing that drugs like Premarin, manufactured by harvesting estrogens from the urine of pregnant horses, prevented osteoporosis, improved cholesterol values, and reduced cardiovascular risk, since preliminary epidemiological studies, not real clinical studies of proper design, had suggested such benefits. Despite the lack of evidence, Wyeth-Ayerst (now part of Pfizer) spent many millions of dollars advertising Premarin and promoted its use to doctors, causing it to be the number-one most widely prescribed drug for years.

After several decades of being accepted as a routine prescription, regarded as no worse than aspirin for a headache, the whole thing fell apart in 2002 with the publication of higher-quality (randomized, controlled) studies, such as the 16,000-participant Women's Health Initiative, demonstrating that horse estrogens increased risk for heart attack, stroke, blood clots, breast cancer, and endometrial cancer.[7] Though still available, Premarin has fallen from its perch as the most widely prescribed medication.

There's more to this story: Premarin is nonhuman, a mixture of various estrogens sourced from the urine of pregnant mares (horses), very different from their human counterparts. (No surprise: Pick a species—frog, chipmunk, horse—and female estrogens and other hormones are going to differ from that of humans. Menstrual cycles, periods of fertility, and birthing methods all vary among frogs, chipmunks, horses, and other species, so it should come as no shock that their hormones also differ.) While human females produce estrogens such as estradiol, estrone, and estriol, horses express equalin, equalinin, estradiene, and a number of other estrogens not found in any human. These horse estrogens differ in structure and effect from human estrogens. The effects of these nonhuman estrogens, when administered to humans, were not fully understood during Premarin's heyday and remain incompletely understood even today.

Why administer such a hodgepodge of nonhuman, cross-species hormones with uncertain effects in the first place? And why chance the uncertainties of nonhuman estrogens when human estrogens—hormones identical to human estradiol, estrone, and estriol—are available? Were

form (as opposed to the ethyl ester form in Lovaza and most other brands), which has been put through additional steps that concentrate the omega-3 fatty acids further and reduce contaminants to even lower levels than the ethyl ester form. The triglyceride form is more potent than prescription there studies demonstrating that horse urine–sourced estrogens were superior to human estrogens?

There are no studies demonstrating superiority of horse estrogens over human estrogens. The reasons for resorting to this nonhuman source was simple: patent protection. Patents play a huge role in the pharmaceutical industry. If hundreds of millions of dollars are spent by a drug company to develop a potential drug, the company needs to make sure Its Intellectual property is protected and a competitor can't just copy it and wipe out any hope of exclusivity. One of the unique estrogens in Premarin, delta 8,9-dehydroestrone sulfate—not naturally found in any human female—is patent-protected and played a big role in protecting this drug franchise. Delta 8,9-dehydroestrone sulfate was absent from generic versions manufactured by several competitors, and Wyeth argued that it was essential to the mix. The lack of delta 8,9-dehydroestrone sulfate was declared by the FDA to be grounds for nonapproval of generic "equivalents" for many years. Horse urine and the estrogens it contains were also plentiful (think about the phrase "pee like a racehorse"), making it cheaper to extract large quantities from horse urine than from comparatively pee-challenged pregnant female humans. Even today, with wide availability of human estrogens at low cost, the majority of doctors have no idea that there are alternatives to horse urine estrogens.

Nobody fights for entities that are not patentable. Natural human estrogens are available but nonpatentable, since they have been part of the informational public domain for many years. Therefore, no drug company wants to touch them unless some manipulation, such as a novel method of administration or a biochemical modification, is exploitable. While millions of women were exposed to the uncertainties of nonhuman hormones, human hormones were available but rarely prescribed. In addition to the disservice committed to all those women, all the money spent on research—over 3,000 studies in total—to validate the use of nonhuman hormones (but not directed toward better understanding the use of human hormones) created an informational void that persists even today. At the very least, the use of human hormones avoids all the uncertainties of administering nonhuman estrogens like equalinin and delta 8,9-dehydroestrone sulfate.

Trying to ride this wild bucking bronco of nonhuman horse estrogens highlights the misguided motivations of health care that lead to pursuit of patent protection and maximizing profit, even when safer, more logical, cheaper solutions are available.

fish oil and better absorbed, yet still at a tiny fraction of the price of Lovaza.

Oddly, few physicians advised patients to take fish oil until Lovaza appeared on the market and persuasive sales representatives started dropping off samples with smiles. While doctors could have easily advised patients to supplement over-the-counter fish oil before the "drug" form came on the market, they instead opted to prescribe Lovaza, reflecting the effectiveness of marketing hocus-pocus and adding several thousand dollars of cost per person under the guise of FDA approval. Of course, the $1 billion in Lovaza sales ends up in the pockets of the drug company, while we all bear the burden of increased costs whether or not the drug was prescribed to us. And all of this from something that you could have taken on your own, easily and inexpensively.

Another way the pharmaceutical companies game the system is with "me-too" drugs (i.e., drugs that are minor variations of those already on the market). Unlike other markets in which competition leads to price reductions, me-too drugs tend to cost more even in the absence of any evidence of superiority. The drug Prilosec, for example, a proton pump inhibitor (PPI), used to treat acid reflux, was followed by Prevacid, Protonix, AcipHex, Nexium, and Dexilant. And each new PPI drug was not accompanied by reduced pricing, despite the competitive playing field. We've seen this play out in the world of statin drugs, blood pressure drugs, anti-inflammatory drugs, asthma drugs, antibiotics, antidepressants, sedatives, and just about every other class of drugs; cheaper to develop, involving less commercialization risks, and serving existing markets, me-too drugs are among the darlings of drug companies. But they further fuel inflated costs.

Partly because of the high prices they command, biological therapies (antibodies, interferons, and other biologically active molecules that require injection) have become a recent focus of drug development. Despite fewer people requiring such agents compared to, say, a drug for something as common as high blood pressure, they are still financial bonanzas for the drug industry. Of the 39 new agents receiving FDA approval in 2012, for example, 11 were biologics priced over $100,000 per patient per year.[8] Such agents are also typically so toxic that an arsenal of medications is required to treat or reduce the side effects. Marketing efforts have made the biological therapies Humira, Remicade, and Enbrel among the top-10 bestselling drugs in the world, with global revenues of $11.1 billion, $9.9 billion, and $8.9 billion, respectively.[9]

The same sort of go-for-the-jugular profit-seeking mentality applies to the world of medical devices, a booming industry growing faster than the pharmaceutical industry. Unlike a prescription drug for which incentives for most physicians to prescribe are modest, medical devices are more widely and systematically incentivized in the medical community. The price tag of a medical device to a patient comes with hefty physician charges, as well as hospital charges, charges for anesthesia, and charges for long-term management (as with pacemakers and defibrillators, for example). The considerable fees for deploying such devices make them irresistible to many physicians and hospitals, who thereby try to perform as many procedures as possible, whether or not they are truly needed.

One example: An analysis of 111,000 people who received implantable cardioverter defibrillators, or ICDs, in 1,200 hospitals across the United States revealed that an astounding 22.5 percent of patients receiving them did not have a legitimate indication of need.[10] In some hospitals, as many as 40 percent of implanted ICDs were put in without need. Receiving an ICD is no small matter, as they are large devices implanted under the skin of the chest: bulky, disfiguring, requiring monthly checks and surgical replacement of the battery every few years—yet we have nearly one in four people receiving them without reason. And they're expensive: Typical costs for hospital admission for an ICD implantation begin at $36,000 (Medicare), higher when private health insurance is involved or complications occur, of which at least $1,100 is the physician's fee for implantation.[11] Defenders of such procedures claim that the professional fee is too small to encourage physicians to implant the devices, but I can tell you from personal observations over more than 20 years of medical practice that it most definitely is a motivating factor, particularly if a practitioner implants several devices per week. Just implanting ICDs can be a several hundred thousand dollar per year activity for a single practitioner, not to mention the considerable favors given to physicians from device manufacturers for being champions of their devices. While there is no question that ICDs can be a lifesaver when implanted in the right person (for which guidelines are clear), people who receive an unnecessary ICD are exposed to the hazards of the procedure and device without any benefit.

During my former life as an interventional cardiologist performing coronary balloon angioplasty and inserting stents, each metal stent implanted cost between $500 and $3,000 from the manufacturers. Implanting two, three, or five in a single patient was not uncommon. The average stent weighs 0.2 gram and is made of stainless steel; the pricing for stents means that you are paying $2,270,000 per pound of steel—hundreds of times more than a pound of gold, but for common steel not that different from the spring in your ballpoint pen. Sure, there are research and development costs to recover, but nothing to justify such wildly exorbitant prices. As with drugs, prices charged for devices have nothing to do with

MORE BETTER HEALTH CARE

More free time is nice. More love among family and friends is wonderful. But more health care is not healthier; it can even be downright dangerous or fatal.

Time and time again, studies have demonstrated that more health care does not yield better health. One study of Medicare patients nationwide showed that the more health care people received in the form of procedures, hospitalizations, and specialist referrals, the worse they did in quality outcomes. This occurs even when the cost differential between lowest and highest is wide. Annual per capita Medicare spending was $3,341 in Minneapolis, for example, but $8,414 in Miami; but the less spent, the better the outcomes.[12] The four states with the highest Medicare spending—Louisiana, Texas, California, and Florida—rank the worst in quality.[13] More health care translates into increased complications and more deaths, not more lives saved.

The research group at the Dartmouth Institute for Health Policy and Clinical Practice at Dartmouth College has been exploring this phenomenon, studying healthcare demographics and costs nationwide for 3 decades. Interestingly, the initial reactions to these efforts 30 years ago were critical, as everyone "knew" back then that of course health care was cost effective and safe. But the many studies they have published over the years have repeatedly borne out the opposite: High-cost regions have 32 percent more hospital beds, 31 percent more physicians, 65 percent more medical specialists, 75 percent more general internists, and 29 percent more

reality. Cardiologists are paid around $1,000 to $3,000 per artery[14] for their work, like with ICD implantation, more than enough to incentivize some to do more than they should. (I've heard colleagues lament that it's a shame that humans only have three coronary arteries.) And, indeed, the evidence suggests that cardiologists perform many more procedures than necessary, including thousands of instances every year in which people without heart disease or minimal disease receive stents. Hospital Corporation of America (HCA), for example, the largest for-profit hospital chain in the world with 163 hospitals, has had repeated run-ins with Medicare, the federal government, and state attorney generals for fraud; many of its cardiologists allegedly performed unnecessary heart procedures, including inserting stents in arteries without disease.[15]

Although the abuses are among the worst in my own field of cardiology, there are plenty of similar excesses outside of heart disease. Arthroscopic knee surgery for osteoarthritis—in which a surgeon passes a narrow scope surgeons than low-cost regions, but outcomes are no better, often worse. Nationwide, the pattern was clear: The more money spent on health care, the higher the mortality rate, even after factoring in variation in health patterns across different regions.

Even though Americans spend twice as much on health care as other modern developed countries, we rank dead last in quality, outcomes, accessibility, and efficiency.[16] The common claim made from within health care that the United States has the finest healthcare system in the world is nonsense. We even rank last among Western economies in preventing deaths from treatable conditions, such as strokes, diabetes, high blood pressure, and treatable cancers. You can obtain better, more accessible, more efficient care in the UK, France, Germany, Sweden, and Switzerland, among others. All countries have to deal with growing healthcare costs, but none have to deal with the extreme costs of US health care, which grows unrestrained, unchecked, and without any relationship to real costs.

We also can't ignore the fact that more people die per year from complications of hospital procedures and errors, estimated at 400,000 annually, than from auto accidents.[20] Increasing access to health care thereby increases the proportion of people who die from complications. Yet the medical system works to grow the availability of specialists, fund more hospitals and clinics, and increase the number of profitable programs, such as heart care and cancer care. To them, more health care is more money. To you and me, more health care means more costs, more complications, more deaths, but most definitely not more better health.

and various tools to scrape away rough edges and loose debris and shaves down knee cartilage in the hope of providing pain relief—has been shown to have no benefit beyond placebo.[17] (This is not to be confused with arthroscopic procedures to repair torn ligaments or meniscus tears, which have been shown to be effective.) There can be early pain relief after arthroscopic knee surgery for arthritis, but it is short-lived, yielding no long-term benefit over exercise and physical therapy, no better than a sham operation. Yet this procedure has been performed on millions of people over 20 years, with several hundred thousand still performed in the United States every year.[18]

Hysterectomies (removal of the uterus) are also a perennially abused procedure. While some are necessary, such as for endometrial cancer, the majority are performed for benign conditions such as fibroids or endometriosis. Up until a few years ago, gynecologists—mostly male—had little hesitation in advising women to undergo hysterectomy, not uncommonly involving removal of not just the uterus but also the upper vagina, cervix, fallopian tubes, and ovaries, increasing the likelihood of complications such as damage to the bladder and ureters and sexual dysfunction. Just 50 years ago, hysterectomies were performed for almost no reason—for depression or anxiety or as a form of birth control. Growing awareness of this cavalier attitude among gynecologists combined with emergence of alternative therapies has reduced the number of hysterectomies, but it remains the second most commonly performed surgical procedure in females. With hospital fees in the neighborhood of $12,000 and gynecologist fees of $2,000 (and anesthesiologist fees of $1,000), there are obvious financial incentives for offering hysterectomies willy-nilly.[19]

Why would drug and medical device companies charge prices that are so far out of line from reality and have nothing to do with the cost of production and pay lip service to how much they invest in research and development while reaping extraordinary profits at both the corporate and individual executive levels? Simple: Because they can. There is no lid on what they can charge, so companies charge any amount they want. Yes, we live in a free-market democracy, but the drug and medical device industries operate more like kleptocracies. Though most of it is legal, it is not ethical and is, in effect, a form of legal extortion. Likewise, healthcare providers, particularly those in procedural specialties, often choose to work in the gray zone, increasing their procedural numbers by performing surgeries and other procedures in which need is at least questionable, if not outright unnecessary. Hospitals condone—sometimes overtly, sometimes quietly—such behavior because they, too, make more money that way.

Modern health care is, for all practical purposes, a zero-sum game: Your loss (in health insurance premiums, copays, out-of-pocket expenses, bankruptcies over medical bills) is their gain. Obviously, health care cannot be free. Somebody has to bear the cost. But the culture and mind-set of health care is to maximize personal profit of insiders regardless of the broader consequences, even if it means crippling economies for personal benefit and inflating total healthcare costs to levels far beyond those necessary.

The Wealthcare Bubble

I won't pretend to have all the answers to fix this deeply flawed healthcare system that we have. Because it is largely built on the greed of its insiders—from hospital executives to ophthalmologists charging unjustifiable fees for minor procedures to pharmaceutical executives jacking up the price of drugs to triple digits per day—I call this the "Wealthcare Bubble"—health care doesn't necessarily provide health, but it sure provides wealth.

When this bubble bursts, the fallout will be ugly. We saw what happened when the mortgage-backed-security-and-banking bubble burst a few years ago, nearly toppling the world's financial systems. The Wealthcare Bubble is so big that as it unravels, we are going to have one heck of a financial crisis on our hands. Driven by the continued release of $100,000-per-year drugs, the overuse of high-priced medical devices, and all the other self-serving behaviors of this profit-driven system, imagine your health insurance premiums double, deductibles grow even bigger—these are unsustainable trends. Most of us would end up working to accomplish little more than pay for our family's health insurance, if we could afford it at all. And remember: The money doesn't just vanish; it goes into the pockets of the people who've rigged the game in their favor: wealthcare.

Thankfully, answers are starting to emerge from a number of directions, though few from within health care itself since insiders remain reluctant to sacrifice revenues. The Health Care Cost Institute launched guroo .com, which lists prices charged by hospitals, allowing people to shop for better prices. The Healthcare Bluebook (healthcarebluebook.com) has launched a similar effort. Emboldened by findings such as those from the Dartmouth Institute for Health Policy and Clinical Practice, policy efforts to control healthcare expenditures while improving outcomes are likely to emerge. The idea of "bundling" care for a fixed price, for instance, a practice that discourages overuse and out-of-control expenses, seems to be slowly catching on, and that may also add some restraint.

I tell you all of this not just to make you wary as a healthcare consumer but to drive home the point that by taking the reins of health yourself, you are not trying to avoid a gleaming, efficient, and charitable system set up to serve you. You are trying to avoid being exploited, abused, and misled by a system driven by perverse motivations, unjustifiable costs, and incomplete protections, shaking you down for money like a Mafia leg-breaker at every opportunity while claiming to follow a "calling" or be your "guardian angel," making you believe that you'd be sunk without them. You should stop viewing this system that fails to provide health as health care, but as wealthcare, or for-profit care, a business that puts its own interests first, not your health. There will be times in your life when you need the healthcare system, and those in it will be more than happy to take your money, but it is our job to minimize those times while you become healthier than ever before.

I do believe that you have part of an emerging solution right here in your hands. As you will see later on in this book, the Undoctored experience restores health at so many levels that it allows you to opt out of much of conventional health care. If you have normal blood pressure, you won't need blood pressure medication. If you don't have acid reflux, then you won't need an endoscopy and years of stomach acid–blocking drugs. If you don't develop osteoporosis, you won't need drugs for osteoporosis or a hip replacement at age 70. If you are healthy, you don't need health care. Accomplish just one of the items listed and you have already saved thousands of dollars in healthcare costs and spared yourself plenty of aggravation and, as you now know, the considerable risks that come with wealthcare operating under the guise of health care. But you don't have to stop at just one condition. Why not spread your efforts across as wide a range of health issues as possible?

Before I begin talking about all the wonderful Undoctored things you can do, let's talk a bit further about how modern life creates much of the sickness treated by modern health care and the lessons we can learn when we start asking tougher questions.

Chapter Summary:
Your Next Steps to Becoming Undoctored

It is important that you view the healthcare system without rose-colored glasses and rid yourself of the traditional notion of it being a system of benevolent healers doing good deeds. Just like Wal-Mart or Exxon, health care is a business. But because of the outdated facade of benevolence, health care is permitted to operate under such false pretenses as being nonprofit or providing "miracles." Once you accept this stark reality, you begin the process of divorcing yourself from the bonds of this profit-seeking business.

CHAPTER 3

With Friends Like These...

A doubtful friend is worse than a certain enemy.

—Aesop's Fables

When you want an honest answer to a health question, who can you turn to? If it's not your doctor, not a nurse working in the hospital, not a help line with your health insurance company, then who? If it's not your Aunt Lillian who once passed a kidney stone after she loaded herself up with dandelion root but swears that chewing tobacco cures earaches, then who can you depend on to answer questions honestly with an eye toward solutions that are safe, inexpensive, and effective?

Perhaps, in our distrust of the healthcare industry, we should turn to organizations that claim to be heroes of health—charitable, nonprofit organizations such as the American Diabetes Association, the Academy of Nutrition and Dietetics, and the American Heart Association as well as governmental agencies such as the US Department of Health and Human Services, the FDA, and the USDA. After all, these organizations professionally certify health practitioners, develop guidelines, and fund research. Can we depend on these organizations to shine a light and help us navigate through the landmine-strewn field that is modern health care? Unfortunately, each and every organization has allowed commercial interests to influence its message.

Before we get to the nitty-gritty of the Undoctored program, in this chapter I'm going to show you that these organizations and others have often engaged in behaviors that aren't necessarily based on the latest scientific research and have even provided advice that *causes* health problems but lines the pockets of their membership and friends. These organizations are false friends whose charitable, supportive public persona conceals deals cut privately to benefit insiders. You should, for the most part, ignore their advice. What may have started out with good intentions has mutated into something entirely different, all by falling victim to the same disease of doing and saying things for money. Lest you think that I've gone off my rocker and have receded into some dark corner of conspiracy theories, hear me out. The evidence speaks for itself. It will become clear that while these organizations do plenty of good, they have also proven to be unreliable sources of health information for the health-seeking public, sometimes even steering us down paths that cause the diseases they are supposed to be protecting us from. Recognize these dangerous paths, however, and you will be on your way to enlightened, Undoctored health.

Let me start with one of the most egregious examples of all: the huge and almost entirely man-made problem called type 2 diabetes.

The Perfect Disease

To you and me, there is no such thing as a perfect disease. Along with snakes, spiders, and being buried alive, we want no part of *any* disease. However, from the wrong-side-up perspective of the healthcare industry, type 2 diabetes is the perfect disease. Unlike, say, pneumonia, which necessitates an antibiotic for 14 days and then it's over, type 2 diabetes starts with one drug, then two, and then three or more, not to mention the drugs used for associated conditions, such as hypertension, heart disease, kidney disease, eye diseases, and accelerated dementia. And all of these drugs are prescribed for years, often a lifetime (albeit shortened compared to those without diabetes), resulting in a pharmaceutical bonanza of profit. To the drug industry, diabetes is the gift that keeps on giving.

You've heard the sobering statistics: There are now 30 million people with type 2 diabetes in the United States, three times this number with prediabetes.[1] So if you wear clothes in public or watch reality TV, the likelihood of type 2 diabetes in your future is high. Costs likewise are staggering: $176 billion in direct medical costs and $69 billion in reduced productivity every year.[2] Being diagnosed with type 2 diabetes adds, on average, $7,900 to an individual's annual healthcare costs. (Before they smartened up, annual reports of publicly traded pharmaceutical companies gushed over the surge in people with type 2 diabetes, hailing the epidemic as an unprecedented opportunity for revenue growth. They recognized recently that this could become a publicity faux pas and stopped using boastful wording.)

For example, among the recent additions to the drug treatment of type 2 diabetes is a drug called Farxiga, approved by the FDA in 2014, with a price tag of $380 per month, $4,560 per year. If a doctor prescribes it along with a new form of insulin called Toujeo at $350 per month, these two drugs to control blood sugar total nearly $9,000 per year for one person. That's not the total cost of health care for a person with diabetes, but the cost for just *two drugs* that might be prescribed, commonly among many more.

But there is a major oversight in all this: Type 2 diabetes is a disease of lifestyle and poor food choices and, to a lesser degree, inactivity, nutritional deficiencies, and other modern disruptions, made worse by the advice of agencies who pose as health advocates. Yes, there can be a genetic predisposition to the disease, but the increase in the number of diabetes cases since 1980 and the even faster growth of prediabetes are almost entirely manmade phenomena.[3] After all, the genetic situation in humans has not changed in a short 30-some years; it's something *we did* in the years since *E.T.* and *Poltergeist* hit the big screen.

Here's a basic fact: Eat carbohydrates and blood sugar rises. Every first-year medical student knows this, every nurse or diabetes educator knows this, every person with diabetes who performs finger-stick blood sugars before and after meals knows this. Eat any food with more than just a few grams of carbohydrates and blood sugar will rise; the more carbohydrates you eat, the higher blood sugar will rise. Everyone also knows that foods like butter do not raise blood sugar, nor will a fatty cut of meat, olives, green bell peppers, broccoli, or chicken liver. And since the 1980s, when the sharp upward climb in type 2 diabetes (and obesity) began, the only component of diet that has increased is carbohydrates, not fat or proteins.[4]

There is no mystery: Carbohydrates raise blood sugar, though more so in those with diabetes, who have lost the ability to control blood sugar levels. Just as the sun rises in the morning and sets in the evening, the more carbs you eat, the higher your blood sugar will rise; the less carbs you eat, the less your blood sugar will rise. Eat no carbs, and blood sugar will not rise at all.

So what do doctors and diabetes educators following the advice of the American Diabetes Association (ADA) tell patients with diabetes? Cut total and saturated fat, reduce cholesterol, and eat more grains and carbohy-drates.[5] Sugary foods are allowed without restriction, though the ADA advises people with diabetes to count carbohydrate grams and adjust insulin dose and/or other diabetes drugs to compensate for the blood sugar rise. In other words, follow a diet that everyone knows will raise blood sugar, and then adjust medications to bring blood sugar back down. (A few years ago, this Q&A was posted in a discussion with ADA dietitians: "Question: I have type 2 diabetes. Can I eat sugary foods like cake, cookies, and candy? Answer: Of course you can! Cake, cookies, and candy contain sugar. Sugar is natural. Just be sure to count your carbohydrate grams and talk to your doctor about adjusting your dose of insulin or oral diabetes drugs." This telling comment has since been taken down, but it perfectly encapsulates the mind-set of the ADA.)

Does this approach work?

If your goal is being free of health problems and prescription drugs, no, it does not, no more than lending a compulsive gambler a thousand dollars helps him pay down his debt. It does not reduce blood sugar, and it does not reduce cardiovascular risk. People with diabetes experience higher blood sugars, higher levels of hemoglobin A1c (HbA1c), the long-term measure of blood sugar, and end up needing more medications at higher doses, eventu-ally requiring insulin at ever-increasing doses. Once the need for insulin injections develops, blood sugar goes even higher due to the substantial weight gain introduced by insulin injections (since insulin promotes body fat growth). The pharmaceutical industry responds by creating new drugs that run the bill up further for treating diabetes, while hospitals and doctors manage complications that develop after a few years of the disease. This is not a win-win; it's a clear-cut lose-win.

Doing the opposite of ADA advice—not limiting fat or cholesterol and severely restricting or eliminating the carbohydrates from grains and sugars—improves the entire picture, reducing and often eliminating the need for diabetes medication.[6] Then why does the ADA persist in broadcast-ing a message that clearly does not work?

Honey Bunches of Oats, Sour Patch Kids, and the American Junk Food Association

Despite the growing tide of clinical evidence that suggests carbohydrate restriction, not fat restriction, is a far better answer, the ADA stood by its stance of unrestricted carbohydrate and sugar intake in its 2004 position statement (emphasis mine).

> Low-carbohydrate diets are not recommended in the management of diabetes. Although **dietary carbohydrate is the major contributor to postprandial [after-meal] glucose concentration**, it is an important source of energy, water-soluble vitamins and minerals, and fiber. Thus, in agreement with the National Academy of Sciences–Food and Nutrition Board, a recommended range of carbohydrate intake is 45–65% of total calories. In addition, because the brain and central nervous system have an absolute requirement for glucose as an energy source, restricting total carbohydrate to <130 g/day is not recommended.[7]

In other words, carbohydrates are responsible for high blood sugars but you need them for vitamins, minerals, and fiber—a statement that has *never* been validated in scientific studies. The brain and central nervous system's "absolute" requirement for glucose is a complete fiction, as well. There is no need for sugar in the diet, whether from grains or sugary foods, by the human brain. The human body and brain are well adapted to obtaining energy from fat, as you'd expect in a creature—*Homo sapiens*—that lived through periods of having *no* fruits or roots (i.e., natural sources of carbohydrates or sugar) for extended periods. This is why we have an absolute need for fat and an absolute need for protein—being deprived of either is eventually fatal—but *no need for carbohydrates*.[8] And if depriving your brain of carbohydrates as a source of glucose was truly dangerous or fatal, we should be witnessing mass graves for all the people who are following Atkins, paleo, ketogenic, and other versions of low- or no-carbohydrate lifestyles, all from depriving human brains of their "absolute" need for glucose from carbohydrates—but we're not.

After urging people with diabetes to cut their fat and cholesterol and include plentiful grains with liberal sugar consumption in its 2004 statement, and then watching the health disasters that resulted, the ADA must be suffering a serious case of remorse. After all, the organization proudly displays its mission: "To prevent and cure diabetes and to improve the lives of all people affected by diabetes." Admitting that they were wrong would invite legal liability on a huge scale, loss of credibility, and a drop in revenues, particularly from generous pharmaceutical companies who love the growing ranks of people with diabetes. But it seems that the ADA is beginning to realize that it made a mistake, judging by its 2013 position statement (emphasis mine).

> Despite the inconclusive results of the studies evaluating the effect of differing percentages of carbohydrates in people with diabetes, **monitoring carbohydrate amounts is a useful strategy for improving postprandial [after-meal] glucose control. Evidence exists that both the quantity and type of carbohydrate in a food influence blood glucose level, and total amount of carbohydrate eaten is the primary predictor of glycemic [blood sugar] response.**[9]

Not fat, not saturated fat, not cholesterol, not a silly discussion about butter versus margarine whether or not you can believe it's butter, but carbohydrates as the "primary predictor of glycemic response." The ADA statement concedes that carbohydrates from grains, sugary foods, and other sources are the primary determinants of blood sugar, despite advocating for their free consumption years earlier. This startling confession, unfortunately, was not accompanied by a retraction, apology, or any other effort to make amends for decades of bad advice. To this day, the "ADA diet" sends blood sugar through the roof. (This is why, for instance, a person with "diet controlled" type 2 diabetes who enters the hospital for whatever reason is placed on an "1,800- or 2,400-calorie ADA diet" typically ordered by doctors and develops out-of-control blood sugars, and is discharged from the hospital with newly prescribed insulin injections or other diabetes drug medications. I witnessed this countless times over the years, but debating diet in a hospital is a fool's battle.)

Readers of my Wheat Belly series of books also understand another basic flaw in logic that led agencies like the ADA down this path of dietary disaster: If you replace something bad (such as white flour products) with something less bad (such as whole grains), and there is an apparent health benefit (less cardiovascular disease, less diabetes, less weight gain, less colon cancer—all true), then you should not conclude that a lot more of the less bad thing must therefore be good. The next step in this sequence of logic should have been to examine the effects of elimination of the less bad thing. (Such studies have been performed and do indeed demonstrate benefits such as not less weight *gain* but weight *loss* and not less type 2 diabetes but complete reversal of the condition or marked improvement of blood sugars.)

It gets worse. Major donors to the ADA? Mostly pharmaceutical companies. Among its biggest supporters: AstraZeneca, Boehringer Ingelheim Pharmaceuticals, Eli Lilly and Company, GlaxoSmithKline, Novo Nordisk—all in the business of developing drugs for diabetes. ADA support from just Eli Lilly and Novo Nordisk totaled around $11 million in just 2014 alone.[10] Support for programs that "build awareness" are especially popular among pharmaceutical supporters, which makes sense since the worst thing that could happen to a drugmaker is to have people not be aware of having the condition in the first place, a lost revenue opportunity. ADA programs, such as Step On Up to educate the public about diabetic nerve pain, provide companies like Pfizer a platform to talk about drugs such as Lyrica, its $350-per-month prescription product for, yes, diabetic nerve pain.

For many years, Big Food companies, such as the Hershey Company, Kraft, Post, PepsiCo, and Coca-Cola, were also among the ADA's most generous supporters. But the ADA turned them away in 2006 because of increasing criticism, especially when it caught flack over a several-million-dollar contribution from Cadbury Schweppes, the world's largest maker of candy and soft drinks. At the time, an ADA press release gushed with news of the association: "We are thrilled to have Cadbury Schweppes Americas Beverages join forces with the American Diabetes Association to help deliver crucial messages to consumers about healthy lifestyle changes. . . . Working together, we can get consumers the tools and solutions they need to reach and maintain a healthy weight and incorporate more physical activity into their lives—all key to the prevention and management of type 2 diabetes."[11]

A candy and soft drink company with wisdom on healthy weight? Yes, the fox promises to do a really good job of guarding the henhouse. And according to the message from this unholy alliance, the problem is not them, it's *you* because you don't exercise enough. If you did, you could reward yourself with a box of Swedish Fish or Sour Patch Kids.

Until recently, you could view the proud declaration of ADA sponsorship, for instance, on boxes of Post's Honey Bunches of Oats and Frosted Shredded Wheat breakfast cereals and many other similar products. The ADA's blatant support of the processed food industry's products led Gary Ruskin, former executive director of the industry watch group Commercial Alert, to remark, "Maybe the American Diabetes Association should rename itself the American Junk Food Association."

Let's step back for a moment and take stock of what has happened:

Whether intentional or inadvertent, misinterpretation or blundering, advice to engage in a diet low in fat and rich in grains with a free pass for sugar was a major contributor to the epidemic of type 2 diabetes and weight gain/obesity. Purported efforts to subdue a disease made the disease worse, and not just by a little, by a lot: We now have the worst epidemic of type 2 diabetes and obesity in human history. Even in the face of science telling us that the ADA dietary approach is wrong, the organization stubbornly stands by old advice. Meanwhile, the healthcare system profits enormously, and the pharmaceutical industry celebrates double-digit annual rates of growth and record revenues due to the man-made financial bonanza of diabetes and associated conditions. Yes, conventional health advice *created* an epidemic that paid off big for those in Big Food, pharmaceuticals, and health care. Upside: The flood of people with diabetes and its complications, such as stroke, heart disease, and kidney disease, made the healthcare system very good at taking care of such conditions. Downside: The majority of people should never have developed type 2 diabetes or its complications in the first place.

Complicit in all this are the doctors, dietitians, diabetes educators, food companies, and people in pharmaceuticals who have supported and propagated this misguided dietary advice. An avoidable disease was not just *not* prevented but was coddled, cultivated, and allowed to flourish, while all those properly positioned profited.

You still think you're safe following the advice of your doctor? You can see that the credo of "First, do no harm" holds as much water as Bernie Madoff promising, "Your money is safe with me." Then how about the people in the dietary community who, after all, are trying to do nothing more than to help you make wiser food choices—right?

The Academy of Eat Anything You Want

While the stated purpose of the Academy of Nutrition and Dietetics (AND) is to support education in nutrition, judging from its activities behind closed doors, the organization spends an awful lot of time and effort working to derive revenues from Big Food while legally squashing anyone who erodes its efforts.

The AND's current stand on healthy nutrition is summed up by its most recent position statement (emphasis mine).

> **Classification of specific foods as good or bad is overly simplistic and can foster unhealthy eating behaviors.** Alternative

approaches are necessary in some situations. Eating practices are dynamic and influenced by many factors, including taste and food preferences, weight concerns, physiology, time and convenience, environment, abundance of foods, economics, media/marketing, perceived product safety, culture, and attitudes/beliefs. To increase the effectiveness of nutrition education in promoting sensible food choices, skilled food and nutrition practitioners utilize appropriate behavioral theory and evidence-based strategies. **Focusing on variety, moderation, and proportionality in the context of a healthy lifestyle, rather than targeting specific nutrients or foods,** can help reduce consumer confusion and prevent unnecessary reliance on supplements.[12]

What? Can you discern anything useful in that statement that could help consumers follow a healthy diet? Don't feel bad if you couldn't; I certainly could not. But one message is clear: Any and all foods fit into the AND's notion of healthy eating—including foods from its sponsors, such as Coca-Cola, PepsiCo, Abbott Nutrition (makers of Ensure), Unilever (I Can't Believe It's Not Butter!, Klondike bars, Hellman's mayonnaise), and the Corn Refiners Association (high-fructose corn syrup), among others—and you will require the services of a dietitian to navigate issues like moderation and portion size.[13] It's this sort of thinking that spawns illogical catchphrases like "everything in moderation"—*all* foods fit into the AND dietary model. (Try the logic of "everything in moderation" out on your 17-year-old contemplating crack cocaine.)

The AND therefore collaborates—on a paid basis, of course—to promote processed foods and help with damage control when there are criticisms waged against, for instance, sugary sodas or excessive high-fructose corn syrup. Most curious is the relationship between the organization and Coca-Cola. Through its euphemistically named Coca-Cola Beverage Institute for Health & Wellness—set up by Coca-Cola to defend against critics of high-fructose corn syrup, aspartame, and sugar—Coca-Cola vigorously promotes, with the assistance of AND dietitians, the "calories in, calories out" concept, the idea that people are overweight because they eat too much and move too little and if they would just get out and move more, they could drink Coca-Cola, Fresca, Sprite, or Mello Yellow and be slender and healthy. As media expert and professor Marty Kaplan of the University of Southern California put it: "The academy has long functioned more like a trade group than a professional society," calling the AND "The National Academy of Sugar."[14]

Corporate sponsorship has also managed to infect the educational process of dietitians and continuing education required to maintain certification. Companies not in the business of education but in the business of selling food products are invited to sponsor and provide educational opportunities for dietitians. President of the consumer advocacy group Eat Drink Politics, Michele Simon, a public health attorney, attended an AND annual meeting in 2012, a meeting purportedly intended for AND member education. She described it as "a truly surreal experience just to walk into the expo hall. You know it's supposed to be a nutrition conference and yet it feels like a food industry event. Junk food expo is really the best descriptor. As you walk in, all you can see are the massive booths of companies like Coca-Cola, Hershey's, and PepsiCo."[15]

The AND's love-fest for industry has created some even stranger bedfellows. In 2013, the organization received money from Elanco, manufacturer of antibiotics for livestock, to fund "education" for dietitians about use of antibiotics to accelerate growth of cows and pigs. Nutrition fact sheets are written by AND dietitians with the assistance of industry insiders for $20,000 per fact sheet, which are then published in AND journals for its dietitian membership to read. Past issues have included "What's a Mom to Do: Healthy Eating Tips for Families" sponsored by Wendy's; "Adult Beverage Consumption: Making Responsible Drinking Choices" with the Distilled Spirits Council; and "The Benefits of Chewing Gum" sponsored by the Wrigley Science Institute.[16] The products of AND sponsors may not be explicitly endorsed, but neither are they criticized, even when they have zero nutritional value and are heavily marketed to children.

It also means that the nice dietitian you've been told to see by your doctor has, in effect, had an education bought and paid for by the food industry. You can no more expect to obtain unbiased, unscientific advice from a conventionally trained dietitian than you can from a salesperson from a soda company—because, in many ways, they are essentially one and the same.

And the AND wants to ensure that you are unable to obtain dietary information from anyone but a dietitian trained by AND methods. Witness what happened when blogger Steve Cooksey from North Carolina shared his experience of losing 78 pounds, reversing type 2 diabetes diagnosed at the hospital when he was nearly in a coma, and then getting off all medications by rejecting the advice of doctors and following a paleo-type diet by removing all grains and sugar. After his recovery, he attended a presentation from a dietitian who advised that people with diabetes should cut their fat intake and eat more grains and other carbohydrate sources. Spurred by what he regarded as a destructive message, Cooksey began a small crusade to share his experience of reversing diabetes by rejecting such advice. After answering readers' questions and offering advice on how to do likewise, the North Carolina Board of Dietetics/Nutrition filed a lawsuit, claiming that he was providing dietary advice without a license, a charge of criminal behavior, never commenting on his experience of journeying from diabetic coma to diabetes-free on his own by going against conventional dietary advice. In the end, Cooksey prevailed and waged a countersuit against the North Carolina Board, claiming that it was a violation of his First Amendment rights. Despite Cooksey's success, similar lawsuits have been filed by state dietetic/nutrition boards against other nondietitians discussing nutrition.

Regardless of what the courts decide, dietitians at the organizational level do not want you to discuss diet without a dietitian, regardless of whether you are right or wrong. You might, after all, decide that a food or drink from one of their sponsors might not really be healthy.

From Heart-Healthy Crisco to Heart-Healthy Frosted Flakes

The ADA and AND are far from alone in cultivating lucrative relationships with industry. Nearly every other health organization is guilty of the same. The American Heart Association (AHA) is no exception.

Heart disease, more than any other health condition, is dominated by money and business. Even over the course of my career, I watched heart disease evolve from a low-tech world with few effective tools to a high-tech flurry of new technology—which is great. But it also "monetized" heart disease, making it exceptionally lucrative. More than most other areas of health, heart health is therefore dominated by money. And organizations built around heart disease, such as the AHA, are no different, now a half-billion dollar per year behemoth.[17] What the Eat Drink Politics president, Michele Simon, observed about the AND is similar to what you see if you attend an annual meeting of the AHA: elaborate displays by pharmaceutical and medical device companies, generous gifts handed out to attendees. It's an over-the-top industry hootenanny.

AHA sponsors are a familiar bunch: Big Pharma companies like Amgen, AstraZeneca, Bristol-Myers Squibb, Eli Lilly, Medtronic, Novartis, and Pfizer, as well as food companies and trade groups such as General Mills and the Idaho Potato Commission, all of whom contribute, in total, tens of millions of dollars every year.[18] The AHA claims to be impartial to the ambitions of sponsors, delivering an unbiased message of heart health. But such indifference does not always play out in real life. As far back as the 1940s, Procter & Gamble, makers of the blockbuster product Crisco, made with hydrogenated oils to replace "unhealthy saturated fat" from butter and lard, bankrolled the AHA, and the AHA urged Americans to replace saturated fats with vegetable oils such as Crisco. (It's now clear, of course, that hydrogenated "trans" fats increase risk for heart disease and cancer, while saturated fats do not.) Additional unwise endorsements for sponsor products were made by the AHA over the years, such as the endorsement of the drug alteplase, used to treat stroke, in clinical guidelines. While the drug does its job as advertised, not mentioned was the $11 million in donations received by the AHA from the drug's manufacturer and that six of eight panel members drafting the guidelines had financial ties to the company.[19]

The AHA, under the pressure of public criticism, has updated its conflict of interest policy, forbidding such relationships, though the policy does not seem to fully translate into action. This policy of indifference to industry ties has operated all the way up to the most recent 2013 cholesterol treatment guidelines that expanded statin drug use to millions more people beyond the 25 million already taking them, guidelines drafted by a committee of 15, 6 of whom had relationships to industry.[20] (The situation is worse among other clinical practice guidelines for heart disease and other conditions, with 80 percent of committee chairs having commercial ties to the companies that would benefit from the guidelines.[21]) Defenders of the status quo of relying on experts with industry associations claim that identifying experts who do *not* have such ties means that there are too few experts to choose from—a damning statement in and of itself.

The AHA provides certification for hospitals that meet specific performance criteria, a collection of programs called Get With The Guidelines. Hospitals seek AHA certification, since heart disease care is competitive and accounts for such a large proportion of revenues, and certification allows hospitals to proudly display the AHA logo. There's nothing wrong with setting guidelines for hospital performance, but who sponsors (and thereby potentially influences) this program to certify hospitals? Yup, our old pharmaceutical and medical device friends: AstraZeneca, Boehringer Ingelheim, Medtronic, Bristol-Myers Squibb, Pfizer, Amgen, and others.[22]

Perhaps more than anything else, it's the world of food that reveals the AHA's hand with greatest clarity. The AHA got into the business of certifying food in 1988, a program that became the Heart-Check program in 1995. Some of the products certified over the years include Berry Berry Kix, Count

Chocula, Cocoa Frosted Flakes, Fruity Marshmallow Krispies, Honey Nut Cheerios, and low-fat Pop-Tarts, all declared "heart healthy" with tens of millions of dollars in certification fees paid for by companies including Cargill, Post, Kellogg's, and Coca-Cola. They won't certify onions, green bell peppers, or organic kale, of course, since that's not where the money is. So go for the money rather than health, and what you get for heart-healthy food is low-fat Pop-Tarts.

The AHA continues to support education and research, but it does so while also enthusiastically advancing the big money agenda of Big Pharma, Big Food, the medical device industry, and doctors. I would no more trust an agency with such divided allegiances than I would trust Wall Street to handle my home mortgage.

Will Do Research for Money

The amount of money flowing directly from the pharmaceutical and medical device industry to physicians—not through health insurance or Medicare charges for services, but direct payment for some service such as being a "key opinion leader" to convince other physicians to use a product—is staggering. In 2014, as part of an effort to pull back the shroud of secrecy and make healthcare economics more transparent (the Physician Payment Sunshine Act, a provision of the Affordable Care Act), the Centers for Medicare & Medicaid Services reported that there were over four and a half million financial transactions from healthcare industries to physicians and teaching hospitals over just the last 5 *months* of 2013, with a total value of nearly $3.7 billion.

Academic medical centers are often viewed as centers of education and research. Indeed they are, but they are also increasingly financially cozy with the pharmaceutical and medical device industries. A recent survey found that two-thirds of academic medical centers own equity interest in companies that sponsor research within the same institution.[23] A survey of chairmen of medical schools and large teaching hospitals showed that 60 percent received personal income and two-thirds received income to their departments from industry.[24] While the drug and medical device industries have a primary responsibility to their shareholders, the majority of medical centers, particularly academic medical centers, do not. Their mission should not involve entering into lucrative relationships, equity stakes, and big payoffs from industry—but they do. Obviously, if an institution or its medical staff employ a technology but also own a stake in it, they are likely to selectively

NUMBERS RACKET

Let's pretend that you are in the business of creating devices for cars that increase safety, perhaps a new kind of harness that improves on modern seatbelts. You test the harness in the cars of several thousand volunteers and track data comparing the number of deaths occurring in cars equipped with standard seatbelts versus cars equipped with the new harness. You find that people with cars with standard seatbelts die 1.42 percent of the time in collisions. (I'm making these numbers up for the sake of making a statistical point; they are not based on any real auto accident data.) People driving cars with your new harness die 1.12 percent of the time—slightly less than the old technology, but not that different. The reduction in fatalities from your harness means that for every 100 crashes, there will be 0.3 percent fewer fatalities; stated another way, you would have to tally up 330 crashes to save one life—meaningful but small. On top of this, your device adds another $700 to the car's sticker price. If you advertise this slight advantage to an auto manufacturer or average driver—that your harness reduces likelihood of death in a collision from 1.42 percent to 1.12 percent and the likelihood of survival increases from 98.58 percent to 98.88 percent with added cost to the consumer—you'd likely get a big yawn.

Ah, but then you have a statistical epiphany. What if your sales pitch to the auto manufacturer went more like this: "My harness reduced fatalities in car crashes by 21 percent"? Well, that sounds a lot more substantial. Your restated pitch causes the human brain to hear "for every 100 crashes, 21 fewer people will die." That is enough to raise eyebrows, but that is *not* what your device accomplishes. So where did you get that more persuasive 21 percent from? Easy—just follow along.

The reduction in risk with the harness is 0.3 percent. The risk of dying in a crash with the standard seatbelt is 1.42 percent. You compare the reduced risk of dying in a car equipped with the harness with the risk of dying in a car without it.

0.3 percent ÷ 1.42 percent = 21 percent reduction

This is called relative risk reduction. As you can see, it is misleading, allowing you to substantially overstate the benefits of your device. Yes, the device provides an advantage in protection, but not to the degree suggested by the misleading manipulation made with the numbers.

choose that technology for the financial advantage it provides to them, a decision that may not always be in the patient's best interests.

While there is plenty of useful health information in the medical literature, it is also filled with bias when the pharmaceutical, biotech, or medical device industries are involved. Respected medical editor Dr. Marcia Angell

But that is how medical data are reported. Let's take a prominent real example, the ASCOT Trial of the statin drug atorvastatin (Lipitor), published in 2003 and regarded as one of the best studies supporting statin use. (Unlike most other statin drug trials, this one was not supported by the manufacturer. It was funded by nonindustry grants, removing at least one potential source of bias.) There were 10,000 participants enrolled in the study. Half were given atorvastatin, the other half a placebo, and then they were observed for 3 years. Of the people taking the placebo, 3 percent experienced a heart attack over 3 years, while 1.9 percent of those on atorvastatin had a heart attack, a reduction of 1.1 percent. Alternatively, 97 percent on the placebo survived, while 98.9 percent survived on the drug—different, but not very impressive. But let's play that same statistical game that we played with the auto harnesses:

1.1 percent ÷ 3 percent = 36.7 percent

By the magic of arithmetic, we convert an unimpressive 1.1 percent reduction in risk into a much more headline-worthy 36.7 percent reduction in risk—in this case, a thirty-three-fold exaggeration.

This figure—36 percent reduction in heart attack—was trumpeted all over ads to the public, quoted endlessly by drug sales representatives and in physician education material, and it succeeded in boosting sales of Lipitor to over $10 billion per year to become one of the most prescribed and profitable drugs in history. Imagine the actual value had been used in ads: "Lipitor reduced risk of heart attack by 1.1 percent"—hardly worth spending hundreds of millions of dollars to broadcast and certainly not exciting enough to generate billions of dollars in prescriptions. Because doctors hear "Lipitor will avoid heart attacks in 36 out of 100 people" when they hear these ads, they are much more willing to prescribe the drug, while the public is much more willing to take it—but it's simply not true.

The same statistical hocus-pocus is used in every statin drug trial, blood pressure drug trial, cancer drug trial, and just about every other drug or device trial, a practice that, in effect, wildly inflates the benefits of a drug or device but equips marketing departments with a powerfully persuasive, however misleading, way to sell the advantages of a product. But that is how health care is sold to you.

remarked that "conflicts of interest and biases exist in virtually every field of medicine, particularly those that rely heavily on drugs or devices. It is simply no longer possible to believe much of the clinical research that is published, or to rely on the judgment of trusted physicians or authoritative medical guidelines. I take no pleasure in this conclusion, which I reached slowly and reluctantly over my two decades as an editor of the *New England Journal of Medicine*."[25]

Bias and deceit in studies can take on many forms. One method is to publish studies that cast a favorable light on a product while studies with negative outcomes are not published. In the world of antidepressants, for instance, 37 out of 38 positive trials were published, while 33 of 36 negative studies were never published.[26] It's difficult to know what you *don't* know. Some negative trials are forced out into the open only during the discovery process when lawsuits are filed against companies.

Another way to game the results of clinical trials is to selectively publish only portions of data that are favorable while concealing the negative. Drug company giant Merck, for instance, failed to report the fourfold increased risk of death that occurred when rofecoxib (Vioxx) was used to treat dementia, but this exclusion was uncovered only when lawsuits were filed against the company.[27] Me-too drugs, meant to be incremental improvements on other drugs from the same class, are typically compared to a placebo, not to the drugs that they are supposed to be an improvement over, but marketing is used to solve that "oversight." Another common strategy: Use company employees or paid research companies (contract research organizations, or CROs, whose job it is to perform clinical trials for money and are thereby entirely beholden to the sponsor of the drug or device) to conduct the trial, and then pay a respected researcher at a university for the use of her name on the study. There is, undoubtedly, some truth in such clinical trials, but it is virtually impossible to distinguish what is true from what is not, or how much has been concealed and unpublished.

The research on bias in medical research is clear: If a clinical trial—no matter how large, no matter how well-funded, no matter how prestigious the principal investigator or institution—is funded by the pharmaceutical or medical device industry, the outcome is likely to be favorable to the sponsor.[28] And, incredibly, physicians often do not review the actual data, relying instead on the quick and convenient information provided by the drug or device sales representative over dinner and drinks or on what they call "throwaways," medical magazines and newspapers reporting medical news that is, yes, sponsored (and often written) by the drug and device industries.[29]

The problem is that nearly all clinical research used to support the use of various drugs in all classes and medical devices of all kinds was bought and paid for by industry, meaning the data are flawed, manipulated, massaged, and selectively reported. Yet such data are widely published and used in drafting guidelines for physicians. You can begin to appreciate what an astoundingly flawed and potentially misleading system we have, all due to financial motivations.

Health: A Federal Case

Getting your health information through government-funded sources is no guarantee that the taint of commercial influence is not present.

We've known for years that highly placed insiders in the FDA and USDA leave for jobs in the drug industry, biotech industry, medical device industry, or agribusiness, or vice versa, the so-called golden revolving door. High-level executives and attorneys have bounced back and forth from, for instance, an executive position at Merck or Monsanto to a post at the FDA or USDA. For example, Dr. Arthur Hull Hayes Jr. served as FDA commissioner for 2 years from 1981 to 1983. During his brief tenure, he personally overruled the 3-3 gridlocked vote for approval of aspartame as a sweetener despite nearly 2 decades of contentious debate and animal studies demonstrating that the sweetener was associated with cancerous tumors, and then he resigned to work as a high-paid consultant for the public relations firm used by aspartame's manufacturer, G.D. Searle, a subsidiary of Monsanto.[30] This industry-government overlap continues today with, for instance, the recent appointment of Dr. Robert Califf as the new FDA commissioner despite having extensive and longstanding financial ties to multiple pharmaceutical companies, including as founder of the Duke Clinical Research Institute, which performs paid contract research for the pharmaceutical industry.[31] The citizen watch group Public Citizen charged that "no FDA commissioner has had such close financial relationships with industries regulated by the agency prior to being appointed. Califf's appointment as FDA commissioner would accelerate a decades-long trend in which agency leadership too often makes decisions that are aligned more with the interests of industry, rather than those of public health and patients."[32]

The extent of industry-friendly activity at the FDA did not become fully apparent until Senator Charles Grassley's several-year-long investigation exposed FDA cover-ups to avoid reducing prescriptions of certain drugs, especially antidepressants in children; the agency suppressed data that showed increased suicide in children taking the drugs.[33] Several years later, insider Dr. David J. Graham, associate director of the FDA's Office of Drug Safety, along with eight other FDA scientists and physicians, wrote a letter to newly inaugurated President Barack Obama claiming that the agency "is inherently biased in favor of the pharmaceutical industry. It views industry as its client, whose interests it must represent and advance. It views its primary mission as approving as many drugs as it can, regardless of whether the drugs are safe or needed," and "many other FDA managers who have failed to protect the American public, who have violated laws, rules, and regulations, who have suppressed or altered scientific or technological findings and conclusions, who have abused their power and authority, and who have engaged in illegal retaliation against those who speak out, have not been held accountable and remain in place." One of the issues raised by the whistleblowers was the danger of the drug Vioxx, heavily marketed by drugmaker Merck, despite data revealing increased deaths from cardiovascular disease. When Graham and his colleagues tried to publish their study demonstrating increased heart attack and death, they were ordered by FDA superiors to withdraw the study. Vioxx has since been pulled from the market and Graham's study was published, confirming that as many as 140,000 heart attacks and deaths occurred because of the drug.[34]

The FDA is also largely responsible for the difficulty we've had as a nation in regulating genetically modified (GM) crops. In 1992, the FDA took the stand that products such as Roundup Ready Corn, the strain of corn created by Monsanto by inserting genes for resistance to the herbicide Roundup (active ingredient glyphosate), are "substantially equivalent" to crops produced via traditional breeding methods.[35] Recent studies have raised questions about the safety of GM crops, including questions raised over the herbicides and pesticides that go along with GM crops. One damning experience from a French research group, for instance, began by trying to reproduce Monsanto's data but with more detailed tissue analyses; they failed to reproduce the same benign findings, instead observing kidney, liver, heart, spleen, and adrenal toxicity with the two forms of GM corn.[36] The first effort to extend the period of observation beyond Monsanto's original 90 days raised even more disturbing questions. Over 2 years of observation, increased death rate, breast tumors, liver damage, and pituitary disruption from both glyphosate-resistant corn and from glyphosate itself were reported.[37]

Glyphosate itself, the world's most widely used herbicide, exerts estrogen-like activity, promotes growth of breast cancer cells, disrupts male fertility, and disrupts endocrine function in a number of other ways. The World Health Organization recently designated glyphosate as a "probable carcinogen" based on studies that suggest that non-Hodgkin's lymphoma can result from exposure.[38, 39, 40, 41, 42] Keep in mind that all these observations were made years after the FDA provided its blessings for GM crops and the herbicides/pesticides that go with them.

Much of the same industry-friendly activity also goes on at the USDA, an agency that enthusiastically endorses GM crops. But unlike other federal agencies, the USDA finds itself in a unique position: While its primary responsibility is the health and safety of US agriculture—an industry dominated by agribusiness multinational corporations such as Syngenta, Cargill, BASF, and Monsanto—it has also been charged by Congress with dispensing nutritional advice to the public. It would be as if Congress had the Securities and Exchange Commission (SEC), already dealing with the financial markets, add providing investment advice to consumers to its portfolio of responsibilities; yes, both involve money, but it would be entirely outside the primary expertise of the agency, virtually inviting conflicts of interest. You can envision deals cut behind closed doors, favors, conversations at the ninth hole of the golf course if such conflicting responsibilities were combined. Of course, the SEC is not sponsored by these companies, but it is the USDA that has been charged with telling you what to eat and how much, while also regulating the industry that produces all of it.

How about the question of how much glyphosate in corn, wheat, or other crops is acceptable and whether GM crops are even safe in the first place? Whose side should the USDA be on—agribusiness with its substantial contributions to Congress, intensive government lobbying, and threats of soul-draining lawsuits, or the public that is not very good at taking concerted action and generally does not play golf with congressmen or make generous contributions to reelection campaigns? You get the picture: It's not entirely the USDA's fault. The USDA should never have been charged with providing dietary advice in the first place. But since the agency has been unwisely charged to do so, it is your job to *not* take it seriously. Let the USDA do what it is good at doing, such as advising farmers on how to fight off the latest pest, but the last thing you should do is let some new pyramid or plate guide your thinking about nutrition.

Even the government-funded National Heart, Lung, and Blood Institute (NHLBI) of the National Institutes of Health feels it must involve corporate sponsorship to fund its message through the familiar Red Dress campaigns, involving sponsors such as Coffee Rich and General Mills. While its goals are noble on the surface (i.e., increase awareness of heart disease risk among women), there are some issues that are not so noble. The campaigns start by urging women to "talk with your doctor, find out your risk for heart disease, and take action today to lower it." What "action" are they referring to?

Beyond the usual "cut your fat," "eat more healthy whole grains," and "everything in moderation" sort of advice (all of which is nonsense, as you shall see, and actually contributes to diseases), much of the activity promoted by these programs centers around encouraging physicians to prescribe statin drugs, dispense drugs and devices for heart failure, and send patients for heart testing. Programs at the local level are supported by the all-too-familiar drug manufacturers AstraZeneca, Novartis, Merck, Pfizer, GlaxoSmithKline, CV Therapeutics, Bristol-Myers Squibb, Amgen, Boehringer Ingelheim, and others.[43]

Among the worst examples of questionable and potentially commercially influenced advice that comes via government programs is the National Cholesterol Education Program, a program established by the NHLBI to educate physicians and the public about cholesterol, conducted along with the AHA and the American College of Cardiology. They do so by issuing guidelines called the Adult Treatment Panel, ATP, the first issued in 1988, the latest in 2013.

The 2001 guidelines, ATP-III, reflected the opinions of nine expert medical panel members. The advice dispensed in ATP-III dramatically increased the number of people prescribed statin drugs by intensifying the cholesterol values set as goals for treatment, and it set the pace for prescription of these drugs for over a decade. But look into the background of the members of this expert panel and you see that of the nine, eight had deep and longstanding financial ties to Pfizer, Merck, Bristol-Myers Squibb, and AstraZeneca—the makers of statin cholesterol drugs. This bit of handwork was responsible for boosting revenues for this one class of drugs to over $20 billion per year.

If you read the panel's most recent 2013 guidelines and their review of clinical studies, you will see that they considered the size of each study, its design, and other factors influencing the quality of the findings, but you will also find that there was no consideration given to *who paid for the study.*[44] The vast majority of new studies are funded by the drug industry, all reporting their data, by the way, in terms of relative risk reduction (see "Numbers Racket" on page 58). In my view, the National Cholesterol Education Program should be renamed the *Pharmaceutical Industry* Cholesterol Education Program since the pharmaceutical industry essentially paid for most of the data, had close ties to experts drafting ATP guidelines, and funded local programs.

Government agencies, for the most part, perform essential and often unforgiving roles in health. Unfortunately, when it comes to providing health information to the public that is unbiased, they have fallen far short. More than health friendly, policies within government are *business* friendly, with commercial interests permeating dietary advice provided to the public, endorsement of GM crops, and the information given to your doctor. Just as certainly as there are death and taxes in your future, commercial interests will continue to contaminate government health information. But unlike death and taxes, this is something you can opt out of.

"Nothing Personal—It's Just Business"

That's how math whiz Otto Berman, who figured out how to rig bets for the gangster Dutch Schultz, viewed the world in 1930s New York. If you had a cinder block tied to your ankles and found yourself at the bottom of the Hudson River, well, that's just business. If you get saddled with bags of prescriptions and crippling medical debt, don't get all weepy and snivel about it—that's just the business of health care.

If the answer to this unfairly stacked deal is to spend more money on health care, then it would be no different than trying to fix a crooked gambling game by placing larger bets. But that is what we are doing if we allow insiders in health care to continue expanding the status quo driven by self-interests.

Money in health care is like trying to wash something awful off your hands: No matter how much you wash, you just can't seem to erase the filth. Whenever money and favors of corporate sponsorship are part of the equation, it inevitably influences the message, no matter how much the recipient tries to stay clean; it's human nature. No person or organization that embraces the easy money of commercial interests is immune to this bias. The ADA, AND, and AHA may claim that they are unfazed by the millions of dollars flowing to them, a researcher may defend his $500,000 of shares in the company whose drug he is testing, or a medical center may claim that it uses a technology only because of its advantages and not because it owns some of the company, but that is not what the scientific data on bias argue, that is not what human nature dictates. Scrub all you want, but you cannot rinse it off; it's everywhere, even under the fingernails. And it smells bad, too.

You have therefore been exposed to health advice heavily influenced by commercial interests for decades, leaving you wondering why you still have problems with high blood pressure, irritable bowel syndrome, or type 2 diabetes. You have them, in large part, because it is profitable for you to have them. Like Dutch Schultz's rigged numbers rackets, the healthcare system is a game rigged in favor of the insiders, leaving you as the sucker at the gambling table. It's time to fold and play an entirely different game, one in which the odds are stacked in your favor because the rules are open to you.

The worst news for a healthcare system rigged for its own financial gain? Healthy people. And that is how you can opt out of this game: by not placing any bets and just being healthy.

I hope that, by now, you have disavowed the idea that the healthcare system only has your best interests at heart, provides only unbiased scientific information, and works for your health. It doesn't mean that the system is evil or out to screw you; it means that its goals are not aligned with yours, despite the public face it provides. You now understand why we must turn to other sources for unbiased, reliable health information—yes, they are indeed out there, though often not as publicly visible or well funded—and why, outside of injury, infection, and some other exceptional situations, you are healthier by opting for the Undoctored path.

Lastly, before we get to the juicy part on the specific steps you take to become Undoctored, let's talk about the role your doctor has in this new world.

Chapter Summary:
Your Next Steps to Becoming Undoctored

Before we begin crafting our program to become Undoctored, it is essential that we know whom to trust for information, and whom not to trust. Unfortunately, many of the people and organizations who purport to provide you with unbiased advice do nothing of the sort, since cozy ties with industry and their deep pockets govern their behavior. Likewise, much medical "research" is really nothing more than thinly veiled marketing, even though much of the medical community accepts such findings at face value.

Undoctored provides advice that is unbiased and untainted by industry relationships, just designed to obtain health—a unique and revolutionary concept, despite its simplicity.

CHAPTER 4

Any Doctors in *Undoctored*?

These . . . are uncola nuts. They grow here, too. But,
as you can see, they are a bit different from cola nuts.
Rather large, for one thing. Rather juicy, too, I'd say.
Marvelous little things, uncola nuts. We use
them, of course, to make the uncola.

—Actor Geoffrey Holder, TV commercial for 7UP, 1970s

If there's no health in health care and the uncola has no cola nuts, does the Undoctored lifestyle have any room for doctors?

The Undoctored approach to health does reserve a place for doctors. But they will no longer be the white coat–wearing, dictatorial "I'm-the-doctor-you're-the-patient" variety. They will be playing a very different role in our world.

Let's drill down to the gritty realities of dealing with doctors who still think it's 1980 and that you feather your hair like Farrah Fawcett and wear velour tracksuits and who scoff at your newly found informational freedom and expect you to submit unwaveringly to their commands, while we explore the empowering and independent world of an Undoctored lifestyle.

Why exactly do modern doctors have such one-sided, my-way-or-the-highway attitudes and expect you to acquiesce so readily to their version of health while choosing to so easily ignore the views of the person who matters the most—you? Let's explore just what makes the doctor such a . . . doctor.

Spin Doctor

In 1955, Mickey Mouse premiered on television, Betty Crocker personified cooking habits of American housewives, and minimum wage was increased to a dollar. Go to the doctor that year and he (males only, of course) would tell you in no uncertain terms what to do. The doctor made a diagnosis, then prescribed treatment. The paternalistic, autocratic relationship left little room to question the course of treatment or contribute your own ideas. This one-sided relationship worked—in its own limited way—because most people were too ignorant about health issues to make a meaningful contribution. The tools to permit any form of self-directed health were not yet available, as far out of reach as smartphone apps and 3-D printers in the age of Dwight Eisenhower and *I Love Lucy*.

At about that time, a man named Martin Salgo, suffering from severe atherosclerosis of his abdominal aorta, underwent an angiogram that resulted in paralysis below the waist, a complication that his doctor had not warned him about. In a subsequent lawsuit, *Salgo v. Leland Stanford Jr. University Board of Trustees*, the concept of "informed consent" was introduced, the idea that a patient must be made fully aware of all risks of a procedure prior to providing consent, a radical shift in the long-held perception that the doctor was all-knowing and to be trusted beyond question.

Informing you as the patient is therefore a surprisingly recent notion, an idea that got started just as baby boomers were born. Up until that time, patient ignorance was expected and the public delivered. For centuries, doctors' practices were guided by the principle that they needed to instill confidence—not knowledge—in patients for the all-knowing power of medical care, reflected in 20th-century TV portrayals of medical care such as *Marcus Welby, MD* and *Dr. Kildare*. Any suggestion of uncertainty was thought to erode patient trust and diminish the healing power of the placebo. It was even regarded as dangerous to inform a patient of the medical unknowns, as blind faith was an important component of medical care.

It wasn't uncommon in those days, for instance, for a doctor to diagnose a cancer but withhold that information from the patient. Physicians were asked in a 1961 poll whether disclosing a cancer diagnosis to a patient was advisable; 90 percent voted no—you would suffer the pain, debilitation, and life-abbreviating effects of cancer, unaware of why, how, or when.[1] Of people diagnosed with cancer in 1976 but not informed of their diagnosis, nearly all admitted suspecting that they had cancer but expressed a wish to *not* know anything more.[2]

Examples of people not wanting to know more is an example of *learned helplessness:* passive acceptance of a situation in which circumstances are perceived to be beyond control. It is a behavior learned not just in health care but also in situations such as incarceration, torture, and depression. Psychologist Dr. Martin Seligman pioneered studies of this effect at the University of Pennsylvania. Dogs given unavoidable electrical shocks stopped looking for escape even when they were subsequently provided an escape route from the shocks. College students given challenging mental tasks interrupted by a loud noise could learn to turn off the noise by pulling a lever, but if the lever had no effect at first, they failed to retry and exert control in future experiments because of their prior experience of helplessness. They, like the dogs, learned to be helpless.[3]

Just as with helpless dogs and college students, the doctor-patient relationship is also defined by learned helplessness: If you know that no empowering information will come from the interaction, only the dictates of the doctor to blindly follow, you no longer expect it or ask questions. If you were told that your uterus needed to come out, that's just the way it was. This one-sided passive relationship worked when expectations were low because most people were ignorant and tools for self-directed health were not yet available. Lest you think that such an autocratic process no longer operates in our day, just think back to the drug prescriptions handed to you without explanation or with the most cursory justification, despite the fact that many common drugs, such as hormone replacement for women or diuretics for hypertension, are marred by deplorable track records of side effects, such as cancer, diabetes, fatal blood clots to the lungs (pulmonary emboli), and sudden cardiac death—not just hair loss, oily diarrhea, or an odd rash.

Dr. Benjamin Rush, the namesake of Rush University in Chicago, summed up attitudes of doctors toward patients: "The obedience of a patient to the prescriptions of his physicians should be prompt, strict, and universal." In other words, you are expected to respond, "Yes, doctor, anything you say" in any and every situation, from hemorrhoidectomy to heart transplantation, since it's assumed that you don't know the difference between a hippocampus and an amphibious, mud-wallowing creature from Africa.

This attitude led doctors to have complete disregard for the rights of patients. In the early 1940s, indigent and mentally ill patients were injected with radioactive plutonium to observe the effects. Patients at the Jewish Chronic Disease Hospital in Brooklyn, New York, were unknowingly injected with cancer cells to determine whether their immunity differed from that of healthy people. The history of medicine is filled with tales of experiments inflicted on the unaware that make us cringe today. It required the revelation of atrocities performed by Nazi doctors at the Nuremberg trials in 1945 to acknowledge that human experimentation should not be conducted freely (though it continued largely unabated for several more decades).

Maintaining the appearance of infallibility, following doctors' orders without question—these are the beliefs that defined the attitudes of both doctors and patients for centuries, the attitudes that modern doctors learned during education and training, portrayed in popular media, persistent even today.

Just as the 7UP uncola campaign introduced a revolutionary idea into the world of soft drinks, upending expectations from a simple bottle of soda, *Undoctored* will discombobulate your expectations for the process of doctoring, regardless of what the doctor may think.

Role Reversal

With our Undoctored shift in relationships, we are going to engage in a limited form of role reversal, not as extreme as a *Freaky Friday* mother-daughter body switch, but one in which you assume many of the roles of the doctor and do it better.

Imagine you walk into the doctor's office. You've already begun your Undoctored program and have improved your health: You've lost 25 pounds, reduced cholesterol and blood pressure without medication, and reversed the pain and joint disfigurement of the rheumatoid arthritis that previously required three prescription drugs. You are now free of all pain and have worked your way down to *no* drugs, recently completing a 10-mile bike ride and enrolling in dance classes while, months before, a walk to the mailbox was a major challenge. However, you could use help obtaining a test of your vitamin D blood level, important to monitor in this situation. Since the cost of the test is covered by health insurance, you ask the doctor to order a 25-hydroxy vitamin D level to assess the effects of your nutritional supplement program; you know exactly what you are asking for, why you need it, when you need it. In other words, while you may still rely on your doctor to provide counsel when needed, for the most part, *you* are in charge of your health. You will also be empowered to recognize bad advice, such as being prescribed drugs for osteoporosis or a cholesterol drug when you are not at risk for heart disease, or being told "You don't need vitamin D anymore" or "Calcium is all you need for bone health," which you will learn is not just ineffective but potentially disastrous advice.

You go to the doctor for an opinion, for assistance, but not to be ordered

ANNETTE IS UNDOCTORED

Ontario, Canada

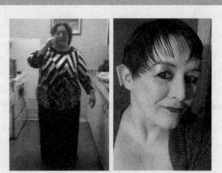

I started August 20, 2014, unable to do the most basic things. I was diagnosed with many health issues, including rheumatoid arthritis, IBS [irritable bowel syndrome], prediabetes, migraines, chronic hives, PCOS [polycystic ovary syndrome], tendonitis, plantar fasciitis, carpal tunnel syndrome, anemia, osteoarthritis, etc., etc. I couldn't walk or stand for more than a few minutes at a time. Bathing or even wiping myself was near impossible. I had to use an electric wheelchair and was taking heavy-duty pain medication (Percocet and morphine), which only made me sick and didn't help with pain much.

I now take no medications, ride a bike 5 kilometers every day, and walk another 10 kilometers. I've lost around 170 pounds so far.

It's been 22 months now since I started. Starting weight 355 pounds, currently 183 pounds. Chest was 60 inches, now 42 inches, waist was 52 inches, now 34 inches, hips were 64 inches, now 48 inches, thighs were 46 inches, now 23 inches, calves were 20 inches, now 13 inches, arms were 24 inches, now 12 inches, neck was 20 inches, now 12 inches. Diabetes gone, blood pressure normal, cholesterol normal, chronic hives gone, chronic pain gone, migraines gone, wheelchair gone. A life that was full of pain, sadness, depression, hopelessness is gone. I am completely pain-free with no health issues. I'm having the life I always dreamt of but never thought possible. Dr. Davis saved my life.

or directed. Your doctor may be operating with attitudes from times when a woman's uterus was removed without permission, but you are participating in a global experience of awareness and information that follows the rules of a new age, empowering you to reject the notion that the doctor is in charge—*you* are in charge. The doctor is working for you. Before you even get to the doctor's office, you have accomplished far more than can be achieved in the usual abbreviated health interaction. And the results you obtain are *superior* to what your doctor could achieve without your help— and you didn't even need a stethoscope or white coat to accomplish it. But you still rely on your doctor for assistance with the occasional unexplained pain or unanswered health question or to facilitate testing you request. There is no need to be timid or apologetic; after all, it's *your* health at stake.

In fact, without seizing the reins of your own medical fate, you will flounder. Left to the whims and neglect of conventional healthcare delivery, you will obtain the minimum allowed by the absurd time constraints and misaligned motivations of your healthcare provider, a situation that ends up causing you to eventually "need" the healthcare system's catastrophic services advertised on billboards. Without all the new knowledge you will be acquiring, you might even fall for all the bad information that comes through dietary counseling, "heart healthy" foods, and other corrupt sources.

You—not your doctor, not your local hospital, not your pharmacist, not your personal trainer—are the most likely person to take the initiative for personal health and ensure that steps are taken to remain healthy and/or regain health.

Can You Outsmart a Teenager?

With attitudes in health care so slow to catch up with modern views on individual rights, can we really expect anyone in health care to cooperate with us? Can you really achieve independence in health without alienating healthcare practitioners who still adhere to an outdated paternalistic model of care?

While much of the world of self-directed health can be achieved *without* doctors or healthcare professionals, there will be times when it will be easier or more effective to enlist their assistance. So how can your doctor be enlisted as an *assistant* or *advocate* rather than a *director* in the health process?

It's easier than it sounds. Start by acknowledging that you should not booby-trap the effort by trying to control the doctor. For instance, if you go to the doctor's office armed with a list of tests and treatments you insist you need, along with copies of studies you found on the Internet, and then demand that he order everything you ask, you will get nowhere. You push, they push back, and you will hear objections such as "I'm the doctor here," "This is unnecessary," "Insurance won't cover this," or "I don't practice Internet medicine," or any of the other common axioms that seem to come so naturally to doctors when their authority is questioned.

Despite their patronizing tendencies, outdated attitudes, and revenue-seeking ambitions, most doctors still wish you to be healthy. Instead of coming on like a bull and insisting that your doctor comply with your demands, approach him as you would a nasty, rebellious teenager. Don't demand, but ask. "I'd like your help. Could you help me understand why I am so fatigued all the time? Some friends who shared their health information with me told me that reducing their TSH to less than 1.5 and addressing their free T_3 levels really turned their lives around and helped them feel much better. Would you add that to my blood work?"

Many doctors will willingly comply with a heartfelt request to seek answers in health, while the same request posed as a demand will almost always end in refusal. Your use of some of the language of health also signifies that this is not a casual request but something that truly concerns you. You are also suggesting that if you don't receive a satisfactory response, you will pursue your answers one way or another. If your doctor does not yield, shows no interest, or ridicules your request, then it's time for a new doctor. You are looking for an advocate in health, someone to facilitate your success, not an obstructionist or dictator. I would estimate that around 50 percent of healthcare practitioners are hopelessly stuck in 1950s-style thinking—still expecting you to comply without question and finding your meddling a nuisance—and are unwilling to change. Minimum wage is no longer $1, and you should no longer tolerate such a one-sided health relationship.

Many of the strategies in *Undoctored* do not directly involve your doctor. But a doctor's guidance can be especially helpful to back down on prescription drugs she has prescribed, especially those for hypertension or diabetes, since some agents for these conditions cannot be abruptly stopped. Inflammatory conditions, such as rheumatoid arthritis, which respond to the Undoctored strategies, will require you to work with a doctor to remove, say, the methotrexate and prednisone, but gradually so that no disease flare-ups are permitted. Know that many, if not most, prescription drugs can be replaced by natural, nondrug strategies with results that often exceed that achieved with drugs. Once again, if your doctor refuses to assist you, empower you, acknowledge that it is indeed possible to achieve results with your new efforts, walk away and find one who will.

People with complex or multiple medical problems, in particular, benefit by having a willing and knowledgeable healthcare provider to adjust medications and monitor changes. If you have type 2 diabetes, for example, and have been taking injectable insulin and three oral drugs, you will need the help of a doctor to taper off the insulin and drugs as you become less diabetic to avoid the extremes of blood sugar, both high and low. Unfortunately, many people develop such complex or multiple problems *because* of the indifference or neglect of the medical system; expecting the same practitioners to help you fix the situation is not often possible. So you may need to

CHOOSING A HEALTHCARE *ADVOCATE*

Let's face it: Many healthcare practitioners, certainly those in conventional medicine, are *dis*empowering, *un*cooperative, and *non*collaborative. You want to avoid those. You can waste an awful lot of time and health with such practitioners, so it is important to seek out a healthcare provider whom you can count on for advice, assistance, or just confirmation when you need it.

It's a shame that nobody has developed a smartphone app like the ones for online dating that make it as easy as swiping left or right to make a connection, so just a bit of clever maneuvering will be required. To identify an effective healthcare advocate, it is important to identify just one individual, as once you identify this one person, she will usually know like-minded practitioners in other specialties. Identify a functional medicine practitioner, for example, who willingly collaborates with you, and he can suggest a like-minded gynecologist, gastroenterologist, or endocrinologist, should the need arise. So we tap into networks of empowering practitioners by just starting with one. (The vast majority of specialists in these fields, by the way, do not fit your bill of needs. So being able to weed through the unhelpful ones by starting with a promising referral can spare you plenty of aggravation and time.)

Empowering practitioners can be found in a number of fields, but the most productive areas to start your search include:

Functional medicine. Practitioners of functional medicine use biochemistry, physiology, and nutrition to understand health issues, and they are more likely to use nutritional or natural solutions to health. They are also more likely to draw from "integrative" or "alternative" strategies and not jump immediately to prescription drugs or procedures. Practitioners can be found from a number of backgrounds and areas of expertise, including medical doctors (MD, DO), chiropractors (DC), naturopaths (ND), nurses (RN), and nutritionists. A listing of functional medicine practitioners certified by the Institute for Functional Medicine (functionalmedicine.org) can be found by selecting the "Find a Practitioner" option on the institute's home page.

Integrative health. Like practitioners of functional medicine, integrative health practitioners are more open-minded and, as the label suggests, tend to integrate methods from various sources, including nutrition, nutritional

identify a health advocate for yourself in such situations (see "Choosing a Healthcare *Advocate*"). Make clear your intentions: You are not seeking more prescription drugs or procedures; you are hoping to reduce or eliminate reliance on conventional medical treatments and replace them with natural, empowering strategies as much as humanly possible. Over time, your reliance on the doctor and the medical system should diminish dramatically.

You may need your doctor or other healthcare provider to occasionally supplements, chiropractic, and biofeedback. The Academy of Integrative Health & Medicine (aihm.org) maintains a listing of practitioners in the United States at aihm.org/find. Practitioners include medical doctors, osteopaths, chiropractors, naturopaths, physician assistants, nurses, and psychologists.

Naturopathy. The practice of naturopathy has come a long way over the past 20 years, from a sketchy past to a modern approach in which practitioners are educated through a rigorous process and practice a natural, integrative approach that favors, but does not exclude, conventional medical care. Having spent a fair amount of time with many of its practitioners, I have developed a new respect for the scientific integrity but open-minded attitude that their training and experience cultivates. The American Association of Naturopathic Physicians maintains a listing of practitioners accessible from its Web site, naturopathic.org, by selecting "Find a Doctor" or by going directly to naturopathic.org/AF_MemberDirectory.asp?version=2. While many naturopaths are general practitioners, an increasing number of specialists are emerging, also, searchable on this directory. Naturopaths are unable to prescribe, change, or discontinue prescription drugs, but many collaborate with medical physicians to do so. One uncertainty: Many states do not yet license practitioners of naturopathy, allowing some with minimal education to declare themselves practitioners. Fully trained practitioners have an undergraduate education, a 4-year period of education and training in a college of naturopathic medicine, and a variable period of postgraduate training and are listed in the association's directory.

Chiropractic. While most chiropractors focus on musculoskeletal and neurological health, an increasing number have expanded their skills into nutrition, biochemistry, and alternative methods. Most chiropractors cannot stand alone as a sole healthcare provider, but they can be very useful advocates, as well as a starting place to tap into provider networks of like-minded practitioners. The American Chiropractic Association (acatoday.org) maintains a listing of certified practitioners under "Find a Doctor."

Undoctored U–certified practitioners. I am in the process of providing training to doctors, nurses, personal trainers, and others interested in delivering Undoctored principles to their clientele. Certified practitioners will be listed in coming years on the undoctoredhealth.com Web site.

order imaging tests you desire. Say your mom had a stroke from carotid disease at age 50. You are 47 years old and would like to know if you have inherited the same tendency and if you have already developed some degree of carotid atherosclerosis that puts you at risk for stroke, too. You therefore need a simple carotid ultrasound. Your doctor can help in obtaining the carotid ultrasound. "My mom had a stroke at age 50. Because I'm approaching the same age, I'm concerned about my own risk for stroke. I'd like to pursue a carotid ultrasound to see if I share this risk." If your doctor resists, once again, vote with your feet and find a new doctor or pursue this testing yourself; the carotid ultrasound can even be obtained in most states without a doctor's order and at a fraction of the cost.

There are also situations in which submitting to the guidance of a healthcare provider is to your advantage. Facing a carotid endarterectomy, for example, you are best following pre- and postoperative advice, provided you have done your homework to ensure the competence of the provider for that service. What that person should not be is your sole source, director, or dictator of health information for the other 95 percent of your health issues. You wouldn't consult the guy changing the oil in your car about what new car to purchase or auto insurance to buy, so don't regard anyone performing a specific service as an expert in all aspects of health—they are not.

An intelligent, informed, and empowering healthcare practitioner will also be able to recognize when natural efforts will not be successful. As powerful as these strategies can be, it would be foolish to believe that every health condition can be reduced or eliminated. I wish this weren't true, but it is. Cancer, genetically determined health conditions, lung disease from smoking, and traumatic injuries are beyond the reach of Undoctored strategies, and expecting, for instance, pancreatic cancer to reverse with these efforts is unrealistic. The Undoctored strategies will not harm you in any way, but they cannot be expected to reverse all conditions. An advocate for your health can help you decide when and how far you can go and what may not respond.

Living your life Undoctored does not mean that you should cancel your screening colonoscopy or annual gynecological exam. It means that when you see the doctor, you will be armed with better information and higher expectations and a better appreciation for what can be achieved on your own, and what cannot. Your job is not to persuade your doctor to join the 21st century and accept the new reality. Your job is to obtain the health solutions you desire by overcoming this temporary stumbling block, even if it means changing doctors. Your new health enlightenment can also help you recognize when the doctor fails to have answers, but *you* do. And to know that you are not helpless.

Echoes of Nuremberg

Unfortunately, in order to get the job done, a polite approach does not always work. There are times when you must demand that certain actions be taken. Such situations arise when you encounter outright ignorance, arbitrary or unlawful rules, or other unjustifiable behaviors. We need not be worried in our world of being experimented on or waking up minus a kidney, but we do need to be concerned that we are often denied information, access, or just a benign helping hand.

About half of all doctors are, after all, self-admitted control freaks with high expectations that you do everything they tell you to do.[4] Many firmly believe that only they know what is best for you and that you will bungle it without them, thereby denying you access to information.

For example, in online discussions a common issue crops up when someone reports feeling inappropriately cold and fatigued all the time, being unable to lose weight, and having thinning hair, symptoms that are classic for hypothyroidism, or low thyroid hormone status. (Later on in this book, I will discuss how obtaining a full thyroid evaluation is crucial.) A person reports that she did indeed have thyroid labs run, but the doctor and his staff advised her that she was not allowed to view the results, as "You wouldn't know what they mean" or "They are the property of the doctor and the clinic." This is entirely false: By law, the lab results are *your* property and the doctor and staff are operating out of ignorance. You should apprise them of this fact. If you still encounter resistance, a call to the state medical board can turn the tides, as the board can provide a brief statement that you can present to the doctor and the staff. Recent changes in regulations also allow you to obtain lab results directly from the laboratory facility itself, whether or not your doctor approves. Thanks to regulations finalized in February 2014 by the US Department of Health and Human Services that replaced a hodgepodge of uneven state-by-state rules, laboratories in all 50 states are now required to comply with your request to provide results to you without your doctor's permission or knowledge.[5] (You may need to sign a statement stating that you are indeed who you say you are, and not a nosy ex-spouse or other persona non grata, but the results are nonetheless yours to obtain.) You may need your doctor to *interpret* the results, but you no longer need your doctor to *obtain* the results. As more clinics and offices convert over to electronic reporting, you may be able to access lab results online, an excellent option with near-immediate availability of results.

You also have the right to obtain other medical records, such as results of various imaging tests (CT scans, x-rays, MRI scans, etc.), narrative results of any procedures (laparoscopy, colonoscopy, pathological studies, etc.), doctors' dictations and interpretations, and other common components of patient charts. Once again, the US Department of Health and Human

Services is clear on this: You have the right to review your health records. The health facility or doctor's office may impose a modest charge for providing the copies of your records, but the records are yours to view. To ensure privacy, a signed statement, once again, proving your identity may be necessary, but *your health records cannot be kept from you*. I stress this because I have lost count of the times people have told me that they were barred from viewing their own medical records. And, by the way, the doctor or other health personnel who tells you that you cannot view lab results or other records is not just wrong but obstructing your health. (And what is that person hiding? You may be surprised at some of the comments in patient charts.) If that health practitioner is ignorant on this important matter, how many other important health matters is he ignorant about?

Also recognize that the doctor-patient relationship is voluntary. It is not a relationship of servitude or blind obeisance. You enter into the relationship willingly but do not have to comply with anything the doctor tells you (barring exceptional situations in which you are mentally or emotionally incompetent or unable, but then you wouldn't be reading this book). It is your choice whether or not to follow any of the advice provided. Despite the doctor issuing "orders," they are not orders to you; they are only suggestions. (They are orders to hospital or office staff, but you don't work for the doctor.) An auto mechanic can help fix your car and offer her best advice, but she cannot make you accept a new transmission. Likewise, the doctor can only offer advice but has no right to make you take a drug or submit to a procedure, thanks to the legal decisions of the last century.

It would be wonderful if you could trust that your doctor or healthcare provider only provided advice that was necessary, helpful, insightful, and empowering, but such advice is, more often than not, tainted by the desire to control your behavior or steer you in the direction of procedures that yield revenue for the doctor or healthcare facility or a simple refusal to acknowledge that you can achieve plenty on your own. Don't allow yourself to be trapped in such unhelpful situations, and identify healthcare practitioners who don't treat you like you are helpless or ignorant.

Goodbye, Dr. Welby

Looking back at the world of just 30 or 40 years ago, it is astounding how much things have changed—but also how much they have stayed the same.

Forty years ago, the warm, trusting smile of Dr. Welby was all you needed. Today, modern health care is still dominated by the doctor, while the patient remains passive. It is not a partnership, nor is it a collaboration.

Think about it: We have been given nutritional advice by "official" sources in the business of dispensing dietary advice that is largely a front for Big Food. We've been told by doctors and the dietary community that nutritional supplements are a waste of money and can only supplement nutrients obtained through the awful diet advised. Because of the misguided design of the healthcare system, empowering health information is not passed on to you or your family, and you are allowed to develop health problems from neglect, such as high blood sugar, depression, reduced bone density, hypothyroidism, muscle cramps, and abnormal heart rhythms. Health problems, once manifested and brought to the attention of the doctor, are blamed on bad genes, bad luck, or *your* poor attention to health. The healthcare providers who permit such a system of blunder and neglect are the same ones we turn to for solutions when trouble develops. This bears repeating: *The healthcare providers who permit such a system of blunder and neglect are the same ones we turn to for solutions when trouble develops.* Imagine a helpless alcoholic, struggling with her addiction, ruining her social and family life, who, in desperation, turns to a bartender, hoping for some piece of wisdom since, after all, he deals with alcoholics every day and, oh yes, there is a two-shots-for-the-price-of-one sale—really not that different from an unprotected, uninformed visit to the doctor's office or hospital.

Healthcare providers who permit such a system of blunder and neglect are the same ones we turn to for solutions when trouble develops.

One important lesson from Dr. Seligman's experiments on learned helplessness was that subjects who just *knew* that control was possible improved performance—just being aware that action was possible was empowering. The first step in this newly empowered Undoctored world is to therefore *know* that you have control, to recognize that you are not helpless; your health and life are not uncontrollable and at the mercy of the system. Make these shifts in expectations and you seize the potential to change, improve, and gloriously outperform your previous helpless level of health.

The notion that you can play an active role in healthcare decision-making is new and surprising to most people. The idea that you should not only be informed but in control of your health care is the next step in the natural evolution of enlightenment and empowerment in health. This is necessary even more today than in previous years since the profit motive has come to dominate so much of modern health care and where concern for your health ends and interest in personal profit for the doctor and health-care system begin is often hard to know—Dr. Welby saddled with a hefty payment for his Maserati.

We are in the midst of a cataclysmic shift in health, a transition from the learned helplessness of traditional health care to the information- and technology-charged individual, further empowered by tectonic shifts emerging from group collaboration. The doctor still has a seat at this table, but she is just one voice among many others.

Contrary to predictions of chaos and irresponsible behavior that defenders of the healthcare status quo may deliver, you will find improved health—often astoundingly improved health—when you decide to take the reins and assign your doctor a peripheral, supportive role, not the controlling, dictatorial role that he expects. You won't find chaos; you will find unexpected and empowering success that will change your life.

In fact, once your doctor observes just how much healthier you've become with your own efforts, she should congratulate you, even thank you, because it means that the doctor can concentrate on the things that she does best, which you now know is not to deliver health but to deliver drugs and procedures for illness and maximize revenue return.

Now that I have reordered your views and opened your eyes to the real landscape of health care, not the idealized semifiction version they'd like you to see, let's now get on to the real business of undoctoring.

Chapter Summary:
Your Next Steps to Becoming Undoctored

Health care has undergone a dramatic transformation from the doctor-as-dictator and learned helplessness to the informed, empowered individual. This situation can only make your individual healthcare position even more powerful.

You will need a doctor in this new age, though one who plays a much reduced role that breaks with tradition and doctors' expectations. It is important to find one who serves as your health advocate, not an obstructionist to health. You may need to diplomatically outsmart your doctor in order to obtain the services you need. But recognize that, bottom line, doctors are humans and subject to human emotions. If the end game is health, you can indeed get the doctor—the right doctor—to help you achieve health goals.

Personal medical information is your property, and you cannot be denied access. Information is, after all, the factor that sets us free, and you need to be able to obtain the information you need to live, Undoctored. Let's begin with laying out the essential tools necessary to begin carving out a life free of the flawed and dangerous healthcare system.

PART II

What are the tools of your trade? If you no longer want to draw from the limited, individual knowledge of one doctor, no longer want to be exposed to the profit motive of modern health care, and desire a level of health that exceeds what doctors and the system can provide, what tools are necessary to navigate this new Undoctored world?

Your Black Bag of Undoctored Health Tools

Unlike doctors of the early 20th century who packed the basic tools of their craft into their iconic black bags, your "black bag" will carry an entirely different set of tools: Undoctored health tools.

Your bag will not contain a stethoscope or emetics or laxatives, and it certainly won't contain placebo tablets (as original black bags did). You won't need to go to the apothecary to have the "chemist" grind up concoctions with a mortar and pestle, nor will you carry a prescription pad to prescribe drugs. Your bag will contain the powerful new health tools of the 21st century that make the doctor's black bag look like an item on the *Antiques Roadshow*, even making your doctor look like a wrinkled relic of a time long past.

Your black bag, like the little purple handbag carried by the Harry Potter character Hermione Granger, which echoed like an airplane hangar and packed magical tents and Harry's cloak of invisibility, contains far more than any real life bag could carry. It holds the collective wisdom of millions of people, thousands of years of human experience, and access to the opinions of both experts and nonexperts, and it draws from the knowledge of hematologists, neurologists, chiropractors, naturopaths, nutritionists, practitioners of Ayurvedic medicine, biologists, toxicologists, biochemists, anthropologists, historians, engineers, computer scientists, teachers, chefs, personal trainers—any and all disciplines that offer a unique perspective, all contributing to a potential fountain of health answers. We are no longer bound by the limited knowledge of one individual or the biased agenda delivered via conventional medical care.

So what precisely is in that little black bag of yours, busting to get out and do its work? There are five categories of health tools in your bag: information, community and collaboration, nutrition, nutritional supplements, and home health tools. These are the tools that we will apply in your 6-week Undoctored program laid out in Parts II and III. Let's begin, though, with information and community and collaboration in the next chapter, followed by nutrition, nutritional supplements, and home health tools.

CHAPTER 5

You've Got Company: Information, Community, and Collaboration

The patient empowerment movement is very young and has spent the past couple of decades learning how to crawl then walk. The internet and social media has accelerated this movement far beyond anyone's expectations. It is exciting and dangerous. The patient is like a teenager with a new Ferrari and too many physicians are driving the old AMC Pacer.

—Carolyn McClanahan, MD, *Forbes* magazine

The immediacy and breadth of information exchange today makes the time-limited, one-on-one doctor-patient interaction of the last several thousand years woefully outdated. And while information is great, how do we sort through and apply all of it? As we dive into this Undoctored experience of limitless information to nonexperts, are we, in effect, allowing a bunch of hormone-jazzed teenagers to get away with speeding their parents' fancy Italian sports car down the highway, texting and beer drinking, loud friends in the backseat egging them on? Or are we empowering a new age of people with

85

REXENE IS UNDOCTORED

Franklin, Indiana

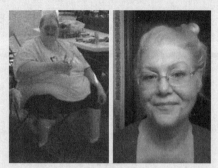

Celebrating 1 year: June 23, 2015, to June 23, 2016.

I lost a total of 106.2 pounds. That's more than 10½ ten-pound bags of potatoes, 3½ thirty-pound bags of dog food, or perhaps a fifth grader! That helps me grasp just how much that is. I was carrying around a lot with me and on my feet, my heart, etc., that in just 1 year is gone. Just doing everyday things has become so, so much easier.

In the past year, I have had no grains, no sugar, no cooked potatoes—none! It's been pretty easy. I take the supplements that Dr. Davis recommends, plus a few others.

I was hardly able to do anything that required exertion. I worked my way totally off of a beta-blocker (atenolol) that I was taking to slow my heart rate down in just 5 weeks of being grain-free. My heart rate was running between 102 to 126 beats per minute (via a 24-hour monitor) when I got put on it. Now it averages 67 beats per minute. My breathing has greatly improved. No more problems with getting short of breath from just brushing my teeth. My blood pressure was running 180/90, and now it's averaging 110/62.

I have had type 2 diabetes for over 18 years. I was able to wean myself completely off of 168 units a day of Lantus (long-acting insulin) by week 9 of being grain-free. I got completely off NovoLog (short-acting insulin). I still take

higher expectations that make the status quo in health care outdated and unnecessary, as out-of-touch as your husband's jean shorts or mom's beehive?

I'm placing my bets on the latter. Accomplishing this all on your own, however, would require you to read thousands of clinical studies, stumble through endless reams of good and bad information, and agonize over false starts and dead ends. This is why it is important to understand that you are not on your own, nor are you unequipped; you undertake this exciting journey as part of a worldwide community of people, all following the same path and outfitted with an unprecedented stockpile of tools.

Information: From Impenetrable to IMHO

Witness what has happened to healthcare information over the past half century.

metformin. That helps with insulin resistance. My blood sugar levels went from averaging 200 on all that insulin to 100 off all insulin. At 7:00 p.m. it was 89! In May 2015, my HbA1c (3-month average blood sugar) was 6.9 percent, and it was 5.7 percent this April. That's at the prediabetic level! I am working hard to reverse my diabetes entirely with very low carbs, low protein, and intermittent fasting. And I will.

I was told in 2002 I had a fatty liver after an ultrasound, and I've had quite a few elevated liver enzyme levels over the years. The CT scan in February reported no abnormalities in my liver, and all blood tests have been normal.

My irritable bowel syndrome and dysbiosis have straightened out, going from severe diarrhea six times a day (a nightmare if you leave the house) to normal bowel movements 95 percent of the time for 8 months. I had 20 years of suffering with this. No more acid reflux. No more sinus infections. I still deal with allergies (although less), but no more colds or infections. My asthma is nonsymptomatic. I do not have to use my inhaler, nebulizer, or Advair Diskus at all—none! No more night sweats either. The turkey skin on the back of my arms, there since my teens, is completely gone. They're soft and smooth! I rarely have headaches anymore. And my energy level is through the roof.

My mood also has greatly improved. I have been a longtime sufferer of anxiety and depression. I was just coming out of a severe major depression episode when I finally had the energy to start this new way of eating. I loved the energy and mood boost I got mid–second week. There are still ups and downs, but so many more good days than before.

I keep sharing all of this so I can appreciate where I've come from and perhaps give someone some hope. I have a long way to go yet, but thanks for helping me change my health around so quickly, Dr. Davis.

1960: You need health information because someone close to you has been diagnosed with a serious illness. You go to the medical library (since there's little more than children's material at the public library) and ask the librarian if you can peruse the medical books for information. She gives you a sharp look up and down, wondering if you're some kind of pervert hoping to look at pictures of naked people. She judges you as honest and grants you entry. But once you start reading the arcane lingo of medicine, much of it in Latin, you slam the books shut in frustration, not a whit better informed for the effort. Maybe your barber offers an opinion, or your uncle who survived a botched appendectomy, but it looks like you and your family member are stuck with accepting the advice of the doctor at face value, hoping for the best.

2017: You need health information because someone close to you has been diagnosed with a serious illness, or because your doctor has written prescriptions for three new medications to treat your high blood pressure, cholesterol, and anxiety based on your last 15-minute visit. You go to your computer, perform a Google search of each condition, and uncover plenty of information. You also discover social media pages, discussion forums, support groups, and data-tracking software documenting the effectiveness of various treatments. You join conversations involving several thousand people, all sharing similar issues and discussing what they have learned, how they dealt with hurdles. You begin to monitor your blood pressure and heart rate with wearable devices, track and graph your data on a smartphone app, and correlate values to situation, time, sleep quality, and nutrition. You perform finger-stick blood tests in your kitchen to track cholesterol values and blood sugar, matching diet changes to the numbers. You also find that you can read actual clinical studies, the same reports read by doctors. During your occasional few-minute interactions with your healthcare professional, you summarize the last 6 months of experience, as well as the steps you've taken to correct any unhealthy deviations. You question the need for medications, and you ask about some simple tests that might offer additional insights. Your doctor comes to understand that you are not going to allow yourself to be mindlessly directed in health care but are eager to collaborate on health issues.

It is truly breathtaking to see how far information access in virtually all areas of life has grown in the space of just one lifetime. Never before has so much information been available, so rich in actionable strategies, from shopping for the best price for a flat-screen TV to schematics to build a wind turbine. It is searchable and categorizable and can be managed and studied by anyone with access to a computer, tablet, or smartphone.

Your black bag is therefore packed with health information. It holds more information than any real physical repository, more than the holdings of the National Library of Medicine, more than all the medical school libraries in the world—certainly more than any individual primary care physician or specialist has in her brain. Access to information is no longer a hurdle, an astounding and unprecedented development in a world that previously prized information but guarded it closely.

Open access to all of this is relatively new. While you may be comfortable booking a restaurant reservation on your smartphone or sharing political views on your Facebook page, your doctor may not be entirely comfortable with your freewheeling access to so much information. After all, until recently, information was the primary factor that separated healthcare practitioners from the public. It seems comical today when we look back at how hard the medical establishment tried to control health information and keep it under wraps over the years, taking great pains to ensure that outsiders did not penetrate the walls of secrecy. Medical texts and libraries were typically off-limits to the public, both physically and in lingo and language. No other profession except the priesthood required Latin to be used in day-to-day practice: *Bis in die* (bid), *pro re nata* (prn), metropathia hemorrhagica (excessive uterine bleeding), and others are common parlance among practitioners but unintelligible to most people. Medical texts traditionally advised that the use of Latin "helps to conceal the kind of medicine being taken, and perhaps the nature of the disease being treated, from the patient himself . . . and also from other inquisitive persons."[1] Only in the last few years has there been a push to write prescriptions in modern English and mostly for safety reasons (i.e., the illegibility of doctors' handwriting), not for the sake of openness.

When guarding information was insufficient, practitioners resorted to artifice—essentially putting on a show. Many of the familiar trappings of medicine—such as the white coat, operating room garb, and stethoscope—may have real purpose but are also used to impress, intimidate, and distance the practitioner from the patient. A telling piece of history: When the nursing profession proposed that nurses should carry stethoscopes in the early 20th century, physicians were outraged that lower-level staff would presume to use the same tools. Nurses won the battle but only after conceding that they would not call their devices "stethoscopes" but "nurse-o-scopes," and they could not be black like those carried by physicians, but had to be red, pink, blue, or other colorful designs, something you see in evidence even today. Despite the tidal wave of information, the attitude of secrecy and contrivance is alive and well.

The Information Age is changing all that. Just as Toto pulled back the curtain on the wizard and revealed a humble, bumbling, common man with no real magic up his sleeve, you can now see behind the masks, white coats, and big words to understand what really goes on in health care.

While we are all now able to access the same information regardless of occupation, skin color, or dress size, we choose our information differently, by different criteria and with different aims. Unlike what presently passes for conventional healthcare information, you are interested in information unbiased by commercial interests. Much healthcare information fails miserably to satisfy this requirement. Healthcare practitioners are oddly unfazed by this fact, following drug industry–sponsored clinical trials as enthusiastically as, even more enthusiastically than, say, a trial paid for with taxpayer money through the National Institutes of Health, largely thanks to

TWO IS COMPANY, TEN'S A CROWD

Under the right circumstances, groups are remarkably intelligent, and are often smarter than the smartest people in them.

—James Surowiecki, *The Wisdom of Crowds*

Let's take Mr. Surowiecki's quote above one step further: "Groups are remarkably intelligent, and are often smarter than the smartest people in them" . . . including doctors.

Mass panic, stampedes, shoppers trampled on Black Friday—crowds in a panic or seized by anger or greed can be frightening. But what about crowds quietly contemplating a question, each individual applying his or her unique insight and experience? Can we obtain answers by harnessing the collective wisdom of crowds?

It's not an entirely new concept. A rudimentary form of crowd wisdom is already part of the legal system that assembles courtroom juries of a dozen peers. We also see crowd wisdom playing out in online sites that, for instance, allow crowds of people to rate hotels, restaurants, or movies. Would you bother seeing a movie rated 7 percent by Rotten Tomatoes?

Collect diverse insights and experiences of groups of people, all weighing in on the same question (putting aside polarizing social issues such as those in politics), and something wonderful happens: We obtain answers that, in many cases, exceed the accuracy of answers provided by individual experts—the wisdom of crowds, or collective intelligence. While the accuracy of answers improves with groups as small as three participants, groups of 10 dramatically improve accuracy, with additional improvements as crowds grow to the hundreds or thousands.[2, 3] The more the crowd allows each participant to express views, the greater the accuracy. And accuracy is also largely independent of the individual intelligence of the participants; smarter groups do not always provide smarter answers.

Mr. Surowiecki recounts the story of the West of England Fat Stock and Poultry Exhibition of 1906 in which a contest to guess the weight of an ox

a well-dressed, well-paid, and attractive sales force schooled in the manipulation of information and physicians, in addition to billions of dollars spent on advertising.

The pace and volume of health-related information, which has been growing exponentially over the past several decades, shows no signs of slowing. But the growth of published medical studies between 1978 and 2001 included a near tripling of studies funded by drug and medical device manufacturers.[4] Witness, for example, the more than $2 billion spent to "validate" was conducted. This was observed with interest by famous British scientist Francis Galton, cousin of Charles Darwin. Galton gathered the 800 written votes cast, expecting to demonstrate how bumblingly inaccurate the guesses were. While few participants individually guessed anywhere near the correct weight, when he averaged all the guesses, to his great surprise, he found that the group as a whole guessed that the ox weighed 1,197 pounds, a pound off from the real weight of 1,198 pounds. A mix of people, some uninformed and unsophisticated, collectively guessed darned close to the exact right answer, more accurate than guesses offered by ox experts.

Do we really always need experts to answer our questions for us? In the case of health care, what if the "experts" are often not really experts anyway but dispensers of outdated ideas, limited by individual abilities, reliant on flawed information sources, swayed by conflicting interests?

The online program PatientsLikeMe is a pioneer in health tracking and health empowerment. The first clinical effort to explore whether lithium carbonate was effective for treating Lou Gehrig's disease, or amyotrophic lateral sclerosis (ALS), as limited preliminary evidence suggested, did not come from a deep-pocketed drug company. It came from 150 people with ALS who collaborated through the PatientsLikeMe online site, took the recommended dose of the drug, and then tracked their experiences using an ALS symptom rating scale. They demonstrated that the drug did not have any effect on the progression of ALS symptoms, a finding later corroborated by four conventional clinical trials—formal scientific methods proved the crowdsourced answer correct.[5]

Imagine what we might achieve as we expand and apply such crowd-powered efforts to other questions in health, all facilitated in unprecedented ways by new information tools. Can we discover answers to individual health questions through group interaction? Can we derive answers that exceed the quality of answers provided by experts? I believe the answer to these questions is yes, and it returns control over many aspects of health back into individual hands and frees us from the limited wisdom of the sole practitioner.

the use of statin cholesterol drugs. You now know that nearly all of it was paid for by manufacturers of statin drugs, "research" that now dominates "consensus" guidelines and day-to-day practice.

Yes, information is exploding, but the growth of proprietary information geared toward drugs and devices is growing fastest. It means that we have a terrific wealth of information to draw from but that we need to be selective in what and how we interpret that information. We are going to choose information that empowers individual health, not lines the pockets

UNDOCTORED INFORMATION: UNBIASED, UNDISGUISED, UNVARNISHED

If you were in the market for a new car, would you rely on a TV sales pitch that shows how smart and sexy you'd be in the company's car as your sole source of information? Or the advice of a car salesman? Probably not. You would look for unbiased reviews from reliable sources, as well as feedback from people who purchased the model you're interested in. Not very sexy, but a lot smarter.

Likewise, in your exploration for health information, it is important to avoid misleading marketing and other pitfalls. First of all, view marketing or advertising as sales pitches that are unreliable; never rely on them as your sole information source. They are trying to sell you something, not provide unbiased information.

After you have dismissed all the obvious marketing being blasted your way, here are some guidelines to follow when processing all the health information you encounter.

● Whenever possible, dig for the primary source of information since news reports and Web sites (secondary or tertiary sources) commonly exaggerate or misinterpret results. For instance, if you are searching for the results of a particular study you heard about on the news, find the actual research report. The National Library of Medicine publishes medical studies on its Web site, PubMed (pubmed.gov). Though you may not fully understand the language of the entire study, the abstract summary is usually easy to understand. (Reading the entire study can be helpful, but only during a very serious effort at exploring a question.) Do this with some regularity and you will learn that what news reports say and what the science says are often two very different messages.

● Should you dive deeply into any medical study, always read the disclosures (i.e., the financial ties held by the study's authors). As you now know, if the drug or medical device industry supported the study or the investigators, be skeptical of the findings of the study and be ready to completely

of industry, a selection process that yields very different answers from those coming from conventional health care.

Open access to information is therefore crucial to the Undoctored approach to health. (Some useful and reliable starting places beyond *Undoctored* are listed in Appendix D, though there is more than enough to get you off to a powerful start just within these pages.) But even all that open access to information is insufficient by itself. The new tools available to us provide *more* than raw information. In addition to the explosion of information, another powerful new trend has emerged over the past decade, the scale of dismiss them. The findings might be true, they might be exaggerated or incomplete, or they might be completely biased and untrue—but you won't be able to tell which. Learn to *not* rely on studies funded this way, even though most doctors do.

• Identify Web sites and information (i.e., secondary) sources that you can trust. You will find over time that there are sites and authors that, time and again, are able to explain health issues clearly and process new information into useful strategies. (I list some useful starting places in Appendix D. *Undoctored* will get you off to a powerful start, but as your curiosity and experience grow, you will indeed want to expand your horizons into new sources.)

• Recognize that there are information sources that are strongly biased in favor of commercial interests and should never be relied on for information, even though the information is passed off as fact, even reviewed by doctors. If ads for prescription drugs or hospitals are featured on the Web site, avoid that site, since the information is designed to increase your consumption of prescription drugs or hospital testing, not provide health. (A very popular Web site, for instance, that begins with *Web* and ends with *MD* is one such site that you should never rely on for unbiased information.)

• If information is tied to a sales offer for a product, reject that site as an unreliable source of information. It might still be a useful source of a product but should not serve as a source for information about the value of that product. For example, if you are exploring whether the nutritional supplement ashwagandha is useful to deal with stress, don't rely on a retailer of the product telling you that this is the best solution for stress on the market. Instead, find a primary or trusted secondary source for information.

I will get you started with much of the information you require to regain or maintain health, particularly through the information and strategies provided in the Wild, Naked, and Unwashed program to come later in the book. But when health issues crop up in your life not fully answered in the Undoctored program, following the above guidelines can help keep you on track.

which was unimaginable until recently: the emergence of community and collaboration, which brings the farmer in rural South Africa or acupuncturist in Kuala Lumpur as close and accessible to you as your neighbor next door.

Community and Collaboration: Safety in Numbers

When you are stumped by something—a financial question, a moral dilemma, how to handle a lazy teenager—do you rely solely on your own personal resources to solve it, or do you turn to others for insight and guidance? If you are like most people, from time to time you seek the advice and support of others. That support can sometimes prove invaluable, the difference between disaster and finding a productive solution.

What if you could multiply the contributions of others by tens, hundreds, or thousands, spreading your net to capture insights across borders and oceans, age and occupation? There'd be plenty of "noise," but buried in that mountain of information, like the collective guess of the weight of an ox, could be priceless answers.

Prior to online search-and-find capabilities, identifying people sharing similar health interests (or any sort of interest, for that matter) was a lot tougher. If you had an uncommon condition such as sarcoidosis and wanted to talk to other people with the same condition, it would be unlikely that you would uncover anyone else with similar concerns by tapping into your circle of friends and acquaintances. At best, you might connect to a handful of people through a hospital or a local sarcoidosis support group, if one even existed in your city. More often than not, you'd rely on the limited expertise of your doctor along with the input of the inexperienced people around you who did not share your condition.

Modern information tools have changed all this. Today, linking up with hundreds or thousands of people, both nonexperts and experts, sharing an interest in your condition, and thereby sharing a deep and personal focus, takes minutes. The immediacy and scale of this resource are unprecedented.

The emergence of online communities that provide the ability to collaborate is a powerful trend that, even on its own, has the potential to transform the landscape of health care. It is a way to harness information, since raw information by itself can be unmanageable. Communities provide a way to learn and teach each other, obtain feedback, and generate new insights. Popular social media sites, such as Facebook and Twitter, as wonderful as they are for sharing experiences, have not managed to harness information in ways that can be focused on solving health questions. You can post a question about health and obtain responses, but that is really only incrementally better than polling friends, family, and acquaintances.

Discussion forums and support groups provide a more focused means to allow people with common interests but varying backgrounds, knowledge, and experiences to share ideas. All levels of discussion, from simple to complex, are entertained, though the level of discussion can reach surprising levels of sophistication. I personally helped create and monitor a forum focused on coronary disease. In a recent post, a businessman asked a question about measuring and correcting sitosterol and campesterol (counterparts of cholesterol in plants) blood levels, particularly in people with the apolipoprotein E4 gene (who absorb more of these compounds than other people), as a potential contributor to heart disease risk. Discussion ensued, with perspectives and opinions offered by a musician, housewife, airline pilot, gynecologist, and retired engineer, all trying to grasp the importance of this issue. (Here's an exercise demonstrating the powerful wisdom of crowds: Ask your primary care doctor or cardiologist the same questions being discussed by this group of everyday people and note the reaction.) Not all conversations achieve this level of sophistication, nor should they, as newcomers to the discussion need to find an easy means of joining in. So "entry level" discussions are also entertained: "What does _____ mean?" "Can anyone help me get started?" Because thousands of people see the request or comment, nobody gets ignored and conversations develop quickly, with plenty of vigorous discussion resulting.

Uncovering a support group or discussion forum is as easy as an online search requiring all of 2 seconds. Search "endometriosis forum," for example, and you will encounter the thousands of women discussing, sharing, encouraging each other in the quest for understanding and taking command of their condition.

It's not just about the numbers of people involved; new ways to rank information are emerging, such that members of a community can vote or "weigh" the value of information so that participants can view a built-in value factor. You can readily see the usefulness of such value factors in non-health Web sites such as TripAdvisor (tripadvisor.com) for rating hotels or Angie's List (angieslist.com) for rating home contractors. The same rating methods can be applied to health questions with results even more impressive than a satisfying experience with a plumber. PatientsLikeMe (patientslikeme.com), originally conceived as a means of helping people with neurodegenerative disease share experiences (founded by James and Ben Heywood, whose brother was diagnosed with Lou Gehrig's disease or amyotrophic lateral sclerosis, ALS), has pioneered data collection methods for its members, now numbering over 400,000. People share diagnoses and symptoms and rate treatment successes and failures, all of which are graphically displayed for others to view (if permitted by the individual). If you share your diagnosis of, say, multiple sclerosis, you will be able to connect to people experiencing the same condition, participate in discussions, view experience with various treatments, see what worked over what time period, and obtain feedback, all within moments.

CureTogether (curetogether.com) provides a similar experience over nearly 700 health conditions, prompting users to enter diagnoses, symptoms, and treatments attempted and rate level of success or failure. The site's founders hope to extract therapeutic lessons as their data collection grows. They recently reported that among the 800 people seeking solutions for arthritis pain, massage and low-dose naltrexone (an opiate-blocking drug that is not part of conventional treatment for arthritis) were among the most effective for pain relief. Crowdsourcing identifies strategies that work, whether or not they are revenue generating for health care. CureTogether has research collaborations under way with investigators at Stanford, the Massachusetts Institute of Technology, and the University of California, Davis; even conventional institutions are beginning to recognize the answer-seeking power of the crowd.

In a blend of crowdsourcing involving semi-like-minded experts, mostly physicians, called CrowdMed (crowdmed.com), founder Jared Heyman, motivated by his sister's struggle to obtain a diagnosis for unexplained symptoms, developed a platform that allows people to submit their medical information, which is then reviewed by hundreds of volunteer physicians from a variety of disciplines. Over 1,000 participants, sick for an average of 8 years, having consulted with eight doctors without answers, with more than $50,000 in medical expenses, obtained diagnoses through this service. CrowdMed is yielding lessons in how to extract wisdom from an expert crowd, so it has only limited application to our situation in which we desire answers that better empower our day-to-day health concerns, not necessarily elusive diagnoses. Nonetheless, the CrowdMed phenomenon adds another interesting dimension to the landscape of self-empowerment.

People in business, academia, and elsewhere are catching on. The Institute for the Future (iftf.org) is a charitable organization devoted to charting coming disruptive changes in health care. It is working to catalyze the connected, collaborative online world into a focused tool to answer health questions. The organization predicts a shift to consumer-driven health, "the well-being economy," referring to the increasing shift away from hospitals and doctors offices and into homes and workplaces, empowered by direct-to-consumer tools and innovative self-monitoring gadgetry.

You may find the collaborative community of the Undoctored program itself (undoctoredhealth.com) helpful, a place where you can discuss, share, and learn along with thousands of other people, all of whom share the common goal of gaining and maintaining health by opting out of conventional health care as much as possible. And as I mentioned earlier, I invite you to

I'LL SHOW YOU MINE IF YOU SHOW ME YOURS

Tit for tat, an eye for an eye, you scratch my back—it's all about sharing.

Many health Web sites permit, even encourage, users to enter, display, and view health data. Users can enter simple measures such as age, blood pressure, blood sugar, or body weight. They can also enter more elaborate data, such as cholesterol values, hemoglobin A1c, or vitamin D blood levels. Symptoms, such as abdominal discomfort or fatigue, can be rated and tracked.

Privacy is not generally an issue as users can choose to use nicknames (a continual source of amusement, many very creative), and they can also choose whether or not to make their data public or keep the data private. Choose a name, no matter how wacky or tacky, take on whatever persona you desire, but share your data and maintain your privacy behind it. No one will know that MacnCheezToGo is really a 48-year-old accountant from Houston, even when you engage in intimate conversations about prostate health.

Most people learn over time that willingness to share data facilitates the experience, as you are able to view the data of others and they can view yours. This allows others to see your blood sugar or thyroid values, for instance, and offer insight into what the numbers mean and what you can do to improve them. You, likewise, can offer the advantage of your unique insight and experience to others, all of whom are eager to hear what you've got to say. You are not being paid to say anything, and you won't drive a Mercedes-Benz because of your participation; you participate because you contribute to personal and collective success.

Site organizers on PatientsLikeMe, for example, encourage users to enter and share their health data, emphasizing how it is essential for everyone to learn: "All that data helps you track how you're doing over time, helps the next person diagnosed learn what could work for them, and tells researchers what people really need so they can develop more effective treatments, faster." They are then able to analyze data collectively, leading, for instance, to improved management of epileptic seizures.[6] It's no longer about privacy; it's about helping cultivate a place where learning, teaching, and sharing are defining themes.

And it's also all about getting better answers involving no high-ticket healthcare insurance or medical procedures, all while keeping your clothes on.

share your health information anonymously so that we can track the results of your Undoctored experience; these discussions are not just idle speculation but a genuine effort to change the world of health care at a very personal level. The first few hundred experiences may not yield much, but imagine what will happen when we assess the experiences of hundreds of thousands of people, add new lessons learned, and add new protocols for other conditions; doctors and hospitals will increasingly be marginalized into the roles they perform best: to provide acute and catastrophic care.

We are shifting from a time when one or a few presumed experts try to provide answers to a time when many more people—from varied backgrounds: scientific, business, educational, or just life, all across the map of experiences—make contributions. It means that the seat of control over health decisions is being taken out of the doctor's office and hospital and being transplanted to your home while you sip coffee or a glass of wine—no waiting room, no scalpels, no crippling medical bills to worry about.

A Clean Slate of Health

As exciting as these new and innovative collaborative Web sites and programs are, with the Undoctored approach, you are going to experience real answers right now.

The Undoctored approach flips the way we think about disease and health on its head. Rather than starting with a health condition such as endometriosis or acid reflux, and then trying to explore treatments via discussion forums or crowdsourced wisdom, we flip-flop the process by *restoring overall health first*. Because virtually everyone's health has been disrupted by factors such as diet, weight gain, industrial chemicals, nutritional deficiencies, and inflammation, we all follow the same starting program to reverse these effects. Head-to-toe restoration of health helps you feel better and lose weight faster, and it reverses numerous health conditions without agonizing over the details, essentially wiping the slate clean and allowing you to start over. Engage in the topsy-turvy, put-the-solution-first Undoctored effort, and *the majority of health conditions recede or disappear completely*. This explains a big part of the reason why we can accomplish so much without the involvement of the doctor. Then, and only then, is it necessary to tackle specific health issues that persist and tap into the wealth of new information and collaboration tools—a much simpler way to become healthier overall, an approach that won't leave you floundering in the details.

The reason this approach works so wonderfully well is that the same efforts that reverse type 2 diabetes also reverse high blood pressure and high cholesterol and triglycerides levels, achieve dramatic weight loss, reverse joint pain and inflammation, and provide relief from acid reflux and constipation within days of starting. The same efforts that yield weight loss also provide relief from migraine headaches, skin rashes like eczema and sebor-rhea, irritable bowel syndrome, fatigue and fibromyalgia, even infertility. The Undoctored strategies also share powerful *synergies*, meaning that the combination is far more powerful than any one component. Each component of the program provides limited health benefits, but put all the Undoc-tored strategies to work at the same time, and a powerful combined effect emerges. Leave just one strategy out or cherry-pick strategies and your results will suffer; you must do them *all* to experience the full synergistic benefit. It means that by engaging in the full program, even if you begin with five health conditions and seven prescription drugs, you may find your-self, within a relatively short period of time, with *no* health conditions and *no* prescription drugs. Obviously, some "scars" of the misguided intentions of the healthcare system cannot be undone, such as having said goodbye to your gallbladder due to gallstones or your thyroid gland removed due to nodules (or for no reason at all) or a prosthetic knee or hip put in place of the real thing. But you can, at the very least, reverse the factors that led you down these paths in the first place and help avert any future health catastro-phes of the sort celebrated by the healthcare system.

It also means that the collaborative conversations that ensue with the Undoctored approach are going to be very different than the ones in pro-grams that search for patterns in disease or quantify collective responses. Rather than begin with questions, we begin with answers, starting with the structured program that everyone follows that I call Wild, Naked, and Unwashed. I then invite you to join discussions, both Undoctored and oth-erwise, to build on the foundation of health you have created and to use the home health tools available to address any residual health issues, as well as to continue to learn new lessons as our crowdsourced wisdom grows.

Blow the Doors Off

So start your engines, put the pedal to the metal in your new informational Ferrari, ignore signs warning yield or danger, and pass the doctor hobbling along in the slow lane in his rust heap. Life in this health fast lane comes equipped with a bag filled to bursting with a lot more than the sad black bag sitting in the doctor's AMC Pacer. You'll pass him in a blur.

To appreciate how far we have come, imagine a world in which the tools for obtaining information or enlisting the help of others are no longer acces-sible and, instead, you are trapped by the limited knowledge of the handful of people around you: Welcome to all of human history—except for the last few years. We now have an unprecedented opportunity to disrupt the system at breakneck speed.

Let's now go on to the three other components of the Undoctored experience: nutrition, nutritional supplements, and home health tools.

Chapter Summary:
Your Next Steps to Becoming Undoctored

Just as technology and the Information Age wiped out entire industries and transformed the way we shop, travel, learn, and converse, they will also bring the same sorts of disruptive changes to health. Wide access to information and the ability to collaborate makes numerous aspects of conventional health care obsolete while putting the individual at the center. It is therefore crucial that you reject the standard rules of health care and adopt an entirely new way of viewing and engaging health information.

The result: dramatically improved health without the doctor.

CHAPTER 6

A Return to Our Grainless Roots

There is definitely life after oat bran. All our nation has to show after years of that is diarrhea.

—Julia Child

W
e must all eat. Failure to eat, like not breathing, is eventually fatal. You might be picky, you might indulge specific tastes like kosher garlic pickles, but in the end, you have no alternative but to consume things to stay alive. Choice is therefore everything. And wrong choices can result in far worse than diarrhea.

Garbage in, garbage out. Poor choices in food have the potential to cripple health, whether in the form of hemorrhoids or ulcerative colitis. As you will see, many, if not most, of the health conditions that make us reliant on the healthcare system are caused by the foods we choose to eat, many of them chosen because we were advised to choose them or because those choices were made available to us. It may have been your doctor, dietitian, or the barrage of information from media, but it is likely—no, certain—that you were given nutritional information that damaged your health. Conversely, smart choices in food empower health and avert hundreds of health conditions. Food is more powerful than any nutritional supplement, any form of exercise, any prescription drug—nothing matches the power of the choices you make in food. I've seen it play out many hundreds of thousands of times, and the science bears it out.

You are not a horse, a lemur, or a tadpole. We walk on two feet, don't generally hang from trees, and spend 9 months inside our mother's uterus rather than as an egg deposited on a rock. As a species, we have unique nutritional needs. Our needs differ from a cat (an obligatory carnivore), a goat (a grazing herbivore), a woodpecker (an insectivore), or an oyster (a plankton-feeder). If we were to feed a cat an entirely grain-based diet, it would become ill, then die. If we fed a horse a diet of insects or plankton, we'd have a very unhappy, hungry, unhealthy, and eventually dead horse. If we tried to feed an oyster a medium-rare cut of filet mignon, it would have no way to deal with it, nor would it even recognize the steak as food. You get the idea: All species have unique nutritional needs to which they have adapted over millions of years of evolutionary history. We cannot rewrite the history of a species, we cannot change its unique collection of nutritional adaptations, and doing so can have fatal consequences.

This third item in your black bag, nutrition, or what I call eating "Wild, Naked, and Unwashed" because we return to a style of eating that humans followed before civilization got much of it wrong, will serve as an indispensable cornerstone of your effort. Even if you think you know a thing or two about nutrition, I urge you to read on, as I am going to throw many conventional ideas out the window along with other woefully outdated concepts, like treating hysteria with bed rest or "everything in moderation." This chapter and the next will grind through a lot of detail, but know that as you come to understand these ideas, you are being given the ticket to opt out of much of health care.

Nutritional advice is handed down to us through vehicles such as the USDA food pyramid or food plate, styles of eating that might get you a nice deal on an early grave, or at least accelerate your need for healthcare services. Given the void in effective nutritional advice created by blundering, disease-causing "official" agencies, there has been no shortage of diets and theories to fill that void and articulate ways to construct a healthy diet. (Ever hear anyone claim, "Wow! I followed the USDA food pyramid and incredible things happened!"?) There are advocates for just about every style of eating imaginable, from a 100 percent fruit diet to complete avoidance of animal products to a completely raw carnivorous diet. There are also people who tattoo every square inch of skin surface on their bodies and inhale various substances up their noses to escape reality.

At first, you may view some of the dietary strategies in *Undoctored* as extreme. But you will learn that it's not the Undoctored eating strategies that are extreme; it's modern eating habits that are the extreme: extremely counter to our evolutionary past, extremely adrift from the realities of human physiology, extremely illogical, extremely unhealthy. You will begin to appreciate how far off course modern dietary habits have wandered as we dive deeper into this way of thinking. It will also begin to make sense why returning to the way humans were supposed to be eating all along reverses an impressive list of health conditions. And I'm only kidding about the "naked" and "unwashed" part; go ahead, feel free to shower and put on some pants.

Don't get too bogged down in the details here, as I will eventually deliver the arguments in this chapter and the next one, distilled down to a step-by-step, blow-by-blow program to get you going. I provide these two chapters to reassure you that these are not crazy, arbitrary, anecdotal, nonscientific arguments. There is a detailed rationale backed up by extensive science underlying the Undoctored nutritional approach, though it requires an interpretation of the science that is different from what you will hear from your friendly neighborhood dietitian or primary care doctor or what you will find in some pyramid or plate. But therein lies the key to extraordinary health success.

I challenge the notion that we can improve on the millions of years of adaptation programmed into our bodies. Can we improve on the quality of grass and forage a horse eats or the microscopic creatures filtered by oysters and make them super horses or super oysters? Given current knowledge, we cannot. The best we can do is recognize the dietary needs to which a species is adapted, meet those needs, and allow functioning and health unimpaired by dietary misadventures. Feed a horse the wild forage and grass it needs, and it can thrive, run at high speeds, cavort with other horses, and reproduce. Allow a woodpecker to find insects and grubs, and the occasional fruit and tree sap while pecking his nest, and he will thrive for a lifetime and create more woodpeckers.

I stress the difficulty in improving on nature's design because, over the years, we have all encountered dietary styles or nutritional supplement programs that purport to outdo what nature alone would provide through food. I've heard it argued, for instance, that we would all do better by taking megadoses of digestive enzymes to better extract nutrients in foods. Well, there may be a germ of truth in this notion if you've developed an impaired digestive process. What if we instead take some simple steps to allow our bodies to recover their natural digestive capacities and extract the thiamine, riboflavin, niacin, B_{12}, flavonoids, fats, proteins, and other nutrients effectively without the need for cartons of digestive enzymes; humans have done so for millions of years quite successfully. Humans who live traditional lives with no access to such enzymes enjoy wonderfully natural digestion and full nutrition without the range of gastrointestinal and inflammatory struggles of modern people.[1] Loading the digestive tract with large quantities of enzymes to improve on human digestion would be like arguing that topping up the gas tank in your car will make it go faster: it does not, of course. You cannot push the process by adding more. Rather than try and overcome poor digestive processes, shouldn't we identify the cause of incomplete digestion, correct it, and then enjoy proper digestion without supplements?

The modern diet, with its unrestrained excess and perverse indulgence of innate impulses such as the desire for sweet, compounded by pseudoscience and misinterpretation, underlies an astounding number of modern health problems, what are labeled "diseases of civilization," diseases that are virtually unknown in primitive societies following traditional diets.

We can put such insights to work. If we re-create the diet of traditional societies as much as possible in modern settings, we can dramatically reduce risk for the long list of familiar diseases of civilization. Like a cat returning to its carnivorous needs or an oyster happily filtering plankton or a human pushing the oat bran aside, when we revert to the foods to which humans have adapted for as long as we have walked the earth upright, we also rid ourselves of all the diseases acquired from the mistakes made by our species. It's as simple as that.

DAWN IS UNDOCTORED

Akron, Ohio

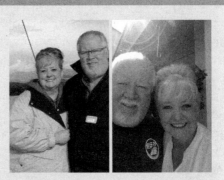

I have always been addicted to breads, crackers, sweets, and potatoes and thought there was no way I could ever give them up for good.

My skin cleared up; the puffiness in my face went away; my headaches, joint pain, and indigestion have disappeared. I no longer have any trouble saying no to all of those things I thought I could never give up. I have lost 29 pounds so far, and my husband has lost 37 pounds. The iodine and Magnesium Water have been two of my favorite strategies. But, best of all, I got my husband to join me in this way of eating, and he totally reversed his diabetes and is on no medications or insulin. His doctor is flabbergasted.

I can't say enough about how this has changed or, even more accurately, has saved our lives.

Wipe Off the Makeup, Lose the Cell Phone—What's Left?

If we were to strip you of your eyeliner and lipstick, wristwatch and class ring, SUV, and GPS-equipped smartphone, what would we have? More than a tree-hugging modern-day hippie: I'd say we have a human with needs unique to its species, nothing more and nothing less. You may view yourself as distinctively modern with fake nails and an American Express card, but your physical needs are virtually identical to the Hadza woman in East Africa carrying an infant while digging in the soil to harvest wild tubers or the Gabi-Gabi native Australian clothed in wallaby skin and hunting in the brush for marsupials for lunch. Don't let your thinking get lost in the clutter.

If modern lifestyles are to blame, what do people who do not follow modern lifestyles look like? And what is their health like?

We've known this for over a century: People living primitive lifestyles in the absence of modern food enjoy extraordinary health. So-called diseases of civilization—diabetes, overweight and obesity, much psychiatric illness, autoimmune diseases, heart disease, colon cancer, constipation, even common skin conditions like acne and skin rashes—are virtually unknown in primitive societies following traditional diets.[2, 3] That's not just the pronouncement of some primitive medicine man but the observations of sociologists, anthropologists, physicians, and other scientists who have studied the health of such populations. The Aché of Paraguay, the Hadza of Tanzania, the Kitavan of Papua New Guinea, the tribes of the Xingu rainforest of Brazil, the Maori of New Zealand, native North Americans, and others—all living in their unique habitats, hunting animals and gathering plants and roots, living the life that humans lived for the past 2.5 million years—have almost none of the conditions we see every day all around us. You will see no deformities from rheumatoid arthritis, no constipation or irritable bowel syndrome, and none of the obvious behavioral peculiarities of schizophrenia, and you will be struck by their slenderness despite having plenty of food—BMIs (body mass indexes) of 20 are the rule. (The average BMI of an American: 26.5, with a growing proportion in the obese range of 30 and higher; we are among the most overweight population in the history of humans on earth.) Blood pressures are normal, heart disease is unknown, cancer a rarity. They have nearly perfect teeth despite having no toothbrushes, fluoridated toothpaste, fluoridated water, dental floss, or dentists. They have no acne without acne creams or scrubs. They have no constipation without loading up on fiber cereal, bran muffins, or stool softeners.

They are slender without limiting calories, restricting fat, or adding another move to their CrossFit routine. They have normal blood pressures without worrying about salt or taking blood pressure medication. They have no acid reflux or the bloating and diarrhea of irritable bowel syndrome without taking acid-blocking or antispasmodic drugs. They have no heart disease despite not taking statin cholesterol drugs or aspirin. And this level of health continues even when they live into their fifth decade, sixth decade, and onward.

A day in the life of a primitive human male, without the USDA or dietitian to guide him, consists of rising to start the day and setting out for the hunt with crude weapons, while females take their young and forage for berries and other fruit, dig in the dirt for roots and tubers with a bone fragment or stick, and grab the odd bird egg or edible leaves, stems, or mushrooms. When the hunters return from a hunt, if successful, they tear the flesh with their primitive stone tools, consuming the organs—every organ, every morsel from snout to tail—and then the meat with gusto.

We ate animal organs and meats raw for much of human history until we understood how to tame fire, at which point we obtained the increased digestive efficiency of cooking our food. (Cooking is part of the human experience and has been so for at least several hundred thousand years, likely longer.) We didn't bat an eye over intake of cholesterol, saturated fat, or calories but ate to our stomach's content, or as much as our share, divided among the others in the clan, allowed. Nobody talked about moderation, limiting portion size, or fat grams; nobody drank protein shakes or ate "superfoods"; yet nobody was obese, no one had diabetes, all had intact teeth, not a penny was spent on prescription drugs, and no dietitians blathered on about restraint.

Primitive populations, living the same lifestyle as our ancestors dating back thousands of generations, may suffer injuries such as breaking a leg tumbling down a rock or infections such as malaria and dengue fever, but not the diseases that plague us. When hunter-gatherers are exposed to modern foods, they develop the diseases of civilization at explosive rates—even faster and more severely than we do, explaining why, for instance, Pima Indians of the American Southwest have the highest proportion of people with diabetes in North America and why formerly slender, healthy South American rainforest dwellers now suffer epidemic levels of obesity, diabetes, depression, and suicide and now need modern medical care. The people of the Xingu rainforest; the Maasai of eastern Africa; the Samburu of Kenya; the Fulani of Nigeria; and the people of the Cook Islands, Tonga, and

Tokelau show flagrant obesity, diabetes, tooth decay, gastrointestinal problems, and hypertension when exposed to Western foods, even while living outdoors and otherwise conducting their lives in traditional ways—all effects of diet, not a change in scenery.[4, 5, 6, 7, 8]

It's as if we've had a "control" group of people living the traditional way humans have lived for as long as our species has walked this planet, with modern people representing the "treatment" group with a "treatment" (modern diet) that has failed miserably. In other words, consuming a Western diets of grains, sugars, and other processed ingredients means that all the diseases we have come to view as unlucky, genetically determined, and everyday phenomena are really products of modern food and lifestyles.

This plays in reverse, as well. Kerin O'Dea, professor of nutrition and public health in the health sciences division of the University of South Australia in Adelaide, asked 10 diabetic, overweight Aboriginal individuals living Western lifestyles to move back to the wild and resume their previous lifestyle of hunting kangaroo, catching wild fish, and digging for underground roots. They began with blood sugars of 209 mg/dL (average), high triglycerides of 357 mg/dL, and high insulin levels. After 7 weeks of living their traditional lifestyle, the 10 Aboriginal natives lost an average of 17.6 pounds, dropped blood glucose to 119 mg/dL, and decreased triglycerides to 106 mg/dL; 5 of the 10 no longer had type 2 diabetes.[9]

Over and over again, we witness this effect: People living traditional lives without agriculture suffer almost no modern diseases. When "Western" foods are added, a long list of chronic health conditions emerge at explosive rates. Go ahead: Apply your eyeliner, Tweet your dinner plans, navigate your next trip on GPS. But eat the foods added recently to the human experience and you will be making an appointment with a doctor who will be eager to write prescriptions and sign you up for the next hospital procedure. There's nothing wrong with the wristwatch or phone, but let's explore your inner untamed human and . . .

Go Put on Your Best Loincloth

Elk skin, beaver skin, or leopard patterned, we can put these crucial insights to work. The diet that dramatically reduces risk of modern disease re-creates the diet of traditional societies predating the appearance of recent man-made additions like breakfast cereals and soft drinks. After all, beneath your yoga outfit, without your hybrid automobile and modern home, you are a primitive, unwashed, hungry member of the species *Homo sapiens* whose nutritional expectations are really no different than our wild predecessors.

In the Undoctored dietary approach, the culprits behind modern disease—grains, sugar, corn syrup, processed foods, food colorings, emulsifying agents, hexane-extracted oils—are eliminated. With their elimination and a focus on real foods such as fats, meats, organs, eggs, vegetables, roots, mushrooms, and select fruits and nuts, appetite diminishes to that reflecting physiologic need, blood sugar and blood pressure plummet, cholesterol (total and LDL) drops like a stone, excess abdominal fat evaporates, acid reflux and irritable bowel syndrome are gone within days, autoimmune conditions retreat, fatigue and depression lift, and skin rashes clear; you mimic the healthy, vigorous physiology of a wild member of the Hadza, Maori, or Yawalapiti people, minus the leg gash received by stumbling across a crocodile or malnutrition from an intestinal worm. And not only are outward signs of disease reversed, but many concealed disease triggers are corrected, as well, such as small LDL particles (the number-one cause for heart disease), the initiating steps of autoimmunity, and abnormal inflammatory processes that lead to cancer, diabetes, heart disease, and dementia. And you will start asking new questions: Rather than asking why you have so many health problems and can't lose weight, you will be asking questions like, "Am I too skinny?" or "I wonder if I need this anti-inflammatory drug or antidepressant any longer now that I feel so good?"

In fact, nutrition provides such a powerful foundation that by *not* following this program, you simply cannot expect to enjoy the full benefits of an Undoctored life. Grain elimination, in particular, needs to be a 100 percent effort, as just modest or occasional quantities trigger long-term, persistent effects: inflammation that can last for days to weeks, autoimmune responses that can go on for months or years, formation of small LDL particles causing heart disease risk that is cumulative, and appetite stimulation for several days, enough to add at least several pounds of weight—just from a single "indulgence." Indulge once per week, or have one off-program meal per week on a "bad" day, and you will have to contend with retriggering, for example, changes in bowel flora and increased intestinal permeability, both of which underlie autoimmune inflammation. The metabolic disruptions introduced by unnatural foods that we are not adapted to are really that bad. Just as there are no half-pregnancies or part-time criminals, there is no halfway, most-of-the-way, or 6-days-out-of-7 in this grain-free lifestyle.

We will, of course, not precisely re-create a primitive diet, since you don't want to spear an elk or drive an ax through the head of a wild boar. We will also factor in a few newer dietary experiences that have emerged along human history that are benign, even healthy, though not found in primitive cultures, such as modest intakes of alcoholic beverages, coffee, domesticated fruit, and harmless natural sweeteners.

The end result: a diet that is rich and varied but based largely on real, whole foods that would be as familiar to your great-, great-, great-, great-, great-grandmother as they are to you, minus all the cellophane-wrapped, just-add-water, order-at-the-drive-thru-window, low-fat or nonfat, pop-the-top sorts of foods that have filled our diet these last 50 years. While adopting this lifestyle means preparing more foods than the typical family, shopping differently, and being acutely aware of ingredients, it is also a big part of your effort to Undoctor your life.

Domestication and Agriculture: The Pushmi-Pullyu of 300 Generations

I can walk with the animals, talk with the animals, grunt and squeak and squawk with the animals, and they can squeak and squawk and speak and talk to me!

—Dr. Dolittle

Dr. Dolittle, in singing about the wonder of communicating with animals, left one thing out: "I can also share their diseases."

For over 99 percent of human time on earth, our species hunted animals using rocks, spears, throwing devices, stone axes, and bows and arrows. Aside from dogs being domesticated around 33,000 years ago, animals were prey or predator, not members of a household, not walking tame around the yard.

While primitive humans targeted the weak, injured, or young in a group of potential prey, the intensity of hunger often dictated how much risk a group of hunters was willing to take with their hunt, a dangerous undertaking, especially with large game such as elk, zebra, or mammoth. But 300 generations ago, our relationship to animals changed. While hunting continued, we also learned that selected species of mostly herbivorous (plant-eating and thereby posing no predatory risk to humans) creatures could be domesticated—corralled, herded, allowed to graze, and then used for food. The process of domestication, over time, changed the appearance of these herbivorous creatures, making, for instance, cows smaller and tamer than their wild auroch ancestors.

Domestication had its pluses, but it also came with some distinct and costly minuses. Domestication of herbivorous creatures made gathering and hunting less important, continual nomadic wandering for richer lands less necessary. This provided the impetus for humans to abandon nomadic lifestyles in exchange for a stationary life, staying put in one area to grow crops and keep animals, the beginnings of villages and cities. But unanticipated effects from our relationship with domesticated animals developed: We acquired many of their diseases.

Domesticating creatures often meant living in close quarters with them. It was not uncommon that you and your family slept in one corner of your adobe hut or cave while your animals slept in the other. This was the birth of an impressive collection of familiar diseases, such as smallpox, tuberculosis, measles, influenza, and anthrax, a list of diseases called zoonoses, diseases passed to us through animals. The Centers for Disease Control and Prevention estimates that 60 percent of all human pathogens originated from animals.[10]

Collectively, zoonoses altered the course of human history. Tuberculosis alone, for example, originally a disease among cows, caused the deaths of Anton Chekhov, Frederic Chopin, President Andrew Jackson, Eleanor Roosevelt, and millions of others around the world. Smallpox first appeared almost immediately with livestock domestication, detected even in Egyptian mummies, and has killed millions of people over the years, as many as 500 million during the early 20th century alone. Zoonoses, by the way, also account for the devastation experienced when members of Western culture encounter primitive cultures without domesticated animals and agriculture. Populations such as native Americans, Amazonian rainforest dwellers, and native Africans succumbed far more frequently to the zoonoses we passed on to them than to guns and swords (since, as with grain consumption, they lacked the partial protection Westerners and Asians have acquired over 10,000 years).

Thankfully, there's no extra room in your nice three-bedroom suburban home or sleek urban condo for goats, and contracting anthrax or tuberculosis from livestock is no longer a concern. But we are left with the legacy of this practice. Ironically, while modern medicine has been quite effective in dealing with zoonotic diseases—flu vaccines for influenza, antitubercular drugs for tuberculosis, a vaccine eradicating smallpox—we are still left with the practice of consuming domesticated livestock, an otherwise fairly benign nutritional means of mimicking our hunting past. While there is nothing wrong with growing, rather than picking, berries or buying modern cabbage and spinach instead of their wild counterparts, the expansion of the roles of grains (i.e., the seeds of grasses) in the human diet in particular has not only persisted but expanded to an unprecedented degree, now providing 70 percent of all human calories.[11] Let's tackle this issue next.

Let Them Eat Grass

There's another dimension to this close relationship with ruminants, creatures that graze on grasses and forage low-lying plants reachable by mouth. Ruminants have no interest in rabbits or mice, nor do they chase birds. They obtain 100 percent of their nutritional needs by grazing because they have evolutionary adaptations that include specialized teeth that grow continuously (compared to yours that grew twice, the last prior to your high-school prom), a four-compartment stomach (you have one), a spiral colon (yours takes only two 90-degree turns), and unique microorganisms (different from those you have) in their intestinal tracts suited to breaking down grasses—none of which humans have.

At about the same time we domesticated animals, geologists tell us that there was a period of natural global warming that caused food to fall into short supply. Observing the grazing behavior of their domesticated ruminants, humans were likely inspired to ask, "Can we eat grass, too?" You already know the answer: Humans cannot consume grasses of the earth and did not do so for the preceding millions of years—but that did not stop clever humans from trying. Just as we cannot save lawn clippings to sprinkle on top of a salad with a little French dressing, we found out the hard way that the roots, leaves, stalks, and husks of grasses are tasteless, inedible, and wreak gastrointestinal havoc like nausea, abdominal pain, diarrhea, or passing through the gastrointestinal tract undigested, if not promptly vomited up. But desperate humans discovered that they could consume the *seeds* of grasses, but only if separated from the husk, dried, pulverized with stones, and then heated with water and consumed as porridge. Several thousand years later, Egyptians figured out how to ferment grains into beer, and then used the beer to make leavened bread. Thus was born the reliance of humans on grains, the seeds of grasses that despite their ingestibility, remain largely indigestible, underlying many health problems resulting from their consumption.

Agriculture and animal domestication abruptly changed human health. In addition to zoonoses, there was an explosion of tooth decay and oral abscess formation, changes in the microorganisms of the mouth and colon, shrinkage of the maxillary bone and mandible resulting in crooked teeth, iron deficiency, and reduction in bone length and diameter resulting in reduced height (5 inches in males, 3 inches in females).[12, 13, 14, 15, 16] What foods were introduced into the human diet by these two innovations of agriculture and animal domestication? Growing vegetables and fruits was not new, of course, nor was consumption of foods from butchered domesticated livestock, little different from those obtained from wild sources. The big changes were that humans learned to cultivate and harvest seeds of grasses, or grains, and consume the products of the mammary glands of animals such as cows and goats (i.e., dairy products). No human 100,000 years ago thought to consume the seeds of grasses for food or approach an auroch to squeeze its mammary glands for its milk. But these two foods became commonplace with the recent innovations of agriculture and animal domestication.

Life would be very different had we not begun to domesticate animals and farm the land. Civilization with cities, transportation, and technology blossomed over centuries from these two innovations; we can only imagine what life would have been like without them.

But I am proposing that we recognize that 300 generations or 10,000 years ago marked the time of a dramatic shift in human eating and living behavior due to the practice of agriculture and domesticating livestock. Both represent departures from a lifestyle that defined human life for the preceding 99 percent of human existence. It also marked the time of a dramatic shift in human disease: The diseases acquired when we learned to grow grains and kept close quarters with domesticated animals. We no longer, of course, share our huts or caves with goats, but we do carry on this practice of consuming grains, the seeds of grasses, and consuming the products of bovine mammary glands. Because we are mammals that drink the milk of our human mothers for our first few years, consuming the product of bovine mammary glands was not entirely unfamiliar, but just a bit different (in protein structure, etc.). But grains represent the most extreme departure from foods that humans eat instinctively. We traded calories, in effect, for deterioration of long-term health. But understand these simple anthropological facts and you have nutritional insight of astonishing power in your hands, so powerful that it allows you to opt out of much of health care—loincloth optional.

Let's now drill down to some of the details behind this lifestyle, starting with my favorite food to bust, grains. Taking a cue from the movie classic *Ghostbusters*: "If there's something weird and it don't look good, who you gonna call?" Grainbusters!

Grainbusters

Maybe you're not afraid of ghosts, but you ought to be terrified by grains.

As you now know, grains were added to the human diet in the relatively recent past. But what precisely can be found in grains that make them such extravagant triggers for human disease? (This section, by the way, is the basis for the Wheat Belly series of books; if you have read the books, then this section is optional reading for you. If you have not read them, read on, as I shall clear up several misconceptions, including the idea that this lifestyle is "gluten-free.")

First of all, the grains of today are not the grains of biblical or prebiblical times, not the grains of medieval times, not even the same grains that your grandmother used to bake cookies. While grains have wrought destructive effects on humans for the 10,000 years we have consumed them, many of the effects have been made substantially worse as geneticists and agribusiness got into the act and genetically changed them. They did not change them for evil purpose, but for agricultural goals such as increased yield per acre or resistance to pests. But the changes have been so extensive that along with the changes in yield and pest resistance, they exert effects on humans consuming them.

Wheat and corn, the two most widely grown and consumed grains in the world, have been extensively changed over the past 50 years by agribusiness. Modern wheat, for instance, looks different: shorter, thicker shaft, larger seeds. The reduction in height—making modern wheat, labeled "semi-dwarf," stand 18 inches tall (not the 4½-foot-tall traditional plant we all remember)—is due to mutations in Rh (reduced height) genes that code for stalk length. That's just one mutation among hundreds of others.[17] The changes introduced into wheat predate the methods of genetic engineering, which has allowed the grain industry to make the claim that wheat is not "genetically modified," GM (meaning no gene-splicing techniques were used), since GM is increasingly becoming a public-relations nightmare for agribusiness, but this is simply a clever word game. Wheat has been genetically changed, but using methods such as multiple hybridizations (mating different strains and wild grasses) and mutagenesis (the use of radiation or chemicals to induce mutations). These last methods, radiation and chemical mutagenesis, can be substantially *worse* than GM since mutagenesis introduces dozens of mutations, rather than introducing one, two, or three genetic changes with GM.[18] And the changes do not end at changed appearance.

Here are some of the other changes introduced into wheat.

GLIADIN—Gluten is often blamed for being the sole source of wheat's problems, but it's really gliadin, a smaller protein within gluten, that is the culprit behind many damaging health effects of modern wheat. More than 200 forms of gliadin proteins have been cataloged, all poorly and incompletely digested by humans, consistent with being a component of the seeds of a grass.[19] A gene for one form of gliadin, called Glia-α9, yields a gliadin protein that is the most potent trigger for celiac disease, the intestinal destruction of the small intestine from wheat, rye, and barley. The Glia-α9 gene was present in only a few strains of wheat from the early 20th century, but it is now present in most modern varieties,[20] likely accounting for the 400 percent increase in celiac disease since 1948.[21]

If you eat, say, an egg, the proteins are degraded into single amino acids. That is the way proteins are normally digested. Not so with the proteins from the seeds of grasses. Many of the proteins of grains are either degraded into small pieces, or peptides (short chains of amino acids), rather than single amino acids, or are not degraded at all. In a peculiar twist, new gliadin variants are partially digested to small peptides that enter the bloodstream and then bind to opiate receptors of the human brain—the same receptors activated by heroin and morphine with effects that include mind "fog," paranoia, anxiety, the mania of bipolar illness, depression, and appetite stimulation.[22, 23, 24, 25] The last effect—appetite stimulation—is common and can be overwhelming, as evidenced by people who struggle with relentless appetite, such as those with bulimia and binge eating disorder. Researchers call these peptides exorphins, or exogenous morphinelike compounds. Gliadin-derived peptides, however, generate no "high" but just increase appetite and calorie consumption, with studies demonstrating consistent increases in calorie intake of 400 calories per day, mostly from carbohydrates.[26, 27] In other words, wheat—along with rye and barley, which share the same gliadin protein structure—are potent appetite stimulants with other mind-altering effects.

GLUTEN—A large protein consisting of gliadin and glutenins, gluten confers the stretchiness unique to wheat dough. Gluten has been genetically manipulated, as the long-branching glutenin proteins determine baking characteristics. Geneticists have therefore crossbred wheat strains, bred wheat with nonwheat grasses to introduce new genes, and used chemicals and radiation to induce mutations in the glutenin component of gluten, breeding methods that are unpredictable. Hybridizing two different wheat plants yields as many as 14 unique glutenin proteins never before encountered by humans.[28] Accordingly, new glutenin protein genes have been identified in modern strains of wheat that are not found in older strains; none, of course, have been tested for suitability for human consumption.[29]

WHEAT GERM AGGLUTININ—The genetic changes inflicted on wheat have altered the structure of wheat germ agglutinin, WGA, a protein in wheat (and barley, rye, and rice) that protects the plant against molds and insects. The WGA of modern wheat differs in structure from that of ancient wheat strains due to fiddling by agribusiness.[30] Ironically, geneticists have tried to increase WGA content of grains to improve pest resistance, thereby amplifying toxicity on the human gastrointestinal tract. WGA, from a class of proteins called lectins, is remarkably tough, completely indigestible, resistant to any breakdown by the human body, and unaffected by cooking, baking, sprouting the seeds, or sourdough fermentation; no matter how you process it, you ingest intact WGA. Undigested WGA lectins are toxic, as they do damage directly without need for genetic susceptibility. WGA alone is sufficient to generate celiac disease–like intestinal damage, disrupting microvilli, the absorptive "hairs" of intestinal cells, even in the absence of gliadin/gluten.[31] It is a perfect example of the unsuitability of grain proteins for human food, given its complete indigestibility, something you will never see with, for example, meats or vegetables.

PHYTATES—Because phytic acid, or phytates, like WGA, resists pests for the plant, grain-breeding efforts over the past 50 years have selected strains with increased phytate content. And because phytate content parallels fiber content, advice to increase dietary fiber by consuming more "healthy whole grains" thereby increases phytate content in the diet. Modern wheat, corn, and millet, for instance, contain 800 milligrams of phytates per 100 grams (3½ ounces) of flour. As little as 50 milligrams of phytates turns off absorption of minerals, especially iron, zinc, calcium, and magnesium. Children typically ingest 600 to 1,900 milligrams of phytates per day, while enthusiastic grain-consuming cultures are exposed to as much as 5,000 milligrams of phytates per day, levels clearly associated with nutrient deficiencies.[32, 33] Phytates are thereby a common cause of iron deficiency anemia, often unresponsive to iron supplementation.[34] Zinc deficiency can cause skin rashes, poor wound healing, impaired immunity, reduced sense of taste and smell, and slowed growth in children. Nutrient absorption is restored upon stopping ingestion of grain-sourced phytates, though deficiencies can be severe and require specific supplementation. (You can also appreciate how advice such as "eat more whole grains for better nutrition" is complete fiction.)

ALPHA AMYLASE INHIBITORS AND OTHER ALLERGENS—Numerous allergens have been identified in modern wheat not found in ancient or traditional forms.[35] A class of proteins called alpha amylase inhibitors are among the most common allergens, responsible for causing hives, asthma, cramps, diarrhea, and eczema. The structure of modern alpha amylase inhibitors differs from traditional strains by 10 percent, representing up to several dozen amino acid differences. As any allergy expert will tell you, just a few amino acids can spell the difference between no allergic reaction and a severe allergic reaction, even anaphylaxis (shock). People in the baking industry frequently develop a condition called baker's asthma. There is also a peculiar condition called wheat-dependent exercise-induced anaphylaxis, a severe and life-threatening allergy induced by exercise after eating wheat. Both conditions are due to allergy to gliadin proteins.[36] Among the other proteins that have been changed over the last 40 years are lipid transfer proteins, Ω-gliadins, γ-gliadins, trypsin inhibitors, serpins, and glutenins, all of which can trigger allergic reactions experienced as asthma, skin rashes, sinus congestion, or gastrointestinal distress.

AMYLOPECTIN A—While most components of grasses and their seeds are indigestible, there is one highly digestible component: amylopectin A, the "complex" carbohydrate of grains. It is so highly digestible by the enzyme amylase in saliva and the stomach (due to a unique branching structure) that it yields some of the highest blood sugars of any food, explaining why the glycemic indexes (the value that describes the blood sugar–raising potential of a food over 90 minutes after consumption) of grains are among the highest of all foods, higher than table sugar.[37] A lifestyle of plentiful "healthy whole grains" thereby causes repeated blood sugar highs, followed by increased likelihood of prediabetes and diabetes. Blood sugar highs are also followed by blood sugar lows accompanied by feelings of fogginess, fatigue, and hunger in a predictable 2-hour cycle.

Don't be fooled, as the nutrition community has, by epidemiologic observations that demonstrate that whole grains cause less diabetes than white flour products; the studies show that white flour products lead to diabetes and that whole grains do, too, just not as badly as white flour—less bad does not mean good, though. That is a crucial distinction: White flour products lead to not only diabetes but also colon cancer, heart disease, and weight gain; whole grains also lead to colon cancer, heart disease, and weight gain—just not to the degree that white flour does. This should not be interpreted to mean that whole grains therefore reverse these conditions, as they most definitely do not. In the Nurses' Health Study, for example, of 74,000 females, those who consumed mostly white flour products gained an average of 10 pounds over 12 years, while those eating mostly whole grains gained 9 pounds—whole grains make you less fat, not skinny.[38]

Adding fiber and B vitamins to table sugar would not miraculously convert it into a health food any more than the fiber and B vitamins retained in grains, rich in gliadin, gluten, wheat germ agglutinin, allergens, and amylopectins, can erase all their other problems.

Wheat and its two most closely related grains, rye and barley, are therefore not just a vehicle for gluten but are packed with dozens of compounds toxic to humans, with adverse effects inadvertently amplified by agribusiness through efforts that have everything to do with agricultural goals and nothing to do with your health.

The worldwide experience of grain removal from the diet (triggered in large part by the Wheat Belly books) has also yielded some new lessons. Abrupt cessation of grain consumption, and thereby cessation of gliadin-derived opiates (exorphins), especially from modern wheat, yields *an opiate withdrawal syndrome:* nausea, headache, fatigue, and depression that typically lasts a week. And just as an alcoholic who stops drinking two-fifths of bourbon on Tuesday is not in ideal health by Wednesday or Thursday, former grain-eaters can require weeks, months, and occasionally years to recover from the range of disruptive health effects of former grain consumption. While many of these effects reverse naturally with the removal of grain, others require your intervention to set right. It requires a specific and purposeful effort, for instance, to restore healthy bowel flora once the disruptive gastrointestinal effects of grains are removed; to correct nutrient deficiencies that developed due to phytates; to restore disrupted hormonal and endocrine health; to fully reverse health conditions such as hypertension, diabetes, and autoimmune diseases initiated and perpetuated by grains and to stop the drugs used to treat them. These considerations are all built into the Undoctored 6-week Wild, Naked, and Unwashed nutritional program.

Another important lesson: Once someone is grain-free for more than a few weeks, any reexposure, whether intentional or inadvertent, commonly triggers bloating; diarrhea; joint pain; mind "fog," anxiety, or anger; appetite stimulation (often uncontrollable); and recurrence of symptoms previously relieved by grain elimination, such as migraine headaches, knee or hip pain, depression, or skin rashes. Such effects can last from hours to days, sometimes longer. One example of how long a grain reexposure can linger can be observed in people with autoimmune conditions, such as rheumatoid arthritis. Say someone is grain-free; has experienced reversal of the joint pain, swelling, and disfigurement; and feels great. That person indulges in a slice of pumpernickel bread or a handful of pretzels, and pain and swelling return within hours and can persist for weeks to months before the inflammation subsides again. And not all reexposure reactions are perceived; some are silent and you will not know that they are bubbling beneath the surface. Small LDL particles, for instance, causing heart disease are exceptionally easy to provoke. The amylopectin A from the wheat in a whole wheat bagel is more than enough to trigger plenty of small, oxidation-prone LDL particles, an abnormal response that lingers for a week and adds to cumulative heart disease risk, unlike the 24 hours of large LDL particles triggered by fat consumption before the liver clears them from the bloodstream.

That covers wheat and closely related rye and barley. Let's talk about other grains now.

Grains: A Zero-Tolerance Policy

In this street gang of dietary intruders, wheat and closely related rye and barley are the worst offenders, the ringleaders who mastermind the bad stuff. But it does not mean that the other gang members (what I call nonwheat grains) are law-abiding citizens; they are simply *less bad*. In busting up this dietary crime of grain consumption, we aim for the death penalty.

Corn (called maize outside of North America), oats, triticale, bulgur, millet, teff, sorghum, and rice (all forms) are, like wheat, the seeds of grasses. Less bad means that a variety of undesirable health effects are provoked with their consumption—just not as badly as those provoked by the worst of the bunch, modern wheat.

For starters, all nonwheat grains share a high carbohydrate content. While sugar is 100 percent carbohydrates, grains aren't too far behind with around 85 percent of their calories coming from carbohydrates, even higher in rice. This makes sense: The carbohydrates stored in the seed were meant to provide nutrition to the sprouting plant as it germinates. But the carbohydrates in all seeds of grasses, amylopectin A, are digested rapidly and raise blood sugar, gram for gram, higher than table sugar.

Like wheat, nonwheat grains also raise blood sugar rapidly and to high levels. For instance, a 1-cup serving of cooked organic, stoneground oatmeal with no added sugar has 50 grams of net carbohydrates (net carbohydrates = total carbohydrates – fiber; we subtract fiber since it does not raise blood sugar), or the equivalent of 12 teaspoons of sugar, giving it a glycemic index (GI) of 55 (misleadingly classified by dietitians as "low" GI, by the way). This is enough to send blood sugar through the roof and provoke all the phenomena of glycation—irreversible modification of body proteins that leads to conditions such as cataracts, hypertension, destruction of joint cartilage resulting in arthritis, kidney disease, heart disease, and dementia. And all nonwheat grasses raise blood sugar extravagantly and provoke glycation to similar degrees.

Corn is often consumed not as corn on the cob or intact kernels but ground into cornstarch or cornmeal. The increased surface area for digestion of these forms compared to intact kernels explains why the glycemic index of cornstarch is 90 to 100—the highest of any food—compared to 60 for corn on the cob and 59 to 65 for sucrose or table sugar.[39] Cornstarch is among the most popular ingredients in gluten-free foods, also explaining why gluten-free breads, muffins, and other products are associated with extravagant weight gain and high blood sugars.

For years, we've been told that complex carbohydrates are better for us than simple sugars, meaning the lengthy carbohydrate molecules of amylopectin in grains don't raise blood sugar as high as sugars with one or two sugar molecules, such as glucose (one sugar) or sucrose (two sugars: glucose + fructose). But this is simply wrong, and this silly distinction has been abandoned: The GI of complex carbohydrates is *the same as or higher than simple sugars*. The GI of whole wheat bread is 72, and the GI of millet as a hot cereal is 67. Neither is any better than the GI of sucrose: 59 to 65. (Similar shenanigans apply to the glycemic load, a value that factors in typical portion size.) The World Health Organization and the Food and Agriculture Organization of the United Nations have both dropped the complex versus simple distinction and rightly so, as grains, from a blood sugar viewpoint, are the same as or worse than sugar.

Some of the highest blood sugars you will ever see follow consumption of grains, even if "whole," organic, stoneground, sprouted, or sourdough-fermented. After a bowl of oatmeal (without added sugar), for instance, I have witnessed blood sugars as high as 200 to 500 mg/dL—incredibly high values for a food regarded by many as "heart healthy."

The amylopectin content of grains explains why corn, wheat, and sorghum are fed to livestock to fatten them up prior to slaughter, yielding

FOOTLOOSE AND GLUTEN-FREE

By now, you surely recognize just how many mistakes have been committed in the name of nutrition. While some mistakes got their start 10,000 years ago, others are more recent. The fat-free, cholesterol-free trend, a powerful and popular modern movement that made a big contribution to the epidemics of obesity and diabetes, was a financial windfall for manufacturers of processed food. Fat-free cookies, ice cream, and salad dressings are landmines of grains, sugar, and high-fructose corn syrup but hugely profitable nonetheless.

The same misguided opportunism is going on in the world of gluten-free replacement foods. You now understand that viewing grains as just a source of gluten is a hazardous oversimplification; there is more than intolerance to gluten involved in human consumption of the seeds of grasses. Nonetheless, many people have fallen into the trap of thinking that if a food lacks gluten, it must therefore be good. And clever food manufacturers sniffed another profit opportunity: create gluten-free foods to replace gluten-containing grains.

Problem: Manufacturers chose four ingredients to substitute for wheat flour and gluten. Cornstarch, rice flour, tapioca starch, and potato starch—because they provide a reasonable facsimile of wheat and gluten in creating bread, muffins, cookies, and other familiar baked products—are now the main ingredients in 99 percent of gluten-free processed foods on store shelves. You now know that cornstarch, due to its small-particle nature, raises blood sugar the highest of all foods, thereby contributing to high insulin levels, weight gain, hypertension, heart disease, cancer, and

"grain-finished" cuts of meat. Ducks are fattened with corn and wheat, often force-fed through a tube passed into their stomachs, to cause the fatty livers for the much-prized foie gras.

Corn, more so than other nonwheat grains, has effects beyond high-carbohydrate content. The zein protein of corn partially resembles the gliadin protein of wheat, meaning it can provoke some of the same health effects. It means, for example, that the zein protein of corn can initiate the first step of autoimmune diseases, conditions as far-ranging as rheumatoid arthritis, lupus, multiple sclerosis, autoimmune hepatitis, type 1 diabetes, psoriasis, eczema, cerebellar ataxia, and some forms of dementia.[40, 41, 42] Corn is also a prominent trigger for allergies. As many as 90 percent of people who deal with cornstarch in the pharmaceutical industry (as filler in pills and capsules), food production, or agriculture develop allergic responses to corn over time.[43]

dementia. The other three gluten-free replacement ingredients are much the same. We now have gluten-free Fruity Pebbles breakfast cereal and gluten-free animal cookies and many others; manufacturers just won't talk about the high blood sugars and other health problems that are associated with gluten-free products.

This is why people who misinterpret the grain-free message as gluten-free typically gain weight, often substantial amounts; expand their waist-lines; end up with prediabetes or diabetes; develop metabolic distortions such as high triglycerides; and acquire inflammatory diseases. Incredibly, this has not slowed the double-digit growth of the gluten-free processed food industry, now approaching $7 billion in annual sales. Yes: Mistakes can be quite profitable because it's all about spin and riding trends. You can appreciate that if we are working toward an Undoctored lifestyle free of as many health conditions as possible, **gluten-free foods made with these terrible replacement ingredients have no place on the menu.** (This does not mean, however, that you will never have pizza again; I shall talk about how to re-create such familiar foods with healthy replacement ingredients in Chapter 10.)

There's nothing intrinsically wrong with the idea of being gluten-free. A rib eye steak and hard-cooked eggs are gluten-free, after all. It's the she-nanigans conducted by food manufacturers—mistakes, poor understanding, ignorance, or just plain dishonesty and deception—that are to blame for the gluten-free fiasco. Let the food manufacturers play their game, let the retailers proudly feature entire shelves of them, but don't let yourself fall into this trap.

Because rice contains less than 1 percent protein, it exerts less potential for effects caused by proteins, such as gastrointestinal toxicity, allergy, and autoimmune diseases. But this does not mean that rice is harmless. With very little protein, much of the rest is amylopectin carbohydrates; 90 percent of rice calories are from blood sugar–raising carbohydrates, the highest of all grains. As food becomes more plentiful and fewer people live on the edge of starvation, rice-consuming Asians are experiencing an explosive epidemic of type 2 diabetes, now surpassing North America and Europe in total numbers.[44]

Rice also has the unique capacity to concentrate inorganic arsenic from the soil, an effect that has been associated with cancer, high blood pressure, neurological disease, cardiovascular disease, and increased risk for death.[45, 46] As with many other grain effects, these problems develop over long periods with chronic, habitual consumption, but not acutely (though the FDA is exploring potential for acute toxicity, as well, in enthusiastic rice consumers).

How can a group of foods be associated with such an extensive list of adverse health consequences? Because the seeds of grasses never belonged in the diet in the first place. Grains are no more food for humans than tree bark or branches.

Ungrained and Unrestrained

If you were starving and desperate and the only thing you had to survive was a loaf of bread, go ahead and eat it; it is, after all, a food that first found its way into the human diet in a moment of desperation. If the only thing between you and an early grave is a stale, moldy bagel, eating it will provide calories and allow you to survive another day, since you are not concerned with long-term health a year or more later. That is the Faustian bargain that modern people have unwittingly made: near-term survival in exchange for long-term health.

To make matters worse, the food of hungry, desperate humans has been held up as the savior of human dietary health, promoted as a solution to a list of human conditions and a source of nutrients. We are urged to make grains the dominant component of diet by government agencies and industry groups alike. The food of desperation now dominates the human diet because of a widespread and widely held misconception, bolstered by commercial interests, while ignoring what human history tells us. If you are not desperate and have the luxury of choice in food, there is no need to make this tradeoff; choose real food in the first place so you don't squander your prospects for long-term health.

Once you recognize the extraordinary and disruptive effects of grains on humans who never should have consumed them in the first place and remove them, extraordinary and unexpected health benefits unfold. Having witnessed health changes and transformations in hundreds of thousands of people since the revelations of the Wheat Belly books, even today I continue to be astounded by the range and degree of health benefits this lifestyle produces. Doing the opposite of conventional advice—not eating more "healthy whole grains" but banishing them completely—is proving to be one of the most powerful solutions for health to come along in 10,000 years.

Grains are so incredibly disruptive to human health that, to a large degree, I regard the healthcare system for chronic illness (not acute illness, such as traumatic injury or infection) as the system largely created to treat the consequences of grain consumption. Understand this fundamental fact and you are empowered to be as Undoctored as possible. Grain elimination is therefore a cornerstone of the diet advocated here in *Undoctored*, an essential process that frees us from reliance on the medical system in an impressive multitude of ways.

Elimination of seeds of grasses therefore allows you to reverse a long list of health conditions over time. But your dietary efforts do not end there, particularly in the modern world in which we don't kill or gather our food but rely on food manufacturers, supermarkets, and restaurants for at least some of our choices. Let's tackle dietary issues outside of grains next.

Chapter Summary:
Your Next Steps to Becoming Undoctored

Nutrition is at the center of your Undoctored efforts. But, like medical advice, most nutritional advice is crafted to suit the agenda of agribusiness and the food industry. If we cast such biases aside and examine what is truly beneficial in diet and what is harmful, we come to very different conclusions. We start our Undoctored journey by banishing all wheat and grains from our lives, reversing a mistake humans made in desperation, ironically now celebrated by all agencies providing dietary advice. But the proof is in the grain-free pudding: the astounding reversal of numerous health conditions.

CHAPTER 7

Meat, Fire, Fat, and Other Essentials

Tell me what you eat, and I will tell you what you are.

—Jean Anthelme Brillat-Savarin

That's enough grain-bashing for now. But if you understand this one concept, that incorporating the seeds of grasses into the human diet was a huge miscalculation on par with enslaving populations or offering human sacrifices to appease the gods, then you are charting a course for health that is unparalleled in the modern experience. Grain consumption may be necessary for survival when nothing better is available, but if you live in the modern world, you have better choices, including many that do not impair health through provocation of chronic diseases, the "diseases of civilization."

The rejection of grains alone is a huge step forward (or backward, depending on your time perspective). But there is *more* to creating a genuinely powerful diet, an essential component of your life to get squared away before we address other factors that get you closer to an Undoctored life. Let's now tackle dietary issues beyond grains that play crucial roles in your quest for health.

The Accidental Carnivore

We are not going to take important lessons on how to live our nutritional lives from dietitians courted by food companies, doctors who have almost no understanding or interest, government agencies cozy with big business, or your mom, whose food experiences came through *The Galloping Gourmet* and Swanson TV dinners. We are going to obtain much of our dietary wisdom from a source you might find surprising: anthropology, the scientific study of human experience of life on this planet. I will be tackling some contentious issues because many popular notions about diet have ignored this critical aspect of nutrition, the lessons of human dietary history.

Far more than a study of skull bone remnants, anthropology has provided us with an impressive reconstruction of human dietary history. How humans hunted, gathered, and ate over millions of years molded the unique physiology of human digestion. We therefore need to eat the foods that we are adapted to eat, not the foods we are told to eat by government food policy or food manufacturers.

As you now know, our needs are different from those of a goat or orangutan. The design of our teeth, saliva, stomach, digestive enzymes, and intestinal tracts are unique to our species. Adopting the grass diet of a goat would be fatal. Follow an all-fruit diet like a Sumatran orangutan, and you will lose your teeth and hair and suffer bone fractures due to nutritional deficiencies. The closer we get to understanding unique human nutritional needs and meet those needs, the better able we are to erase the diseases acquired due to dietary mistakes. You will also begin to understand that many health conditions you previously thought were genetic or due to bad luck are really manifestations of diet gone wrong. To gain this understanding, we've got to go back, *way* back.

Before Harry met Sally, before human civilization got its start, before humans learned to plant seeds, before use of fire and cooking, before any member of the *Homo* species roamed and hunted the savannas of Africa, there were australopithecines, 3-foot-tall, chimpanzee-like primates that stood upright and whose only tools were rocks and sticks. *Australopithecus afarensis* (among which was the famed Lucy discovered in Eastern Africa) was an herbivore, eating fruits and nuts and digging in the dirt for roots, foods suiting the species' large molar teeth and powerful jaws. If they consumed the organs or flesh of animals, they did so by scavenging carcasses killed by other creatures that possessed the natural tools of carnivory: large canine teeth, sharp claws, and digestive systems that efficiently broke down organs and meat, none of which our pint-size predecessor possessed.

Unlike politics, evolution is the story of the replacement of one species with another species that is more successful in adapting to an environment. *Australopithecus* died out 2.5 million years ago and was replaced by *Homo habilis,* which began the path toward larger-brained primate species that were increasingly skilled at toolmaking. *Homo habilis* appears to have also started as an herbivorous meat- and organ-scavenging species, cracking open long bones left by carnivores to extract fatty bone marrow or seizing whatever else remained of organs and muscle.[1]

Anthropologists tell us that harnessing fire and collaborative hunting were two other innovations that changed the course of human life. Changes in anatomy suggest a life on the ground rather than in the trees. Life on two feet was dangerous, as the world was filled with large predators that humans, without large canine teeth or sharp claws, were helpless against—until they had fire and weapons. A progressive increase in brain size resulted as humans increasingly feasted on animal organs and flesh and then learned that cooking—roasting over a fire, burying foods in hot sand near a fire, rolling meat in leaves and placing it on top of hot coals—not only improved flavor but also dramatically increased digestive efficiency, reducing caloric needs.[2, 3, 4] (We witness the digestive inefficiency of eating uncooked foods in modern people who, by choice, eat most of their food raw: constant hunger, a need for frequent meals, weight loss to unhealthy levels, eventual loss of muscle mass and teeth.)

Large creatures, such as wooly mammoths and giant peccary, were indeed dangerous but also tasty. This led to collaborative hunting, as a group of, say, six hunters proved deadlier than one alone. Imagine trying to kill a creature the size of a modern elephant that could, with a single stomp of its foot or swipe of its tusks, put an end to your carnivorous ambitions. It demanded collaboration that could only occur through *communication,* which required the development of a vocal apparatus for speech and the purposeful use of sounds (i.e., language—"Og, you circle around mammoth from behind and use ax to cut rear leg while I distract in front with spear") as well as a frontal lobe of the brain that could plan ahead. Early humans became so effective at hunting large game that anthropologists blame human hunters for their extinction, despite lacking the natural tools of carnivory.

The most advanced primate, *Homo sapiens,* the largest brained yet, first appeared around 180,000 years ago. While less powerful than their predecessors, *Homo sapiens* were smarter, faster, nearly hairless, and capable of running long distances due to the capacity to sweat; our species of clever, lithe primates was so successful that it expanded onto all of the earth's continents except Antarctica.

This shift in dietary fortunes was accompanied by transformations in anatomy to accommodate change in food choices. We no longer needed massive molar teeth or powerful jaws to grind large quantities of fibrous tubers, our small intestines lengthened to better extract nutrients from animal organs and flesh, and our colons shortened because a reduction in plant material meant less effort was required to degrade fibrous components of plants, freeing up energy for our expanding brains.[5] In other words, human anatomy evolved to that of a less herbivorous, more carnivorous, large-brained creature who hunted and cooked its food.

At different times on different continents, though roughly 10,000 years ago, humans learned that some wild animal species could be domesticated, as we've discussed. Because most carnivorous creatures, such as lions and leopards, were not agreeable to such practices, humans succeeded in domesticating mostly grazing, herbivorous creatures, such as aurochs (cows), ibex (goats), red junglefowl (chicken, a bit of an exception as an omnivore), and the llama and camel. Domesticated animals thereby took the place of wild creatures and reduced the need for hunting.

We became dependent on nutrients obtainable only through consumption of animal organs and meats, whether wild or domesticated, such as omega-3 fatty acids from consuming the brains and organs of animals, as well as fish and shellfish; iodine from consuming thyroid glands; vitamin B_{12} from liver; iron from blood, organs, and meat; and zinc from meat and organs—physiologic needs, as well as digestive anatomy, adapted to the consumption of meat and organs.

The human experience in diet is unique in that we originated from herbivorous primates but evolved over the ensuing 2.5 million years into opportunistic scavengers and then skilled, successful group hunters despite lacking the anatomical weapons of carnivory (you don't apply nail polish to your claws or bare sharp canine teeth when your husband swipes your french fries, do you?).

Consumption of animals and then cooking—a practice not followed by any other species—fueled growth of the human brain, accompanied by digestive adaptations that helped create the anatomically modern human. Animal organ and meat consumption is therefore programmed into our digestive health, now causing us to be reliant on nutrients from this source.

As a former vegetarian and animal lover, I wish this wasn't true, but the science argues otherwise. We are the cumulative product of a several-million-year-long process of adaptation, complete with anatomical and metabolic changes allowing us to adapt to this lifestyle. We aren't born with the outward tools of carnivory, but we retain the brainpower, the capacity for collaboration and communication, and the digestive systems and needs of a carnivorous hunter who also gathers nongrain plants. Don't feed a woodpecker a bowl of plankton or a lion spinach and kale. Likewise, don't defy cumulative dietary adaptations that led to the modern 21st-century human, or else you risk disruptions in health.

SUE IS
UNDOCTORED

Houston, Texas

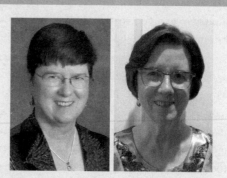

I feel so much better than I did before. I am a 5-year ovarian cancer survivor. All my gastrointestinal issues have gone, arthritis is almost nonexistent, rashes and rosacea are gone except when medicines activate them. My allergies are much better, and I have not had bronchitis since going on the grain-free diet. Best part was getting off all diabetes medicine and lowering my HbA1c to 5.6. Also, my triglycerides have always been a concern, and now they are down for the first time ever.

In 2012, my cholesterol total was 263, HDL was 41, triglycerides were 312, LDL was 160. I was a type 2 diabetic with rosacea and lots of skin rashes, sinus infections, and bronchitis all the time. Gastrointestinal issues from one extreme to the other.

As of June 15, 2016, total cholesterol was 175, HDL 47, triglycerides 100 (lowest it has ever been), LDL 108. All other labs in normal ranges. I am off metformin, Lyrica, Miralax, propranolol, a statin drug, Finacea for rosacea, Lovaza, Dexilant, Zantac, and omeprazole for gastrointestinal issues/gastroesophageal reflux disease.

Before I never thought about mood, but the diet does seem to make you feel more mellow, in my opinion.

Although I did not go on the diet to lose weight, I did end up 30 pounds lighter in the process. My reasons for changing were for my existing health issues that my nutritionist promised would go away if I stuck to the program. After seeing the results, I finally made a believer out of my endocrinologist, and she was asking me for more information. A year ago she thought I was going against medical wisdom with my diet. I saw my oncologist for my 6-month checkup. After she looked at my labs, she started asking about the diet, etc., and wrote it all down this time. Before, she has always said, "Everything is okay in moderation." I guess watching me change has impressed her.

Mrs. Sprat Was Right

If Jack Sprat could eat no fat—well, he's going to be one sick, hungry guy. Fats, unlike carbohydrates, are essential, as necessary as water or oxygen.

If we are, at the core, carnivorous creatures, a product of our unique evolutionary past, it's easy to recognize that consuming the fat of animals is also part of our natural physiology. You and your hungry clan spear a wild boar, but no one declares, "Just cut off a piece of lean meat for me and throw the fat, brain, and liver away." Humans consumed everything from snout to tail, all but the squeal, and fat was savored.

Yet we've been told over the last 50 years that fats, especially animal fats, are the worst for health. Conventional wisdom tells us that fat, particularly the saturated fat of animal flesh and organs, makes us fat and causes diabetes, cancer, and cardiovascular disease. While grain consumption was a mistake we made 10,000 years ago, limiting fat consumption was a mistake we made starting 50 years ago, a man-made blunder based on misinterpretation, misrepresentation, the leanings of dietary zealots, and politics. The evidence used to advance the low-fat message was incomplete, epidemiological (which should almost never be used to generate firm conclusions, only hypotheses; see "Of Horses and Women" in Chapter 2, one disastrous example of using epidemiological observations as "proof"), and riddled with methodological flaws—none of which stopped overenthusiastic dietary fanatics sold on the low-fat message in the 1970s and 1980s. Such fanatical leanings reached the ear of Senator George McGovern, chair of the United States Senate Select Committee on Nutrition and Human Needs, who decided that all Americans should engage in a low-fat lifestyle. (The drama of this entire tragic episode has been recounted in meticulous detail by journalists Gary Taubes in *Good Calories, Bad Calories* and Nina Teicholz in *The Big Fat Surprise*, both "must" reading if you wish to understand the history of how this awful situation got so awful. The documentary film *Fat Head* by filmmaker Tom Naughton, genius for educating while entertaining, provides a lighter version of the history, as well.) The McGovern committee pushed through legislation, written by a staff member with no background in health or nutrition, that charged the USDA, an agency whose mission had been to support agriculture and monitor food safety, to lead the charge in providing dietary advice to the public. This created an odd collision of responsibilities: regulating an industry while also promoting consumption of the industry's products.

Despite resistance from the scientific community over the potential hazards of government-driven dietary advice, the USDA proceeded to fulfill its charge. In addition to delivering McGovern's pet agenda of limiting fat consumption, the grain and processed food lobby was allowed to weigh in on the details of the USDA's final draft, doubling grain intake over that recommended by USDA nutritionists.

The low-fat movement gained further momentum when the processed food industry recognized what a financial bonanza had been thrown into its lap, paving the way to create thousands of foods to suit the reduction in fat created by government advice. Revenue growth at Kraft, General Mills, and companies represented by the Corn Refiners Association leapt to double-digit annual rates as they introduced low-fat cookies, low-fat yogurt, and margarines made with corn, soybean, and other processed oils (you'd better believe it's not butter). It made the 1980s and 1990s an era of unprecedented growth in Big Food. Low-fat products proliferated, even gaining health endorsements from the FDA, the American Heart Association (AHA), and the Academy of Nutrition and Dietetics. It meant that products that contained liberal quantities of sugar and high-fructose corn syrup but were low in fat could acquire the *appearance* of health with, for example, the AHA "heart healthy" Heart-Check mark endorsement affixed to them (Berry Berry Kix, Count Chocula, and Cocoa Puffs breakfast cereals, to name a few)—for a fee, of course.

Any trip to a neighborhood mall or supermarket will quickly reveal the consequences of 50 years of misguided dietary advice, compounded by food manufacturers: the worst epidemic of overweight and obesity ever witnessed in the history of the world. The world of Big Food was built on the bellies—and lives—of Americans, now a contagion shared by increasing numbers in the rest of the developed world.

Government advice, industry profiteering, and the innate human love of anything sugary (a genetically programmed survival mechanism taken to perverse extremes during times of plenty) all combined to create epidemics of disease that go beyond weight gain, with conditions such as diabetes (both type 1 and 2), autoimmune diseases, joint deterioration, and dementia. Incredibly, even while the USDA and other agencies continue to promote the low-fat, plenty-of-grains message and food companies continue to sell tens of thousands of low-fat products, the science has become clear: There are no clinical trials demonstrating that limiting fat or saturated fat provides any health benefits or reduces cardiovascular risk.[6, 7] Likewise, red meat consumption has no relationship to cardiovascular risk if the effects of cured processed meats (salami, sausage, lunch meats, hot dogs) are factored out.[8]

Recent pronouncements that red meat is a "carcinogen"? Yet another unfounded conclusion suggested by epidemiological observations, but far from conclusive, much as horse estrogens were believed to promote female health.

And as this experiment in cutting fat and increasing grains and carbohydrates has played out on a worldwide stage, the data revealing how destructive this advice has been are now overwhelming. But as in many things in health care, this scientific revelation has not yet graced the ears of John Q. Primary Care, who still manages to obtain most of his ongoing medical education from the drug industry. Even in the face of societal and scientific evidence that contradicts the low-fat message, most of the medical community still sends their patients to the dietitian (i.e., the dietary professional whose "education" was largely subsidized with support from Big Food) for counseling on cutting fat and eating more "healthy whole grains"—you know, a "balanced" diet, all in "moderation."

This dietary pyramid has begun to crumble. After decades of dietary misinformation, the latest 2015 dietary guidelines concede that restricting total fat and cholesterol is not beneficial, thereby removing that woefully outdated and destructive advice, though the saturated fat limitation remains.[9] The number of servings of grains recommended every day was also reduced from the 6 to 11 servings per day to just 6. (Such a slow and stepwise backpedaling on previous bad advice, by the way, is how you manage damage control and avoid the liability that could result. Imagine if all the guilty agencies admitted that their dietary advice not only did *not* provide health or reduce cardiovascular risk but also *contributed to* the nationwide epidemics of obesity and diabetes? Liability, loss of credibility, and loss of revenues would be huge.) However, how much faith can you put in advice that has been flawed for so long, having made substantial contributions to the deteriorating health of the public? Should we suddenly accept that they were wrong on such a colossal scale, only now to have finally gotten it right? I think you'd have to be nuts, or at least incredibly naive, to believe anything they say.

Beyond exposing the political shenanigans and unscientific manipulations of a nutritional message, my litmus test for considering whether a nutritional strategy makes sense is to ask: How have humans approached this aspect of diet over eons of adaptation to life on this planet? If humans have been doing it ever since we abandoned life in the trees, then it is highly likely that we are well adapted to this aspect of lifestyle. If it was added only recently and, even worse, because a few authorities said so, then we need to question that advice, with intolerance to a new strategy potentially showing as various disease conditions.

With animal fats, the answer is obvious: Hungry, desperate humans would enthusiastically eat the entire kill of a hunt and not waste a moment being concerned about fat intake. Therefore we know that the fats humans are adapted to consuming are the components of animal fat: monounsaturates, saturates, and some polyunsaturates, such as linolenic acid. Throw in the added fats and oils from nuts, seeds (nongrass), shellfish and fish, and modest quantities of linoleic acid from vegetables and fruits. Natural fats and oils do not include fats created by modern humans such as hydrogenated ("trans") fats. A return to a natural pattern of fat consumption also does not include replacing monounsaturates and saturates with large quantities of polyunsaturates from corn, or oils that require extreme processing that alters fatty acid structure, such as canola.[10]

Fats are satiating. They provide a feeling of long-lasting freedom from hunger. Inadequate fat intake is a common reason for people just starting out on this lifestyle to complain of hunger, since many people struggle to get beyond their deeply ingrained fat phobia. Well, get over it. And I mean that quite seriously. Don't buy lean cuts of meat; buy fatty cuts. If you eat a steak, eat the fat. Pork? Eat the fat. With poultry, eat the dark meat and skin. Have liver, liver sausage (uncured), and other organ meats. (Consider choosing organs and meats from sources that employ humane practices, don't rely on antibiotics or hormones, and allow their animals to graze freely rather than stay penned in large factory farms.) Choose healthy oils such as coconut, olive, avocado, and, should you choose to consume dairy products, organic butter or ghee.

If weight loss is among your goals, one especially powerful strategy is to purposefully load up on fats to induce satiety, thereby reducing your desire to take in more calories. (Don't confuse this with loading up on proteins, which does indeed cause some less-than-desirable health consequences, such as distortions of blood sugar.) Taking in healthy fats and oils is liberating, does not promote cardiovascular disease, and helps you break the bonds of grains and sugars. Of the 6,000 generations that *Homo sapiens* have walked on this planet, we made the low-fat mistake no more than two generations ago. It's time to go back to the way we did it for the first 5,998 generations.

As part of the Undoctored nutritional approach, we will not only *not* shun healthy fats—including the fat in your beef, pork, lard, or tallow—but *celebrate* them. And I'm sure that Mrs. Sprat saved up a big "I told you so" for her husband, Jack.

Sweet and Sour

Imagine a diet loaded with bowls of sugar, some added sugar on top, sugary drink on the side, then licking your fingers in anticipation of a dessert of—sugar. Absurd, of course. But that is not too far off from how many people conduct their modern diets. This overload of sweet ends on a sour note.

While Americans consume the equivalent of 300 loaves of bread each year (representing enormous exposure to the amylopectin A carbohydrate that behaves like sugar or worse), they also consume 200 pounds of sugar. It is not uncommon for sugar alone to comprise a quarter of all calories taken in over the course of the day—some of it out in the open, some of it hidden.[11]

To understand the adverse effects of sugars—sucrose, high-fructose corn syrup, and other fructose-rich sweeteners, such as agave, honey, and maple syrup—we need to understand two phenomena: (1) insulin resistance, and (2) glycation.

When blood sugar rises, insulin is released by the pancreas. Repeated over and over again, the cells of the body fail to respond to the insulin; they become "insulin resistant." This leads to further rises in blood sugar and inflammatory responses, failure to respond to normal appetite signals, and growth of visceral (deep abdominal) fat. The cells of the body—deprived of glucose for energy due to the failure of insulin (which allows entry of glucose into cells)—resort to fat and protein for energy, resulting in rises in blood triglycerides from fats released into the bloodstream, along with loss of muscle.

The essential first step that creates insulin resistance is therefore a rise in blood sugar. Any rise in blood sugar above fasting levels (90 mg/dL) will, over time, provoke insulin resistance: The higher the blood sugar and the more frequently it occurs, the more insulin resistance is provoked. Fructose worsens the effect: inflammation, growth of visceral fat, increased blood triglycerides and fatty acids, and fatty liver—all powerful blockers of insulin that worsen insulin resistance (see "Fructose Feeding Frenzy" on page 142).[12]

The conventional medical solution? Sugar "in moderation," increased whole grain consumption, lots of low-fat foods—disastrous dietary advice,

(continued on page 138)

NO BOLOGNA: DEFICIENCIES OF VEGANISM AND VEGETARIANISM

If a lifestyle results in nutritional deficiencies, sometimes severe and in ways that impair health, then we'd have to question the wisdom of that lifestyle—agreed? If you followed, for instance, a potato-only diet that resulted in fat and protein malnutrition, joint deterioration, skin rashes, and bone fractures and left you toothless, we could only conclude that a long-term spud-fest was an unwise choice.

Following a vegan or vegetarian lifestyle can be a decision made for humane reasons, entirely understandable given the cruelty involved in modern livestock operations, but it also means having to compensate for the multiple deficiencies of this lifestyle. No free-living population through-out history has adhered to a vegan or vegetarian lifestyle until recently, thanks to a handful of modern proponents. If adhering to needs programmed into human adaptation is part of the wisdom of crafting a nutritional pro-gram, then it is very difficult, perhaps impossible, to justify a dietary program that does not include animal products. It makes no more sense to eliminate animal products than it does to eliminate sun exposure or essential nutrients like iodine or magnesium; there will be a health price to pay for going against a need adaptively programmed into human health.

There are obviously people who argue otherwise, citing studies that have suggested that a vegan/vegetarian lifestyle is superior, with less cancer, less cardiovascular disease, and a longer lifespan. First of all, the bulk of data do *not* report such findings. Beyond the flaws inherent in epidemio-logical studies, such studies show no difference in mortality between meat consumers and nonmeat consumers (i.e., no difference in "all-cause mor-tality").[13] Media reports about such studies often blare headlines such as "Red meat causes heart disease" or "Red meat causes cancer." But these headlines are simply not true.

What *is* true is that there are fundamental, and perhaps insurmounta-ble, difficulties with such studies. People who choose a vegan/vegetarian lifestyle are younger, are less likely to smoke cigarettes, drink less alcohol, exercise more, and are more likely to take nutritional supplements—in other words, people who are more likely to join social causes and follow trendy practices, not the auto mechanic who smokes, who drinks too much, and whose idea of trendy is to try the newest IPA. Are the small differences in various diseases due to avoiding animal products, or are they due to the fact that people who make the sacrifice are different? The fact that vegans/vegetarians, on the whole, adhere to healthier lifestyle practices is indis-putable, as it has been shown in every study of the vegan/vegetarian life-style, but it cannot be interpreted to mean that meat consumption per se explains any differences.

Worse, the headlines typically favor news that casts vegan/vegetarian lifestyles in a positive light. The news surrounding the release of the 2016 study from the UK of 60,000 people analyzed for quantity of meat consumption focused on the modest reductions in pancreatic and blood cancers with less meat consumption but failed to report that vegans/vegetarians also experienced higher rates of mental and behavioral disorders, cerebrovascular diseases such as strokes, heart disease, and colorectal cancer.[14] The same study revealed no difference in all-cause mortality, regardless of how much or how little animal products were consumed, suggesting that the data dissected down to each condition likely were statistical anomalies and not real; there are probably no differences, or at least no large differences, in disease occurrence regardless of whether your idea of a Saturday night dinner is a medium-rare steak or a tofu veggie burger.

With a 2.5-million-year heritage of consuming animal products programmed into human anatomy and physiology, choosing to avoid all animal products leads to nutritional deficiencies that pose health complications, though not necessarily resulting in death or other major catastrophes. In particular, some raw vegans (i.e., people who consume no animal products and select foods uncooked or minimally cooked) need to address deficiencies of fat-soluble vitamins, or else experience gingivitis, tooth decay, tooth loss, osteoporosis, skin rashes, depression, and anxiety. Because many vegans/vegetarians are also overly reliant on grains, the nutritional deficiencies of grain consumption, especially iron, zinc, magnesium, and vitamin B_{12}, are greater.

Here are the most important nutritional deficiencies that must be addressed with these lifestyles.

VITAMIN B_{12}

Vitamin B_{12} is especially problematic for vegans/vegetarians since it is completely absent from plant foods and thereby obtainable *only* from animal-based foods, and it must therefore be supplemented.[13] Deficiency is present in up to 90 percent of vegans, with health implications that include megaloblastic anemia, neurological impairment, and psychiatric difficulties.[16]

IRON

Iron is present only as the less-well-absorbed (nonheme) form in plant products, compared to the more efficiently absorbed (heme) form in animal products, resulting in lower body iron stores in vegans and vegetarians.[17] If phytate-containing grains are part of the picture, the prospects for iron absorption are even worse, making correction of iron deficiency more difficult, as well. Iron supplementation is a frequent necessity in people who shun animal products, even after wheat/grain elimination.

OMEGA-3 FATTY ACIDS

Low levels of omega-3 fatty acids are associated with increased cardiovascular risk, abnormal heart rhythms and sudden cardiac death, depression, and dementia. Intake of omega-3 fatty acids, EPA and DHA, is nearly zero

(continued)

NO BOLOGNA: DEFICIENCIES OF VEGANISM AND VEGETARIANISM *(CONT.)*

in vegans and vegetarians, given the absence of fish, shellfish, and animal organs and meat in their diets. Likewise, intake of linolenic acid, another omega-3 fatty acid, is lower.[18] A small quantity of linolenic acid is converted to DHA, so consuming more linolenic acid–rich foods—such as flaxseed, chia, and walnuts—helps a bit with raising DHA levels, raising them to that of moderate deficiency.[19] The average American has 2.5 percent of all fats in their red blood cells as omega-3s, while at least 6 percent is required to reduce risk for sudden cardiac death and 10 percent or more to reduce risk for heart attack and for optimal brain health.[20, 21] The best that a vegan or vegetarian can achieve with plentiful intake of linolenic acid from plants is 3.5 percent—better than average, far from ideal.

Lacto-ovo vegetarians can consume more egg yolks, which contain a small quantity of DHA. DHA can also be sourced from algae and is therefore consistent with a vegan/vegetarian lifestyle, though expensive. Supplementation with 200 milligrams per day of DHA can raise blood levels to that of the average meat-consuming individual but not to levels associated with reduced cardiovascular and other health risks.[22] The best that can therefore be achieved in a vegan/vegetarian lifestyle, even with rich intake of linolenic acid and DHA supplementation, is a level below that associated with protection from cardiovascular events, correctable only by breaking commitment to the lifestyle.

VITAMIN D

While vitamin D deficiency is an issue for everybody, not just vegans/vegetarians, people who avoid animal products have 75 percent less dietary intake. This puts them at risk of the most severe degree of deficiency, given the avoidance of eggs, liver, and seafood that contain modest quantities of vitamin D that augments the quantity activated by sun exposure of the skin.[23, 24] While the human-equivalent D_3 form, cholecalciferol, is preferred, some less-effective nonhuman D_2, ergocalciferol, can be obtained by consuming mushrooms.

VITAMIN K_2

The necessity of this less-well-known form of vitamin K, to be distinguished from the K_1 found in green vegetables, has only been recognized recently.[25] K_1 participates in blood coagulation, while K_2 modulates calcium metabolism, with deficiency contributing to loss of bone calcium leading to osteoporosis, hip and other fractures, and abnormal deposition of calcium in arteries, part of the atherosclerotic process leading to heart attacks. Deficiency may also contribute to cancer risk, especially prostate cancer.

Vitamin K_2 is obtained from consumption of meat and organs, egg yolks, butter (from grass-fed animals only), and foods that undergo some forms of bacterial fermentation, especially cheeses and natto (fermented soybeans).[26] A small quantity is obtained via bacterial conversion from K_1 to K_2 by human bowel flora; it therefore raises the question whether cultivation of selected species of bowel flora that perform such a conversion may result in achieving favorable levels of K_2, even replacing that obtainable from diet, but this has not enjoyed sufficient exploration yet.

A vegan/vegetarian can obtain K_2 by purchasing a vegan/vegetarian form of vitamin K_2 supplementation. But this is, again, a workaround to compensate for the deficiencies of the vegan/vegetarian lifestyle.

There is a real-life laboratory of the vegetarian lifestyle. Of the billion people in India, 30 percent are vegetarian. Vitamin B_{12} deficiency is present in the majority, not uncommonly resulting in neurological dysfunction, psychiatric issues, and underdevelopment in children. Severe vitamin D deficiency and osteoporosis are also common issues, as is zinc deficiency resulting in impaired cognitive function and distortions of taste, and iron deficiency resulting in impaired cognitive performance, childhood underdevelopment, and anemia.[27, 28] Because Indians of the Hindu faith follow a vegetarian lifestyle for religious reasons, not health reasons, they have addressed widespread deficiencies with public health programs to supplement nutrients, rather than revert back to the diet their ancestors followed prior to vegetarian spiritual practices emerged 2,000 years ago.

There is, however, one health advantage of vegan/vegetarian lifestyles that has nothing to do with the absence of animal products, per se, but is due to favorable alterations in bowel flora from increased intake of prebiotic dietary fibers that nourish bowel flora, especially from legumes, since vegans/vegetarians typically consume plenty of legumes for protein. Omnivores can readily address this issue by simply increasing intake of such fibers—voilà: Problem solved.[29] (We will discuss this issue at length later; such fibers should not be confused with cellulose fibers in, for instance, bran cereals that provide stool "bulk"; truly beneficial fibers are *prebiotic* fibers that are metabolized by bowel flora species.)

Iron, vitamin B_{12}, omega-3s, vitamin D, and vitamin K_2—all are commonly deficient in the vegan/vegetarian lifestyle, telling us that there is something unnatural and incompatible with humans trying to survive without animal products. Vegans/vegetarians hate hearing this. While a vegan/vegetarian lifestyle is unlikely to affect your likelihood of death from cancer or cardiovascular disease, a lifestyle without animal products requires specific efforts to address nutritional deficiencies that develop and impair health but do not result in death. Departing from the lifestyle programmed into human genetics is a sacrifice best made for humane reasons, but it is on thin ice as a lifestyle adopted for health reasons.

followed by drugs that come to our "rescue," handily explaining why the diabetes drug industry is growing at unprecedented rates along with booming executive salaries.

The Undoctored solution? Eliminate foods that start the process in the first place. If we eliminate foods that send blood sugar and insulin to high levels, the entire collection of abnormalities reverse. We also slash fructose intake to only fruit—no high-fructose corn syrup or other sources. Yes, do the *opposite* of conventional dietary advice and eat no "healthy whole grains," don't restrict fats but *increase* their consumption, and never rely on low-fat or other fructose-containing foods.

While most people are able to reverse blood sugar and insulin levels back to normal, also undoing insulin resistance and diabetes, some people have progressed so far down this path and have irreversibly damaged beta cells of the pancreas that produce insulin (high blood sugars and high triglycerides damage the pancreas). People in this situation may not return to normal. This situation is suggested by failure to enjoy fasting blood sugars of 70 to 90 mg/dL after ideal weight is achieved and despite doing everything else right. Drugs may indeed be helpful in this uncommon situation. The key is to therefore follow this lifestyle *before* pancreatic beta cell damage sets in.

Let's now shift our focus to that of glycation. Glycation refers to the glucose- and fructose-modification of proteins that occurs when glucose or fructose levels increase, a reaction between sugar and body proteins. Glycation occurs at a natural low rate just from normal blood sugar levels, even while fasting, but it occurs at increasingly greater rates with any rise in blood sugar above 90 mg/dL.[30] Primitive people had limited exposure to sugars: seasonal fruit, tropical fruit in some environments, honey. They certainly did not have around-the-clock, everyday access to sweetened foods and soft drinks, nor were they advised by government agencies to load up on amylopectin-containing grains. It means that modern sugar consumption, made worse by the grain domination of the modern diet, exposes you to repetitive waves of protein glycation.

Once it occurs, the glycation reaction is irreversible. Glycation alters the properties of proteins, making them nonfunctional, essentially creating cellular debris that gums up the function of whatever organ they reside in, much like rust interferes with smooth functioning of the gears in a motor.

All of this has serious health consequences. If glycation of the proteins of the lenses of the eyes develops, opacities accumulate, leading to cataracts. Glycation of skin proteins gives you brown-colored "age spots" and wrinkles. Glycation of cartilage proteins makes cartilage brittle, eroding and leading to inflammation and the pain of arthritis. Glycation of kidney tissue leads to declining kidney function. Glycation of LDL particles in the blood-stream makes them more likely to contribute to atherosclerosis (heart disease). Glycation of brain proteins contributes to dementia. Those with diabetes experience high blood sugars throughout most of the day, therefore glycating more vigorously than the rest of us, explaining why, for instance, they have heart disease, cancer, cataracts, and dementia earlier in life than those without diabetes.

You may recognize the phenomena of glycation as sounding an awful lot like the phenomena of aging, reflected in the advanced glycation end-product, or AGE, theory of aging.[31] Yes: To a substantial degree, aging is a consequence of diet that proceeds faster due to sugars and grains, regardless of whether they are "organic," "sprouted," or any other label designed to pull your attention away from the sugar.

Any time blood sugar rises above normal, glycation occurs at an accelerated rate. What foods raise blood sugar the most, triggering the greatest degree of glycation? Grains and sugar. Gluten-free foods made with corn-starch, tapioca starch, potato starch, and rice flour are guilty of the same. And whatever you do, don't be tricked by talk of "low glycemic index."

Fructose follows a different set of rules. Ingested as, say, the high-fructose corn syrup in a soft drink or ketchup, it provokes the glycation reaction even without raising blood sugar, a stealth reaction that is difficult to detect. Even without the immediate rise in blood sugar, fructation—glycation by fructose—is *eight- to tenfold worse* than glycation by glucose.[32] And as with glucose-induced glycation, it is also irreversible.

The Undoctored solution is to stop overstimulating the processes of glycation or fructation in the first place by eliminating, or at least managing, all the foods that are responsible for these reactions. Removing the appetite-stimulating effects of wheat and grains via gliadin-derived opiates also helps bring the feeding frenzy of sugar in all its various forms to a halt.

We also amplify your chances of fully reversing insulin resistance with the Undoctored Wild, Naked, and Unwashed nutritional supplement program, to be discussed. Add it all up—minimize glycation/fructation, reverse insulin resistance—and you are equipped to reverse or prevent an impressive list of health conditions. You will age, but at the slow, natural rate that allows you to reach your eighth decade and onward without arthritis, heart disease, diabetes, and autoimmune diseases and with dramatically lower risk for conditions like cancer and dementia—with no sour taste in your mouth.

GOLDILOCKS AND
THE THREE GLYCEMIC FICTIONS

In the story of "Goldilocks and the Three Bears," Goldilocks found the "just right" porridge and bed before the bears returned to their cottage. With glycemic index (GI), we are advised that there is also a "just right"—but it simply isn't so. Behind every level of GI hides a big, bad wolf.

GI is a value that describes how high blood sugar rises after consuming a standard quantity (50 grams) of a given food. High-glycemic-index foods raise blood sugar to high levels, low-glycemic-index foods raise blood sugars to low levels, and moderate-glycemic-index foods would be intermediate.

It would be nice if it worked that way—but it doesn't. As occurs over and over again in nutritional thinking, we find that *less bad* has been equated with *good*. Just as the tobacco industry claimed that "lite" and low-tar cigarettes were healthier while they were, in reality, every bit as harmful, so it has gone in the world of glycemic index; there is no just right. Blood sugar works more like this: High-glycemic foods raise blood sugar to high levels, and low-glycemic foods raise blood sugar just a little bit lower than high-glycemic foods. (The same also applies to the related concept of glycemic load, in which portion size is factored in.)

The problem is not with the concept of GI. The problem lies in how the categories of high, medium, and low are defined: bad, a little less bad, a little bit more less bad—*none* of it good. Whenever blood sugar rises, even to the less high levels experienced with consumption of low-glycemic foods, it still yields insulin resistance, irreversible glycation, and weight gain, with blood sugar *highs* followed by blood sugar *lows* in 90- to

Tricks Are for Kids

Remember the Trix cereal commercials from the 1970s? "Ah, Trix, in raspberry red, lemon yellow, orange orange," the rabbit sings. The kids then chime in: "Silly rabbit. Trix are for kids!"

You all recognize what processed foods look like. They're the foods marketed with colorful packaging, sports figures, cartoon characters, and health claims like "heart healthy" or "low-fat." This is how the consumer's attention is diverted. And it's a huge financial success. The General Mills' Trix brand is still around as Trix and Trix Swirls breakfast cereals and as Trix Yoplait yogurt. Even the modern new and "improved" Trix breakfast cereal is made with corn, sugar, cornmeal, corn syrup, rice bran and/or canola oil, and colorings that, until recently, consisted of Red 40, Yellow 6, and

120-minute cycles of mental fogginess, fatigue, and hunger. A blood sugar of, say, 150 mg/dL after consumption of a low-glycemic food such as oatmeal does nearly the same damage as a blood sugar of 170 mg/dL after consuming a high-glycemic food such as a 16-ounce sugary soda. In this fairy tale, Goldilocks might as well eat all three bowls of porridge and sleep in any bed she chooses since the wolf will get her regardless.

From the glycemic index viewpoint, you will find that it is not until you get to single-digit GI values that you begin to have *little to no effect* on blood sugar. For ideal or total health, we can then view glycemic index as useful if the value is in the single digits, such as a value of 7 for peanuts or a 6 for hummus or zero for a piece of salmon, baked chicken, or avocado.

Your doctor might advise you otherwise, discounting the consequences of consuming anything with less than a high GI. But what she is really telling you is that having blood sugars after eating of 200 mg/dL or less is fine because you don't need insulin or medications to control blood sugar (the definition of "health" for physicians is generally based on whether or not you require medication, not on whether it is genuinely healthy or not). We know with confidence that blood sugars after meals of even 140 mg/dL— well within the range provoked by foods with low GIs—still cause all the same problems as, say, much higher blood sugars of 210 mg/dL.[33, 34]

As with the "healthy whole grain" message, the dietary community has misled the public by encouraging the consumption of low- or moderate-glycemic-index foods, failing to understand that this advice was little different than telling us to eat candy, ice cream, and cake.

In the world of dietary advice, fairy tales can indeed come true.

Blue 1, complete with "whole grain" emblazoned prominently on the package front.

Of the 60,000 products on the typical supermarket's shelves, only a handful are truly healthy and safe. It's a striking display of how, when misguided dietary advice and profit seeking converge, unhealthy foods proliferate, growing the profits of Big Food. It's our job to push aside the tricks and pick out the 1 percent of items that remain on our shopping lists.

Processed foods are landmines of sugar, high-fructose corn syrup, wheat and corn, hydrogenated oils, sodium nitrite, herbicide and pesticide residues, genetically modified ingredients with Bt toxin and glyphosate, bovine growth hormone, antibiotic residues, acrylamides, aspartame, synthetic food colorings, even arsenic. You can examine each and every label of the processed foods you pick up off the shelf and choose only those without

FRUCTOSE FEEDING FRENZY

While sugar in processed foods comes as sucrose, a 50:50 mix of glucose and fructose, it also comes as the ubiquitous high-fructose corn syrup, containing as much as 66 percent fructose. High-fructose corn syrup is the sweetener of choice among manufacturers, whether in low-fat salad dressing or Bloody Mary mix.

Fructose is the source of many of the problems of these sweeteners. While glucose, the same as the glucose of blood sugar, also has adverse consequences, fructose has greater potential to wreak havoc. This did not become clear until the processed food industry began loading up on high-fructose corn syrup, an inexpensive, cost-cutting, shelf-stable sweetener, putting it in virtually everything while not understanding the consequences, making you the human version of a fat lab rat. And as consumers got used to everything being sweet, it caused them to expect even greater degrees of sweetness, an appetite satisfied by increasing intake of high-fructose corn syrup—a vicious cycle, a feeding frenzy that even has kids desiring that everything be sweet and rejecting foods they should be eating.

Ironically, fructose was originally billed (and still is) as a problem-free sweetener because it did not raise blood sugar immediately following consumption. It was even thought to be the perfect sweetener for those with diabetes for that same reason. But more recent studies are clear: Fructose raises insulin and blood sugar dramatically, but the effect is *delayed by several days* (only prolonged monitoring uncovered the delayed effect). By an odd metabolic twist, liver processing of fructose causes an increase of triglycerides, which, in turn, trigger distortions in all other lipoproteins (fat-carrying proteins) in the bloodstream converting, for instance, large and benign LDL particles into small and heart disease–causing LDL particles. This means that fructose increases the particles in the bloodstream that lead to heart disease (despite fructose being a major ingredient in many "heart healthy" products, such as low-fat yogurt). Fructose also increases visceral fat, blood pressure, levels of uric acid (that lead to gout and heart disease), and inflammation, and it contributes to fatty liver.[35, 36]

In short, fructose is a lot worse than it initially appeared. Consuming it at the rate most people are consuming it—whether as sucrose, high-fructose corn syrup, other sweeteners, or even excessive quantities of fruit—is a death trap, a spinoff of the effort to reduce dietary fat that provoked a carbohydrate feeding frenzy. The Undoctored program therefore aims to minimize fructose exposure, reduced to that contained naturally in fruit.

such unwelcome ingredients, but there will be almost nothing left. It is testimony to the cleverness of Big Food that various combinations of wheat flour, cornstarch, inexpensive oils, sugar, food colorings, flavorings, and preservatives can be presented as breakfast cereal for kids, fiber-rich bran cereals, "heart healthy" products, ready-to-eat dinners, instant soups, granola bars, snacks, and thousands of other products, all created from the same ingredient list. By avoiding them, you are really just avoiding the thousands of variations on the same theme.

A better solution: Choose real, single-ingredient foods as close to their natural forms as possible. An avocado, for example, is just that: an avocado. How about olives, beets, pecans, blackberries, and pork chops? No aspartame, high-fructose corn syrup, or glyphosate here. Healthy foods can require some degree of processing, such as pressing to yield extra-virgin olive, coconut, and avocado oils; grinding nuts and seeds into meal or flour; and dehydrating foods like apples, onions, or beef. Benign forms of processing tend to leave foods and their components intact: The oil in olive oil is much the same as that occurring in olives, and dehydrated onions are just onions with the water removed. Whenever budget permits, choose organic, pasture-fed, and non-GMO certified foods to further minimize hazards. And avoid anything with a leprechaun or tiger or that goes snap, crackle, or pop.

Cooking, of course, is a form of processing. Cooking varies in its potential for introducing unhealthy effects while increasing the efficiency of digestion, as well as improving taste and texture. Aim for the least disruptive forms of cooking: steaming, boiling, baking, and sautéing, all relatively low-temperature processes. High-temperature processes, especially deep-frying, broiling, and—I hate to say it—barbecuing (i.e., direct exposure to the flame with charring), introduce unhealthy reactions in foods, much more so than the low-temperature processes, and they are best minimized.[37]

Though it may sound restrictive at first, you will discover that a bounty of wonderful, delicious choices remains. You will also find that a fascinating heightening of taste emerges with this lifestyle of grain elimination, such that foods you may have found objectionable in the past, like Brussels sprouts or broccoli, may now taste wonderful with explosions of flavor. And you will find that treats you craved in past are intolerably sweet. These phenomena help shape your new taste for food, and you will find that you actually come to prefer real foods over highly processed ones.

You will also find that you have little need for the inner aisles of the typical supermarket. Nearly everything you need will be found in the meat or butcher section, the produce aisle, and the dairy/egg refrigerator, the areas typically around the periphery. You may need to venture into the danger zone of processed foods when you need laundry detergent or dog food, but for the most part, you will have almost no need for those sections. Frequent farmers' markets and greengrocers that give you access to the best produce, including organic choices. Consider buying meats, eggs, dairy, and produce directly from farmers. This way, you avoid most of the advertising, prominent product displays, featured endcaps, and other methods grocers use to entice you into purchasing processed foods, as you will never see kale or radishes featured that way. But that is the nature of real food: no hype, advertisement, or deception required. No tricks here, silly rabbit.

Count Your Blessings, Not Your Calories

"Calories in, calories out." "A calorie is a calorie." "To lose weight, eat less and move more."

You've heard all these gems of conventional dietary wisdom aimed toward controlling weight. All share one feature: They are all untrue, misleading aphorisms that lead you to believe, for example, that 1,000 calories of doughnuts are the same as 1,000 calories of olive oil. When it comes to calories, I suggest you forget that you can count at all.

It is true that extremes of calorie reduction (e.g., starvation) will result in weight loss. It is also true that when the macronutrient (carbohydrate, fat, protein) composition of a diet is held constant but total calories vary, lower calorie intake can achieve weight loss (as well as create hunger and misery). But striking differences develop when the relative *proportions* of macronutrients within those calories are varied, so that a diet of 1,000 calories per day of one macronutrient composition may achieve the same weight loss as another diet of 2,000 calories per day of another composition.

Clinical research has already disproven the notion that all calories are equal. Studies have demonstrated that if calories are kept constant, slashing carbohydrates but leaving fat and protein results in substantial weight loss, while cutting fat that leaves a preponderance of carbohydrates and proteins results in either less weight loss or even weight gain depending on the number of calories. In other words, *carbohydrate content* is the variable that determines whether a dietary approach permits weight loss or not. When were such meticulous and confident studies first performed? In the early 20th century. That's right: We knew over 75 years ago that calories in/calories out is not entirely true, a calorie is not a calorie, and taking in fewer calories and burning more, while it works in the extremes, is not a practical path to weight control.[38, 39] These studies, impressively meticulous for their time, made some startling observations. In one British study, even when calories were limited to a near-starvation level of 1,000 calories per day, if those calories were 90 percent carbohydrate, weight would *increase*, while 1,000 calories as 90 percent fat or 90 percent protein would result in substantial weight *loss*. (A diet of pure carbohydrates, by the way, is also associated with extreme hunger, while a diet of nearly all fat is not.)

The differences hinge on whether or not insulin is provoked, and far less on the calories themselves. Carbohydrates, of course, oblige a vigorous insulin response, while proteins provoke a modest insulin response, and fat none at all. Insulin causes sugars (glucose) to enter cells and be converted to fat, while suppressing mobilization of fat from fat cells.[40] Foods that trigger insulin the most are therefore the most potent for weight gain, while their absence allows weight loss; the equation is quite simple.

The political shenanigans and misguided ambitions of a small number of people that led to legislating dietary fat restriction, along with advice to eat more "healthy whole grains," caused the lessons learned in these and other carefully conducted studies to be forgotten in the low-fat frenzy of the latter half of the 20th century. Public focus turned to cutting total and saturated fat to reduce cardiovascular risk, ignoring the inevitable increase in carbohydrate intake to satisfy calorie needs. This led to the astounding array of new diseases of our age, or at least diseases on a scale never before seen. Conditions such as morbid obesity; diabetes; uncontrollable hypertension; epidemic levels of dysbiosis (severe alterations of bowel flora); fatty liver (nonalcoholic fatty liver disease); male breast enlargement; endocrine disruption at the hypothalamic, pituitary, thyroid, adrenal, testicular, and ovarian levels; and arthritis of the knees and hips from excessive weight-bearing stress—all results of the dietary misinformation of the last 50 years.

The weight-loss advantages of cutting carbohydrates therefore needed to be relearned and have now been corroborated by modern clinical studies.[41, 42, 43] In study after study, eliminating grains and sugars via a low-carbohydrate dietary restriction while not limiting calories not only generated greater weight loss than other macronutrient manipulations, such as cutting fat, but also led to better cardiovascular profiles (higher HDL, lower triglycerides, reduced blood sugar and HbA1c). (Earlier studies comparing low-carb vs. low-fat diets *with calories restricted to low levels* failed to show such sharp distinctions, as reducing calories below that of physiologic need blurs the differences. But calorie restriction is difficult or impossible for the majority of people and therefore has limited practical relevance,

CARB-LOADING IS FOR
GRAIN-CONSUMING SISSIES

It's become a familiar scene at athletic events: sugar and carb-fests before and during marathons, triathlons, swimming competitions, and other sports among amateurs and professionals, even high school athletes and grade school soccer players. They do it for energy and enhanced athletic performance, having been told that loading up on carbs is the ticket to winning.

This common practice is based on decades-old flawed studies that reported that athletes experienced reduced performance when deprived of carbohydrates, performance restored upon restoration of carbohydrates. Thus was born the notion of "carb-loading" (i.e., consuming large quantities of grains and sugars prior to exercise to improve performance). That simple observation has since become a universal practice. It means runners have pasta feasts the night prior to a marathon in the United States, South African triathletes eat bananas and drink sugary energy drinks during workouts, and even aerobic-exercising mothers in Sydney, Australia, load up on energy bars prior to putting on their Spandex. It is common to see participants in athletic events gorging on pasta, fruit, desserts, and a mind-boggling variety of "energy" bars and drinks from sponsors. They then deal with the "wall" of low blood sugar that results after high blood sugar, as well as abdominal distress and diarrhea from the osmotic load created by the exceptional intake of sugar. (This is why dozens of Porta Potties are familiar fixtures along the route at these events.)

Contrary to popular perception, athletes are not impervious to all the problems presented by overconsumption of carbohydrates and sugars; they are just as prone to all the problems associated with both grain consumption and carbohydrates, such as provocation of autoimmune diseases, impaired digestion, high blood sugars, and the phenomena of glycation, and they are not necessarily spared the visceral fat–provoking effects, either, though their extreme exercise habits blunt it. (Go to any athletic event and you will see it: Easily a third of athletes, including serious athletes, are overweight.) The phenomenon of glycation alone can be responsible for prematurely deteriorating joints from cartilage glycation and cataracts from lens glycation, among other health problems.

A fundamental mistake was made in the studies that purport to prove

and it is also not necessary. Nonetheless, this does not stop critics of low-carbohydrate approaches to use these earlier studies as evidence that cutting carbohydrates carries no advantage.)

Factor in the peculiar appetite-stimulating effects of grains, effects from partially digested by-products of gliadin and related proteins.[46, 47, 48] Throw into the mix the exceptional capacity for grain amylopectin A to send blood that carb-loading is beneficial for athletic performance: If athletes who have relied to a moderate degree on grains, carbohydrates, and sugars are deprived of them, there will indeed be a decrement in performance upon their removal: reduced endurance; slowed running, biking, or swim times; and a premature feeling of fatigue. This is due to reliance on glycogen stored in the liver as a source for glucose sugar for energy. The glycogen supply in the liver is depleted after 40 to 60 minutes of high-intensity physical effort, and then the athlete will experience a marked reduction in energy and performance unless sugars are made available to replenish glycogen, accomplished via ingesting carbs and sugars. This phenomenon has been observed over and over again after depriving athletes of carbs and sugars for up to a week.[44]

What was not appreciated in these studies is that if carb and sugar deprivation is extended to 4 to 6 weeks, performance is restored and then *exceeds* that achieved during carb/sugar-consuming days (yes, athletes do *better* without carb-loading, though the effect is delayed due to peculiarities of human physiology).[45] This obligatory delay is due to the slowed conversion from glycogen-dependence to an increased capacity to mobilize energy stored in fat. While liver glycogen can provide less than 1 hour of energy for high-intensity exercise and forces the athlete to continually seek more sugars, body fat—even in a slender person with little excess body fat—*provides energy for weeks*. And the energy derived from body fat stores involves no loading up on energy drinks, energy bars, or pasta. It means just eating healthy and living off the, well, fat. And that's how humans have done it for millions of years, running for hours without such modern carbohydrate crutches. The capacity for long-distance running is built into human evolution without the need for sugary drinks or energy bars (though hydration and electrolytes are necessary).

It means that someone who expects to run, bike, swim, or engage in other prolonged, intensive physical activity will need to endure an obligatory 4- to 6-week period of reduced performance before things get better again, and often better than before. But it also means that you will no longer be exposing yourself to the destructive health consequences of carb-loading before and during demanding physical exertion, including fewer visits to the delightful Porta Potti.

sugar higher, ounce for ounce, than table sugar, with blood sugar highs inevitably followed by blood sugar lows with shakiness, mental cloudiness, and hunger, a 2-hour cycle that sets the poor grain-consumer in an endless 2-hour hunt for food. The combination provides a perfect formula for weight *gain*, effects that have caused me to accuse wheat and grains of being "perfect obesogens"—foods that are perfect for causing weight gain and obesity.

JAMI IS
UNDOCTORED

Louisville, Kentucky

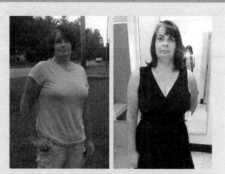

I have been overweight since my midtwenties. I'm 44 now. I've tried to lose weight for years and nothing would work, even long gym sessions.

I had chronic migraines, joint pain, muscle pain. I was always tired. I didn't want to get out of bed most days. A doctor diagnosed me with "chemical" depression and said the only way to treat it was with antidepressants. I was following conventional diet suggestions of more healthy carbs, low fat, and exercise. I couldn't lose weight no matter what I tried.

I developed carpal tunnel. In 2012, my back pain became so bad that I couldn't get up from a seated position. If I was lying down, I couldn't roll over and it took several minutes to get up. I was diagnosed with degenerative disc disease. I was taking gabapentin for my back, various pain medications for my other pains: over-the-counter migraine medicine, Advil, Tylenol, Motrin. I honestly felt like I was dying.

My hemoglobin was normally around 7 [normal is 12 to 15.5 g/dL; a level of 7 represents anemia]. I suspected an underactive thyroid, but my doctor said it was normal.

I only gave up gluten to begin with. I ate gluten-free foods that contained grains. I felt a lot better and started losing a small amount of weight. Within 3 weeks of cutting out all grains, I felt like a new person.

Eight months later, I'm 45 pounds lighter and off the medication. My mood has drastically improved. My hemoglobin is 11. I somehow missed taking iodine until a few months ago. That has made a huge difference, and I'm losing again. Iodine took my TSH from a 3.03 to a 1.5 [lower TSH (thyroid-stimulating hormone) levels reflect improved thyroid function]. I take vitamin D and magnesium. I try to always eat single-ingredient foods. I have also been able to cut out most of my allergy medicine. In previous years, I was taking two Zyrtec a day during the spring and one a day after that. Now I only take it occasionally.

I am a server at a restaurant, and I carry heavy plates and trays. I didn't have a lot of strength in my wrists and forearms, and I had a lot of pain. Now, I have more strength and all of my pain is gone. I have more energy, and I'm living my life again.

Despite the fact that I am telling you to *not* count calories or restrict portion size, when you remove grains from the diet while not restricting calories or fat, calorie intake drops effortlessly by 400 or more calories per day, often much more.[49] By removing sources of gliadin protein–derived opiates, addictive relationships with food dissolve, while the period between, say, lunch and dinner is no longer filled with anxiousness over the next meal. You will find that you rarely even think about food between meals. Hunger even *feels* different, a soft reminder that it might be a good idea to eat something, entirely unlike the desperate scramble that grain-consuming people experience. It is very common in this lifestyle to actually forget to eat. (I've lost count of the times, for instance, that I found myself just a bit hungry after several hours of working before breakfast in the morning only to realize that I forgot to eat dinner the night before.)

Calorie intake therefore drops effortlessly and naturally with grain elimination, and food intake reverts back to that of providing sustenance; you eat what you require, nothing more, nothing less. So calories in, calories—who cares?

Don't Have a Cow, Man

If there's a gray zone in this lifestyle, that's where you will find dairy products. It is an area that overlaps with the grain question, though dairy is not as bad—but remember: Less bad should not necessarily be interpreted as good. Dairy products can cause bothersome, though generally benign, issues like lactose intolerance, but they can also cause more serious illnesses, some irreversible, such as type 1 diabetes in children.[50] It does not necessarily mean that, like grains, we should wipe dairy products entirely off the menu, but it does mean that they should be consumed with caution. It is a group of foods that you can make an individual decision about once you grasp the issues.

Unlike the seeds of grasses for which there was *no* human precedent for consumption, there is a precedent for the consumption of the products of mammary glands, but from human breasts, not from bovines or other creatures. So it's not milk and related products that are new to the human diet; it's *nonhuman* milk that is in question.

Ironically, of all the uncertainties surrounding consumption of dairy products, the one component that is clearly beneficial with no health downside is the fat, the one thing that health authorities urge us to avoid or minimize. Fears over saturated fat and cholesterol content of cheese, full-fat milk, and butter we now recognize as unfounded. If there are problems with dairy, they originate with the proteins, sugar (lactose), processing manipulations, and the fact that the products of bovine mammary glands may be suited to the nutritional and hormonal needs of growing calves but not necessarily to adult, perhaps not even infant, *Homo sapiens*. To understand how and why dairy may or may not fit into the human dietary experience, as we did with grains, we need to go back and examine the history of its consumption.

The ideal human food for up to the first 4 years of life is human milk—not cow's milk, not goat's milk, certainly not soy milk or synthetic formula. The product of human mammary glands is perfectly created to meet all the nutritional needs of a growing infant and toddler (including hormones, antibodies for immune protection, and microorganisms and prebiotic fibers to populate the infant's gastrointestinal tract), not to mention the emotional bond. We know that young humans are well adapted to consuming the products of human breasts for growth and sustenance. Potential problems arise when we turn to milk from nonhuman breasts and continue to consume it beyond those first 4 years.

The consumption of mammary gland products from species other than humans coincides with the history of consuming the seeds of grasses. In addition to mimicking the grass-eating behavior of newly domesticated grazing creatures, we also used some of these creatures for their breast milk.[51] Domesticated cows, goats, sheep, and camels yielded milk that could be drunk, as well as provide skins and wool and serve as beasts of burden. As no refrigeration was available, a variety of fermented products emerged, such as cheese and yogurt, foods naturally modified by microorganisms that can be kept for longer periods.

Human adults did not naturally take to consuming the products of ruminant breasts, encountering difficulty with the lactose sugar after losing the ability to express the lactase enzyme after age 4, not to mention the formidable task of taking on the underside of a 1-ton female auroch with large, curved horns. Imagine trying to approach this creature and then harvest the milk from her when pregnant or while nursing a calf. (Full domestication of the males of the species also required castration—you've got to wonder how they figured this out—that made them docile and amenable to being put to work pulling a plow or load.)

Humans migrating from the Middle East to populate southern Europe acquired a gene mutation that allowed them to continue to digest lactose after the first 4 years of life and into adulthood by maintaining expression of the lactase enzyme beyond childhood. This single development, a mutation that first appeared among inhabitants from modern-day Austria or Hungary, provided a substantial survival advantage in that it opened up an entirely new source of calories.

Anthropologists now believe that this single development allowed dairy-consuming humans to gain an advantage over hunter-gatherer populations that did not consume dairy.[52] It especially yielded an advantage to children who sometimes suffered a calorie shortfall when weaned from human breast milk, now able to rely on an alternative food supply. Your ability to digest lactose depends on whether or not your ancestors developed that capacity. For example, 95 percent of modern people of northern European descent have the ability to digest lactose, but only 5 percent of people of southern African descent share such an ability.

Lactose intolerance can also be acquired through unhealthy changes in bowel flora, such as that developed with grain consumption.[53] Some people with lactose intolerance are able to consume small quantities of fermented cheeses, since the fermentation process reduces lactose to low levels. Raw milk products (i.e., unpasteurized and unhomogenized), however, do not seem to offer any advantages in this regard, contrary to many anecdotal claims implying otherwise.[54] Probiotic supplementation with the species *Bifidobacterium longum* and lactose-fermenting bacteria found in yogurt (with live cultures) may convert some people from lactose-intolerant to lactose-tolerant, at least sufficient to tolerate small to moderate quantities.[55] I've also witnessed reversal of presumed lactose intolerance after several weeks of wheat and grain elimination. And there are products with the lactose removed, so-called lactose-free milk, cheese, and other products, that simply sidestep this issue.

Beyond struggles with lactose, there are issues with the dairy proteins casein and whey and, to a lesser extent, alpha-lactalbumin and beta-lactoglobulin. (Casein comprises nearly 80 percent of dairy proteins, whey around 20 percent, with the others occurring in minimal amounts.) Over half of people who believe they have lactose intolerance actually have intolerance to some other component of dairy products, typically casein.[56]

Some of the struggles with casein originated with an unintentional shift in casein genetics in cows that appeared several thousand years ago following domestication with the appearance of a gene mutation coding for a form of casein called A1 beta-casein, different from the traditional form, A2 beta-casein, the form in human milk, as well. A1 beta-casein is common in cows in North America and Western Europe, where strains such as Holstein and Jersey have been selected over the years for their taciturn demeanor, but is not found in most cows from New Zealand and Australia or in sheep or goats. A1 beta-casein consumption has been linked to increased risk for type 1 diabetes in children, an effect suspected to be from a unique opiatelike compound (similar to, though weaker than, those in wheat) called BCM-7, a casomorphin, or morphinelike compound from casein.[57, 58] There is also worrisome evidence that such casomorphins from dairy milk are present at increased levels in infants with SIDS (sudden infant death syndrome), obtained by consuming an infant bovine dairy formula or the breast milk of a mother consuming dairy products.[59, 60]

It appears that at least a few of the problems associated with A1 beta-casein may be alleviated by only consuming dairy products containing A2 beta-casein. This would include goat and sheep products and A2-labeled dairy products from New Zealand or Australia. Because there is no practical way for a consumer to make the distinction outside of New Zealand or Australia, it means minimizing dairy products. An interesting trend has just gotten under way with some dairy producers who are working to breed cows expressing A2 beta-casein, such as Snowville Creamery in southern Ohio, which may expand choices in dairy. Fermented dairy products, such as cheese and yogurt, may be safer, as the casein is denatured, or broken down, by the fermentation process; this may reduce, but not entirely eliminate, problems from the casein.

The amount of whey protein in dairy—occurring in high quantities in whey protein powders, variable quantities in cottage and ricotta cheese, and lower quantities in fermented cheese (in which the whey is skimmed off) and ghee—poses some different challenges. Whey has the peculiar capacity to stimulate the pancreas to release insulin, as much as doubling its output.[61] Recall that insulin promotes conversion of sugars to fats in fat cells, while also blocking the mobilization of fat into usable energy. Higher insulin levels therefore facilitate growth of fat. For some people, this whey protein effect blocks the ability to lose weight, evident when all dairy products are avoided and weight loss ensues.

We also have to factor in changes introduced by modern production methods, issues that include use of bovine growth hormone (BGH) to stimulate milk production, long-term antibiotics to stimulate growth, homogenization, and pasteurization. BGH administered to lactating cows to increase milk production and extend the lactating period has been shown to increase mastitis, or udder infections, necessitating antibiotics more frequently and possibly playing a role in generating antibiotic resistance. Increased levels of the hormone IGF-1 have been documented in dairy products from BGH-treated cows that, contrary to the claims of the drug's manufacturers, survive human digestion and are suspected to increase risk of gastrointestinal cancers, as evidenced in animal models. In response to such criticisms, a growing number of major food retail chains are only selling dairy products free of BGH.

Let's face it: Cows are somewhat filthy creatures. Without showers, bath soap, or just a warm washcloth, their undersides can get pretty rough. There are natural risks with harvesting the fluid that emits from their udders, dangling from their bellies, swatting away flies and, in modern high-volume commercial operations, standing in paddocks of mud and feces. Pasteurization was introduced in the late 19th century to reduce the load of bacterial contaminants, such as listeria, the mycobacteria species responsible for tuberculosis, brucella, *Staphylococcus aureus*, and campylobacter, contaminants that flourish in the fertile medium of milk and dairy products, particularly during the delay introduced by delivering these products from farms to urban centers. Pasteurization involves heating milk to 161°F for 15 seconds, called "flash" pasteurization (labeled "pasteurized" on the carton), or at even higher temperatures for a few seconds, called "ultra-heat treatment" (labeled "ultra-pasteurized"), both effective for near-complete elimination of potentially pathogenic organisms.

Homogenization is the process of using heat and high pressure to reduce the size of fat globules that are naturally present in cow's milk, a process meant to prevent separation into a cream layer and improve digestibility, as well as to further reduce bacterial counts and extend shelf life. Homogenization is therefore primarily practiced for aesthetic issues and to allow dairy producers to remove fat to create the familiar 2 percent fat, 1 percent fat, and nonfat/skim products. Some people claim that both pasteurization and homogenization modify fat and protein structure, or at least bring dairy proteins casein and whey to the surface of the homogenized fat globules, which is responsible for undesirable effects such as increased allergy, though a blinded comparison did not bear this out and demonstrated no difference in perceived tolerability.[62]

The question that some people pose is whether some health benefits are sacrificed in the pasteurization and homogenization processes. Advocates of consuming raw milk argue that the grass-feeding practices of farmers willing to provide it (often via barter, since selling raw dairy products is illegal in many states) reduce the presence of pathogens while increasing beneficial bacterial populations in milk, such as lactobacillus, and providing improved nutrition and better taste and texture. The problem is that while risk of bacterial contamination, especially from grass-fed, pastured, non-high-volume family operations, is low, the consequences of infection can be devastating, especially in children who consume a greater quantity for their

(continued on page 156)

ISN'T THIS JUST THE PALEO DIET?

With all the talk about reverting back to the dietary roots of our species, some may ask: Isn't this the same as the paleo diet, the popular interpretation of diet prior to agriculture?

Well, sort of. First, put down that bone fragment you were digging with and let's grapple with a basic fact: You are a human born 10,000 years after the close of the preagricultural Paleolithic era, a period that dates back 2.5 million years—that is indeed true. The Undoctored lifestyle and the popular notion of a Paleolithic diet overlap substantially, but there are differences. So let's discuss the points of difference.

First of all, what I am not doing here is bashing the ideas promoted by followers of the paleo concepts. The ideas they follow are a damn sight better than conventional notions of healthy eating, and wonderful results can indeed be achieved on a paleo diet. Many authors from the paleo community are among my friends.

We both agree on this notion that reverting to the dietary habits and foods that molded us evolutionarily for 2.5 million years is logical, representing a return to habits to which our bodies have adapted. We both reject all grains, for instance, the biggest issue of all, given their relatively recent introduction 10,000 years ago. Bad enough if consumed in their natural state, the fiddlings of agribusiness made wheat, corn, and other grains much worse, so there are no points of contention here. We both also reject the use of refined sugar; sweeteners such as agave nectar and high-fructose corn syrup; oils such as corn, soybean, and canola; and highly processed commercial and genetically modified foods. So we agree on more than 90 percent of dietary issues.

But there are indeed differences. Let me list them item-by-item.

In the Undoctored approach, we limit digestible carbohydrates. In most popular versions of the paleo diet, carbohydrate/sugar sources like honey, maple syrup, and fruit are consumed ad lib. We limit carbs because the majority of people starting out on this lifestyle have type 2 diabetes, prediabetes, or some degree of insulin resistance. We limit carbs because a lifetime of drinking soft drinks and eating breakfast cereals and other sugar/carb sources may have damaged some of the beta cells in your pancreas that produce insulin; any more damage and you may lose control over blood sugars forever. We limit carbs because you likely have acquired inflammatory consequences of the modern diet, such as higher levels of inflammatory interleukins, tumor necrosis factor, and C-reactive protein, all of which contribute to heart disease, cancer, and dementia. We also limit carbs because your bowel flora is different than Paleolithic human bowel flora. This means that you digest carbs and other nutrients differently and struggle more with insulin resistance. (Perhaps this issue will recede as we get better at re-creating the bowel flora of primitive cultures in years to come.)

We limit carbs because we want to slow the deterioration of aging provoked by glycation since we live longer than Paleolithic humans (though it is a well-established fact that people in the Paleolithic era could reach old age, such as age 60 or older; but we live longer than that and hope to maintain optimal functioning until the end). Note that the worst form of glycation is fructation (i.e., fructose modification of proteins), which is 10 times more vigorous than glycation by glucose. This means that ad lib consumption of honey, maple syrup, and fruit—all rich in fructose—will accelerate development of cataracts, hypertension, heart disease, cancer, and dementia. (Nobody knows exactly where a safe level of fructose consumption falls, but it is likely low—no more than that contained in one medium-size apple, for example, or about 10 grams.) We also limit fruit because modern fruit has been hybridized for large size, sweetness, and reduction in fiber content to encourage consumption.

In my view, not limiting carbohydrates and sugars in a modern human is a big mistake for the above reasons. And these are effects that cannot be "worked off" by, say, running an additional mile or another 30 minutes of Zumba. Combining carbohydrate restriction with grain elimination is an exceptionally powerful way to address these issues.

Unlike the paleo diet, we include consumption of legumes and tubers, although we adhere to a strict carb limitation in doing so. You now know that consumption of these foods dates back more than 2.5 million years. Observations of the Hadza, !Kung, Yanomami, aboriginal Australians, and other hunter-gatherer people reveal enthusiastic consumption of tubers obtained by digging, at least seasonally. The fact that our intestinal lining is heavily dependent on the fatty acid butyrate (to be discussed later) suggests that the human digestive tract requires fibers that yield butyrate upon microbial digestion. Underground fiber-rich tubers, such as raw potatoes, and cooked legumes, such as beans and lentils, are rich in fibers that yield butyrate when bowel flora consume them. Denying yourself such prebiotic fibers by eliminating all legumes and tubers therefore guarantees that dysbiosis, or health-impairing distortions of bowel flora composition, will develop, accompanied by long-term deterioration in blood sugar, blood pressure, triglycerides, and even mental health and increased risk for colon cancer.

Unlike the paleo lifestyle in which all dairy products are shunned, in the Undoctored lifestyle, dairy products are conditional (i.e., we consume them on a limited basis and are selective). Because many dairy issues are "dose-dependent," meaning effects worsen with consumption of greater quantities, I believe that some people are fine consuming small quantities of dairy. Nobody is safe consuming unlimited quantities of nonorganic dairy, as it will invite issues with hormone overexposure, the insulin-provoking effect of whey, and immune disease–activating effects of A1 beta-casein protein. Fermented cheeses, yogurt, and kefir are among the least problematic, given the denaturation (breakdown) of casein and reductions in whey and lactose introduced by fermentation. Of course, only full-fat, organic cheese, yogurts, and kefirs should be chosen (or made yourself).

(continued)

ISN'T THIS JUST THE PALEO DIET? *(CONT.)*

Also, the butyrate contained in butter is a powerful anti-inflammatory and intestinal health–maintaining factor. Butter and ghee are also nearly entirely fat with little casein or whey proteins and are also among the more benign forms of dairy. But we've got to be careful with dairy: small quantities; organic; favoring fermented cheeses, yogurt, kefir, butter, and ghee.

There are other differences, such as with issues of saturated fat consumption and use of salt. I encourage consumption of saturated fat or at least discourage limitation, and I believe that higher levels of salt are perfectly safe, provided they are not the obscene levels obtained by eating at fast-food restaurants and drinking carbonated soft drinks that are responsible for intakes of over 10,000 milligrams per day. One of the difficulties with the paleo diet is that there are as many variations as there are proponents (there is no one paleo diet). Some limit saturated fat, others do not. Some limit salt, others do not. Some say oats, quinoa, and buckwheat are okay, others say they are not. Think of it: The Paleolithic diet of the African savanna was different from the Paleolithic diet of northern Europe was different from the Paleolithic diet of southeast Asia was different from the Paleolithic diet of the Amazonian basin, and so on. Rather than thinking about a "paleo diet," I think it makes more sense to ask: What was common among all preagricultural human eating habits regardless of location and climate? Several common behaviors emerge: All humans hunted and consumed the flesh and organs of animals, all consumed nongrass plants, all relied on some source of intestinal butyrate, and nobody consumed the seeds of grasses (grains). Nobody limited fat or saturated fat, and salt was something we needed and sought.

And, of course, in the Undoctored Wild, Naked, and Unwashed program, we do not just re-create the diet of primitive humans; we also work to restore nutrients lost by living modern lives, something not addressed in paleo diets. Failing to address nutritional deficiencies would be like getting your car washed and cleaned, with a new set of tires, but forgetting to change the oil and spark plugs; your car will not run correctly, even fail in time. Addressing the nutritional deficiencies of prior wheat and grain consumption, as well as other nutritional blunders, will take you yet another big step closer to ideal health.

body size. Consuming raw dairy products therefore requires knowing the farmer's practices, as well as accepting a small risk of serious health consequences. One study of 18 dairy farms using raw, unpasteurized milk found that half of the samples had detectable *Staphylococcus aureus* contamination from the animal's skin that persisted even through the process of making cheese.[63] The Centers for Disease Control and Prevention (CDC) reported that in the 13 years between 1993 and 2006, there were 4,413 illnesses,

239 hospitalizations, and 3 deaths attributable to tainted dairy products, 60 percent of which were due to consumption of raw, unpasteurized dairy products, mostly by children, contaminated with *Escherichia coli*, campylobacter, salmonella, or listeria, despite the relative rarity of raw dairy consumption.[64] Because organisms in raw milk differ from those in pasteurized milk, hospitalization from raw milk contamination is thirteenfold greater and often due to dangerous pathogenic bacterial strains, such as *E. coli* O157:H7, associated with kidney failure and death. A recent detailed survey conducted in Minnesota, where consumption of raw dairy products is legal if purchased at the farm, suggests that sporadic infections are more common than previously suspected, more common than the larger outbreaks tracked by the CDC; this analysis uncovered over 20,000 cases in the period between 2001 and 2010, with much of the underreporting due to occurrences within farm families consuming their own raw dairy products.[65] In other words, even knowledge of the cleanliness of the facility may not fully protect the consumer.

A recent compromise just getting under way involves a blending of pasteurized milk with the postpasteurization addition of one or more bacterial species believed to be beneficial, such as *Lactobacillus lactis*, which may provide health benefits and suppress pathogenic bacteria. This and similar efforts may gain popularity as the consuming public becomes comfortable with the notion of probiotic-like products.

As you can appreciate, the issues surrounding dairy are complex, vary with the source, and differ from individual to individual. If you choose to consume dairy products, make your choices organic; the animals were not fed genetically modified feed (e.g., Bt toxin corn and glyphosate-resistant soybeans and alfalfa), were more likely to have grazed on grass and forage, were not administered BGH, were less likely to have experienced mastitis, did not receive antibiotics (or less likely in Canada and the European Union), and have a healthier profile of fatty acids, meaning greater quantities of omega-3s, including linolenic acid, eicosapentaenoic acid (EPA), and docosapentaenoic acid (DPA)[66, 67] If you live in New Zealand or Australia, choose products with the A2 beta-casein form (generally prominently labeled "A2"); if you are in North America or Europe, look for manufacturers who are just beginning to respond to this issue—as consumer demand increases, supply will increase. Goat and sheep products eliminate the risk introduced by A1 beta-casein.

Should you consume dairy products? Obviously, if you have known or suspected lactose intolerance, you should not, or at least take some of the precautions discussed above that minimize this reaction. It is wise to always choose products that are organic and full-fat. Given the latest evidence, while risks are relatively small (though underestimated), raw dairy products are potentially hazardous with uncertain benefits, with some of the benefits likely obtainable via prebiotic fibers obtained from other foods (to be discussed later). And because they are almost entirely fat with minor quantities of protein (including A1 beta-casein), organic butter and ghee are among the most benign forms of dairy. With a margin of safety provided through fermentation, cheese and yogurts are also a reasonable compromise.

Bon Appétit

After this lengthy discussion of the dos and don'ts that set you up for a life Undoctored, you may be wondering just how you might navigate this lifestyle. You may also wonder whether, in order to reclaim control over health, you will have to sacrifice familiar and tasty foods you have come to enjoy—and then snatch up your hatchet or rifle, track wild game, and forage for edible plants and mushrooms while wondering whether there will even be a next meal.

Don't worry: None of this is true.

Even strict adherence to this lifestyle does not mean that you will have to resign yourself to a life of deprivation, jealously watching everyone else having fun and enjoying meals; plenty of tasty, healthy foods fit into this lifestyle while maintaining the use of modern conveniences. It means that you can have all the pizza you want on Friday night or a big bowl of ice cream topped with chocolate chunks and not worry about gaining weight, sending blood sugar sky-high, suffering through a case of heartburn or constipation, or any other health consequence. You can just eat and enjoy it. You will find that even foods formerly regarded as indulgent, such as cheesecake or chocolate, can, because we remove all unhealthy ingredients, become health foods—yes, cheesecake and chocolate as health foods. Cap'n Crunch and the Pillsbury Doughboy will no longer be there to keep you company, but you can still enjoy food just as much, if not far more, since you will be back in charge of appetite and enjoying the heightened taste sensitivity unique to this lifestyle. And you shall do so while reversing or preventing a long list of health conditions.

This lifestyle is therefore not restrictive; it is liberating. You will be liberated from the appetite-stimulating, willpower-destroying, blood sugar-raising, inflammation-provoking, weight-increasing, disease-causing effects of conventional foods, even many labeled "healthy," while getting closer and closer to a life free of disease and Undoctored.

Chapter Summary:
Your Next Steps to Becoming Undoctored

Part of the Undoctored way of thinking is to never accept "health" advice on blind faith. This is especially true of nutritional advice.

So much of what is passed off as modern nutritional advice is nothing more than industry marketing and/or stumbling misinterpretations of science. We therefore reject several cornerstones of modern dietary advice: We do not limit fat or saturated fat, we do not limit calories or portion size, and we do not subscribe to the "everything in moderation" falsehood when it comes to sugars. It also means that we need to reconsider what it means to be vegetarian, the carb-loading practices of athletes, what it means to be "paleo," and consuming the products of bovine mammary glands.

CHAPTER 8

From Herbs, Enema Bags, and Pliers to Apps, Smartwatches, and DIY Genetics

The first time I had an ECG e-mailed to me by a patient
with the subject line "I'm in atrial fib, now what do I do?"
I knew the world had changed. The patient's phone
hadn't just recorded the data—it had interpreted it!
A smart algorithm was now trumping one of
my skills as a cardiologist.

—Eric Topol, MD, author of *The Patient Will See You Now*

Buggy manufacturers were angry and befuddled as the appearance of horse-less carriages crushed their world, leaving them wondering if making better buggies might be the solution, until Henry Ford delivered Model Ts to the public for $400 each. People invested in the healthcare status quo will likewise be slamming empty operating room doors in anger as the newly empowered public realizes just how much health power it commands. I feel sorry for those trapped by conventional notions of health, continuing to believe that hospitals are benevolent institutions, drug companies have our best interests at heart, and doctors' pay is based on how good a job of healing they do.

MARILYN IS UNDOCTORED

Grand Rapids, Michigan

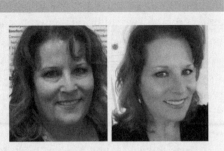

I'm the daughter of a grain farmer. We grew wheat, oats, and barley on our family farm. Homemade bread was part of every meal growing up. Mom could stretch the meal with bread and butter. Sauces were thickened with flour, baked goods welcomed us home from school, and we started our mornings with porridge.

Flash forward 45 years: My weight started to creep up, and I often had the sniffles and regularly succumbed to respiratory infections. My joints ached. Out of nowhere, my elbows starting hurting. In my fifties, I felt like I hit a wall. Weight loss was short-lived. I've counted points on Weight Watchers. I've choked down Nutrisystem. I've taken over-the-counter metabolism boosters. I followed Atkins and was cranky, hungry, and annoyed. My body ached for no reason whatsoever. I'd go through bursts of energy/feeling good, working out, and eating "right," including "heart healthy" whole grains. Then I'd hit a point of complete and utter exhaustion.

My pharmacist suggested thyroid medication and that helped somewhat. I woke up one morning to a muffin face, that tired, puffy, you-look-like-hell moment. Worse yet, I felt it. Going up and down stairs became painful. My wrists started to ache. I was restless at night. I was running on empty.

On January 3, I took the picture on the left. I started January 4, and the second picture was taken 10 days later. I felt a difference in 3. My skin is happy and less inflamed. My face literally shrunk. I lost 5.5 pounds and more than an inch off my waist. My eyes are brighter. I sleep like a tree. I have gotten off the albuterol rescue inhaler. After about 4 days, I found I was no longer a chipaholic. I no longer planned my dinners around what I could snack on later. After 6 days, I rarely felt hunger and my joints no longer ached. You eat real, delicious, yummy food—real, not out of a wrapper or box. I've made fettuccine Alfredo with spiralized zucchini noodles instead of pasta. Low-fat is a no-no on this way of eating—healthy fats are in.

My first picture is me living on grilled chicken in a whole wheat wrap, eating whole oats for breakfast, and sipping a light beer at night. My second is me eating salmon seared in coconut oil, sautéed vegetables, and grain-free cheesecake with a glass of wine! The transformation I see is from existing to living.

I share my muffin face to encourage you. Maybe, like me, you're sick and tired of being sick and tired. Maybe your weight is stuck, too. If I can do it, you can, too.

We now reach again into our make-believe black bag of health tools and come up with two additional components of your Undoctored program: nutritional supplements and home health tools.

The proliferation of nutritional supplements, while wonderful, has also soured many people because of sketchy science and false promises. We are going to take advantage of nutritional supplements, however, in an entirely different way: We don't use them to treat diseases; we use them to reverse the factors that allowed disease to materialize in the first place—a critical difference. Likewise, home health tools have boomed beyond anything you may have imagined, and awareness of them is going to make your life easier and health efforts more effective. *Undoctored* is not just promising to help you lose 10 pounds or loosen up arthritic joints; it is trying to free you from the bonds of conventional health care by restoring health from head to toe, a far more ambitious goal. So brace yourself for some revolutionary ideas that get you closer to a world Undoctored.

As recently as the early 20th century, nutritional supplements were unknown, although Coca-Cola containing alcohol and cocaine was gaining popularity as a treatment for headaches and "an invigorator of the brain." Information tools consisted of, at most, grandma's life experience and a handbook of home remedies, while home health tools typically meant a collection of self-gathered herbs, an enema bag, a mercury thermometer, and a pair of pliers to pull bad teeth. We are going to do far better than that.

Let's start by talking about how far nutritional supplements have come since little Johnny sat at the soda fountain to drink a 5-cent bottle of cocaine.

Nutritional Supplements: Wild, Naked, and Unwashed

A century ago, it became clear that foods contain factors essential for health that could be isolated and taken independently of food. It began with identification of thiamine (vitamin B_1) from rice husks, vitamin A from butter, and vitamin E in green vegetables. Some lessons got their start with dietary disasters, such as the epidemic of diarrhea, mouth sores, and dementia in orphanages and prisons during the early 20th century. First treated without success as a mysterious infection, it proved to be due to overreliance on corn, as corn lacks the B vitamin niacin, resulting in a condition called pellagra. All symptoms reversed with increased consumption of niacin-rich foods, such as meats, poultry, and fish, or taking niacin as a supplement.

The world of nutritional supplements has since exploded, and over half the US population takes at least one, if not dozens, of them.[1] Choices include those with relatively trivial benefits, such as multivitamins; powerful agents such as vitamin D, methylfolate, creatine, and probiotics; nonsense preparations that do little or nothing, such as chrysin and policosanol; and even a handful of supplements that are potentially dangerous despite their popularity, such as calcium, ma huang, and sitosterol. A quick stop at any health food store gives you an idea of the scope of products available, numbering in the thousands. Choices now include minerals, amino acids, cofactors, enzymes, hormones, herbs, and botanical preparations. Nutritional supplements have become nearly as broad and varied as prescription drugs.

Despite their popularity, "official" sources tell us that nutritional supplements are fraught with hazards and should only supplement a "balanced diet." According to the National Institutes of Health, "Dietary supplements are products intended to supplement the diet. They are not drugs and, therefore, are not intended to treat, diagnose, mitigate, prevent, or cure diseases."[2] It's an odd stand to take, as we know with certainty from the lessons of history that niacin *can* be used to treat pellagra, vitamin C *can* be used to treat scurvy, iodine *can* be used to treat goiter from iodine deficiency, and omega-3 fatty acids (EPA and DHA) *can* be used to treat omega-3 fatty acid deficiency, associated with dry skin, cardiovascular death, and dementia. And *nothing else can take their place.*

The "official" stand also means that iron supplements cannot be used to correct iron deficiency anemia or low ferritin (iron stores) levels. Nor can vitamin D be used to enhance memory, ameliorate seasonal affective disorder, or increase bone density, even though clinical studies demonstrate these effects. In other words, in an effort to draw a line between drugs and nutritional supplements, government agencies have, in effect, made the regulatory decision that drugs are the only therapeutic option for human disease, while casting nutritional supplements into the role of being nothing more than a complement to a "balanced diet." From a scientific and health perspective, not a regulatory viewpoint, this is obviously not just a misleading oversimplification but flat wrong—yet widely practiced by doctors.

What about the common warning to "talk to your doctor about the safety" of this or that nutritional supplement? The dirty little secret is that the majority of doctors *know almost nothing* about nutritional supplements and typically dismiss them offhand as useless, a waste of money, or dangerous, even belittling you for taking them. True to the FDA's stance, doctors view prescription drugs and medical procedures as the only effective solutions to disease, while nutritional supplements are fluff. Recommend a program of diet and nutritional supplements when a drug is available to accomplish something similar? Not a chance. Worse, doctors work in healthcare systems that have instituted "quality control" systems that penalize doctors for not prescribing enough drugs for conditions like hypertension or high cholesterol, with no allowance for dealing with health issues by other means.

This outdated regulatory attitude disempowers the public. Much more so than drugs, most nutritional supplements can be applied safely and effectively. This is because, unlike drugs, most nutritional supplements are normal components of human metabolism. Magnesium, for example, deficient in most Americans due to water filtration, reduces blood pressure, reduces blood sugar, and subdues abnormal heart rhythms when supplemented, and the effects are powerful because supplementation corrects the deficiency of an essential nutrient. Fibers such as inulin or fructooligosaccharides nourish species of gut flora in the human intestine, leading to powerful effects such as reduction in triglycerides and LDL cholesterol values, reduction in blood pressure, relief from gastrointestinal complaints such as constipation, and reduced colon cancer risk.[3] This strategy alone can help you avoid use of statin drugs, blood pressure drugs, and laxatives, while contributing to overall health without side effects and at minimal cost—but we are not allowed to claim that they "treat" anything.

Can nutritional supplements be therapeutic? Absolutely. Can they prevent disease? Yes, powerfully. Can they reduce pain, suffering, future debilitation from bone fracture, weakness, heart disease, cancer, and dementia? Without question. But these claims will be flatly disavowed by the FDA and by most doctors.

In addition to being effective parts of the solution to many health issues, nutritional supplements are generally benign and inexpensive, with only a few exceptions. Why not use such strategies as the default solution, the one we reach for first?

Not all the caution is misplaced, unfortunately. While lax FDA regulation stretched the definition of dietary supplements widely, it also encouraged unscrupulous companies to game the system with exaggerated, sometimes fraudulent, health claims and testimonials and other marketing deceptions to make you believe that you will be healthier, thinner, or sexier. We've all seen too-good-to-be-true ads and media reports about the newest weight-loss craze, for instance. Remember the hoopla over hoodia and green coffee bean extract? Neither of these supplements accomplishes much beyond falsely raising hopes and wasting money. There are also preparations with druglike names that have long lists of ingredients, many never or rarely encountered before. (I once had a discussion with a well-respected nutritional supplement–formulating biochemist who had designed hundreds of commercial preparations for national companies. At the time, he was formulating weight-loss meal replacements for a multibillion-dollar nutritional supplement company. When I asked him why I had never heard of many of the ingredients he used even though I prided myself on keeping abreast of such things, he admitted that they were nontherapeutic botanicals added to confuse the competition, not for consumer benefit.) The FDA recently clamped down on a weight-loss "supplement" called New You that contained the *drug* sibutramine (Meridia), which had been voluntarily withdrawn from the market by its manufacturer in 2010 because its use was associated with heart attack and death, and the laxative phenolphthalein, which was removed from the FDA's "generally recognized as safe" (GRAS) list because studies linked its use to cancer—all contained in this purported "nutritional supplement."

Caution, fraud, outrageous or unfounded claims, ignorant doctors—how can a nonexpert interested in health navigate such a tangle? Is it possible? Is it worth the effort?

It is most definitely worth it. On the flip side are successes like vitamin D. We were told for years that the few hundred units of vitamin D added to dairy products, along with modest intake of vitamin D from egg yolks and fish, were sufficient for health and there was nothing to worry about. "You don't have rickets, do you?" Anyone following the conversation of the last several years now understands that this advice was disastrous: Because of modern lifestyles, we need far more vitamin D for ideal health. Correcting vitamin D deficiency reverses the situation that allows depression, seasonal affective disorder, autoimmune diseases, arthritis, heart disease, cancer, and dementia. A "supplement" to round out a "balanced diet"? Not even close, as only trivial quantities are obtainable through diet. Vitamin D is a powerful therapeutic tool when managed properly. Take your "balanced diet" and toss it in the trash along with the food pyramid.

Despite the dark side of the nutritional supplement world, adding the right mix of nutritional supplements to your life can be life-changing. Some you can even make yourself, getting around uncertainties of purchased preparations. For instance, you can make your own lactate-fermented vegetables at home, which are packed with high counts of healthy probiotic bacteria, and you won't need to purchase expensive probiotic capsules for a lifetime (though we will use probiotics at the start for reasons discussed later). You can also make an excellent magnesium supplement at home, better than anything sold in stores.

Because the world is changing, our lives are changing, and our use of nutritional supplements needs to change along with them. Iodine is a perfect example. A trace mineral, iodine is required by everyone, or else peculiar effects develop that impair health. Up until the first half of the 20th century, 20 percent of people in North America (as much as 70 percent of children in parts of the Midwest) experienced iodine deficiency resulting in goiters, enlarged and disfiguring thyroid glands from lack of iodine, earning states like Michigan, Illinois, Iowa, Wisconsin, Ohio, and others the label "goiter belt."[4] This was not just a cosmetic issue but also associated with death from asphyxiation and mental impairment in infants born to iodine-deficient mothers. This was effectively solved through a successful public health campaign that encouraged salt-producing companies to add iodine to table salt, followed by public encouragement to use more salt. (The original slogan for Morton Salt was "Use more iodized salt—keep your family goiter-free!" years before "When it rains, it pours.") Over the latter half of the 20th century, with the public's appetite for salt stoked by such advice, overuse of salt resulted in negative effects in some people, and the FDA responded by urging Americans to cut back on salt and sodium. Many Americans cut back drastically on salt intake. The result: iodine deficiency, even goiters, both making a comeback. The solution: about $5 worth of iodine per year. Understand this and you are empowered. Yes, iodine can be a supplement to diet, but it can be so much more than that, particularly as habits change. But don't expect such life-changing health advice from your conventionally minded physician who just tells you to cut back your salt.

I am going to vastly simplify this world of nutritional supplements for you. I am going to focus on supplements that serve an existing human need, play a critical role in human metabolic processes, and are not foreign to your body, yet are commonly deficient in modern life and thereby allow numerous health conditions to emerge. These are the components of what I call the Wild, Naked, and Unwashed program, replacing nutrients that reverse an impressive list of problems by helping your body not allow such health problems in the first place. We won't treat type 2 diabetes, for instance, but we correct the nutritional factors that allow high blood sugars and insulin resistance to develop. That subtle but powerful distinction puts *you* back in control over your health. I call this "Wild, Naked, and Unwashed" because it re-creates the experience of wild-living humans who, despite not having high-tech OR suites or a drug for every condition, enjoyed freedom from virtually all of the modern diseases of civilization. These are nutrients that fit perfectly into the way that humans have lived for the last 2.5 million years; they are necessary for human adaptation and survival. You will learn how, for instance, vitamin D was a natural part of the lives of primitive humans—and thereby should be a part of yours, too—because they lived outdoors with plenty of skin surface area exposed to the sun, but you do not. You will also learn that vitamin B_{12} commonly becomes deficient following conventional dietary advice and can result in depression, irritability, and anemia but is easily restored by the Undoctored lifestyle. Or that because you cannot sip water from a stream or river flowing over rocks and minerals, instead getting your water from a tap or bottle, you need to get magnesium by another route.

I distinguish such Wild, Naked, and Unwashed nutrients familiar to your body that provide outsize benefits from those that are often used to "treat" a condition, such as turmeric for joint inflammation or aloe vera for gastrointestinal irritation, but do not fill a basic human need. You will find the first category of nutrients incredibly powerful, sufficient to help reverse numerous health conditions, and the second category of supplements used to "treat" conditions as helpful, but only in modest and limited ways. We are going to focus on the first category and only touch on some aspects of the second in this book.

As you can see, nutritional supplements play a crucial role in your self-directed health efforts. The ones we will be focusing on serve more than a "supplement to a balanced diet" role and, whether regulatory agencies like it or not, allow you to prevent or reverse a range of conditions that would otherwise have been "treated" using drugs or surgery. As you venture outside of our basic but crucial list of supplements in the Wild, Naked, and Unwashed approach, caution and knowledge will indeed be necessary as there are simply too many companies eager to sell products to you with overblown claims or ineffective ingredients. But there are also many excellent products and powerful agents to choose from. And remember: The advice for extreme caution from official agencies comes alongside advice such as "cut your fat and eat more healthy whole grains," some of the most disastrous advice ever offered in nutrition. Be skeptical of some of the claims that accompany nutritional supplements, but also be highly skeptical of advice from agencies purporting to be on your side.

And don't fall into the trap of believing that if supplements are so powerful, diet does not matter. As we will discuss, and as readers of my Wheat Belly series of books have come to understand, the foods you put or don't put in your body are not just important, but *critical*—though this often involves doing the opposite of conventional dietary advice. Nutritional supplements can be wonderful, but they cannot replace what you can achieve in health with food choices. Follow official advice in diet and your health can be ruined. Follow official advice regarding nutritional supplements, and you will be reliant on the healthcare system. Get the picture?

In Chapter 12, I will discuss the use of Wild, Naked, and Unwashed nutritional supplements that everyone should consider to reestablish a base of health.

Home Health Tools: Technology Comes to Self-Directed Health

Sensors ranging from wearable devices that measure health states to sensing tools embedded in our floors, computer screens, and cars are . . . transforming health measurement from an occasional activity performed in health care settings into a constant, passive activity performed anywhere and driven in large part by individuals and organizations not traditionally associated with health.

—The Institute for the Future

While grandma's version of self-testing might have included combing through her hair to uncover lice before rinsing her scalp in kerosene, our version of self-testing will be more advanced and hopefully not smell as bad. Our tools have progressed as much as a 1953 Studebaker has been replaced by an electronically equipped Tesla, perhaps more. (And kerosene doesn't kill lice, anyway.)

Technology is fueling the healthcare shift away from hospitals and doctors and into your kitchen, living room, bedroom, treadmill, and other personal spaces. While technology is not yet as omnipresent as described by the Institute for the Future quote at the start of this section, we're getting awfully close. Go to your nearest department store or pharmacy and you can purchase a home blood pressure monitor, blood sugar monitor, blood cholesterol monitor, body fat monitor, or blood oxygen monitor. You can wear a portable EEG monitor to manage stress. An assessment of cortisol hormone levels is just a few samples of saliva away, a full assessment of sex hormone status is obtainable with a finger-stick, and an assessment for thousands of single-nucleotide polymorphisms, or SNPs, that pinpoint genetic characteristics is available for under $200. You can quantify common, everyday activities such as tracking steps walked or calories expended, and then graph your activity on a tablet. With a smartphone, you can monitor sleep phases and identify sleep disorders, perform an electrocardiogram, distinguish normal heart rhythm from atrial fibrillation, monitor something called heart rate variability to assess emotional states and health, and assess and track nutritional intake. Smartphone and tablet applications (apps) for health crop up as fast as Bill Gates can say "the world is going mobile." The tools have all become available just over the last few years as microchips and other technologies have entered the consumer market and costs have plummeted. Can we put them to use to empower health easily, effectively, and safely?

I absolutely believe we can. We are able to apply such tools in unique personal ways, ways not typically used in conventional health care. Blood glucose measurements are, of course, commonly used by people with diabetes to manage blood sugars. With a slight change in the "rules" we follow, for example, an individual can use a personal glucose meter to reverse diabetes or to accelerate weight loss. You can monitor efforts to manage your spouse's blood pressure, track seasonal variations in blood vitamin D levels with a finger-stick, pinpoint factors responsible for recurrence of abnormal heart rhythms, and uncover anxiety triggers. Because your business is health, you will learn about unique applications of these tools that your doctor may not comprehend—but that's okay, because it means that you are heading in the direction of being Undoctored.

This brave new world of health tools has launched a movement called the "quantified self," reflecting booming interest in tracking individual health parameters. Though still the realm of nerds and early adopters, much like those camping out in front of Apple stores the night before the newest iPhone release, the number of people joining this movement, and the lessons being learned, are rapidly gathering momentum. Tap into the online conversations at Quantified Self (quantifiedself.com) to get an idea of some of the new and extraordinary observations emerging. Individuals from varied backgrounds—engineers, teachers, biochemists, college students, and the curious—apply self-observation and quantification to solve health problems in unexpected ways. People track a mundane but common problem area like blood pressure over time; import the values from their blood pressure measuring devices to their computers; graph the values; and then correlate them to various parameters, such as food choices, time of day, sleep duration, exercise within the last 48 hours, and stress levels—all leading to better control over blood pressure without medication. The information is shared and discussed, and new insights are obtained.

New applications are cropping up with astounding frequency. Scent expert Jenny Tillotson, PhD, for example, is applying insights from something called aromachology, the study of various scents on mood, to stress and mood management. She has helped propel this technology into a microchip-enabled process, having tested it on herself to gain better control over bipolar illness. She is pioneering the use of a device, coupled with a smartphone app, that delivers scents when the emotional need (e.g., stress) is biologically detected (e.g., cortisol stress hormone content of sweat), releasing scents known to have physiological effects, such as lavender for relaxation, sweet orange to reduce anxiety, or peppermint to stimulate wakefulness and attention.

A device called Muse (choosemuse.com) monitors brain waves with an electronic headband linked to your smartphone, generating visual and auditory feedback (e.g., waves on the ocean, chirping seagulls) reflecting your mental and emotional state. Although just another form of biofeedback, the use of this novel parameter (EEG) holds the potential to introduce some new personal insights into mood and mind management.

Surely, some of this is nothing more than a high-tech version of navel-gazing. But as more and more people engage in such self-observations, as the tools get better and the menu of measurable parameters expands, I believe that we will witness a wave of new and exciting uses for such devices.

The phenomenon of crowdsourcing is beginning to play a role in self-testing by collecting and analyzing data from large numbers of people to extract new lessons. The Parkinson's Voice Initiative (parkinsonsvoice .org), the brain child of Max Little, an applied mathematician at the Massachusetts Institute of Technology, has been recording voices of people affected at various stages of the disease to develop voice tools for diagnosis and to track improvement or deterioration. To date, it has proven astoundingly accurate at diagnosing the condition—99 percent—a dramatic improvement over conventional diagnostic methods, such as blood tests or MRI brain imaging. In other words, crowdsourcing of recorded voices, analyzed for specific features, now leads to a service that can become available to the public as a diagnostic and tracking tool. If a potentially better tool to track progress is available—inexpensive, painless, quantitative, and accurate—it holds potential to guide development of more effective and trackable treatments, whether conventional medical treatments or those implemented by individuals.

A direct-to-consumer genetic testing service, 23andMe has tested more than one million individuals, the "23" referring to the number of chromosome pairs carried by humans. Getting the test is as simple as providing a sample of saliva in a tube and then mailing it to them. Originally priced around $1,000, this test has bucked the rule of continually escalating healthcare costs and reduced its price—still direct-to-consumer—to less than $200. The service makes available, for instance, analysis for the factor V Leiden gene carried by 5 percent of the population that increases risk for blood clots. With your permission, the company also collects health data you provide, correlates specific genes to various conditions, and then reports new lessons learned. The power of these data has not gone unnoticed, with the company acquiring partnerships with universities, pharmaceutical companies, and biotechnology companies. Unfortunately, in November 2013, the FDA forced the company to cease reporting health and disease associations pending further review by the agency. But once the legal hassles have been sorted out, this approach appears to be among the most exciting catalysts to the personal concept of health, as genetic analysis is truly an individual concept—no other person has your unique genetic code. The power of such collective data analysis is being recognized by people like Sergey Brin, the billionaire cofounder of Google who carries the LRRK2 gene on chromosome 12 that substantially increases the risk for Parkinson's disease. Brin has called the pace of conventional medical research "glacial" and hopes that the new collective awareness of risk, coupled with Google-like rapid data collection, will yield answers at a much faster pace.

The company uBiome (ubiome.com) collects data on the human microbiome (i.e., the composition of microorganisms in the human gastrointestinal tract and other body sites) by providing direct-to-consumer testing of stool and other body sites. (The process is as easy as getting a swab of stool off toilet paper and inserting it into a tube.) Linda Avey, 23andMe cofounder, is contributing to this project that, like its genetic testing counterpart, correlates microbiome data with various health conditions. This service employs the same cutting-edge technology used in the Human Microbiome Project, the extraordinary government-funded project that has spawned many formal research projects and has made substantial contributions to understanding the human microbiome, especially bowel flora.

Direct-to-consumer blood tests are another category of empowering testing available to us. More people are becoming aware of the additional information available through such testing but not pursued by doctors—a huge swath of health measures that can yield health insights and solutions. Increased exposure to healthcare costs is also fueling the growth of home blood tests. It is common, for example, for lab testing of simple measures—such as cholesterol levels, complete blood count (CBC), and electrolytes—to add up to many hundreds of dollars and to now come directly out of your pocket. More advanced forms of testing can add up to thousands of dollars.

CAR BUYING, CT SCANS, AND CAVEAT EMPTOR

While the growing world of direct-to-consumer imaging is exciting with huge potential, it also has some potential hazards you should know about. Just as buying a new car means investigating the reputation of both the dealer and the car you are considering, so it goes with direct-to-consumer imaging services.

Be aware of what facility is offering the service and why. While most direct-to-consumer imaging services are offered by companies independent of hospitals in free-standing or mobile imaging facilities, even hospitals have gotten into the act, though they often view such services as "loss leaders" (i.e., low-cost services performed at no profit, even a loss, in the hopes that there is an abnormal finding that leads to further investigation and additional revenue). Doctors can also own imaging equipment, thereby double-dipping for both facility fees and professional fees, abuses that have sparked government and regulatory scrutiny. Be wary when a doctor recommends such testing.

Testing based on x-rays, such as CT scans, has the potential for radiation overexposure. This was one of the justifiable criticisms of the full-body scan, which was briefly popular a few years ago. The radiation required to scan the brain, neck, thorax, abdomen, and pelvis adds up to the equivalent of a thousand chest x-rays of radiation. Such radiation exposure adds to cancer risk, particularly on top of the other sources of medical and ambient radiation (e.g., flying in airplanes). Any radiation-based form of testing should therefore come with questions about radiation exposure. Radiation exposure is more important the younger you are, since activation of cancer generally requires decades to manifest. Newer technologies have also introduced methods that have dramatically reduced exposures, so it may pay to shop.

Medical imaging, whether applied conventionally or in our Undoctored approach, raises the issue of *unanticipated incidental findings,* the discovery of potential abnormalities that trigger further, often costly, some-

Curious thing: If you go to a lab and ask for the direct-to-consumer price, not the price charged to health insurance, it is typically much lower, often 70 to 80 percent less, since direct-to-consumer lab testing lacks the added layer of costs introduced by health insurance. As with other direct-to-consumer products, competition keeps prices low, unlike the prices charged to health insurance. It means that you can often *save* money by dealing directly with the lab.

The wide variety of health measures available through blood tests is among the most empowering Undoctored health tools. Knowing, for example,

times invasive, investigation. This is among the most criticized aspects of all forms of medical imaging. I have personally interpreted tens of thousands of CT heart scans, a simple test to measure calcium in the coronary arteries that indirectly quantifies the atherosclerosis present. In the typical heart scan image, the cross-sectional image shows the heart in the center and the lungs on either side of the heart. While the scan is designed to focus on the heart, it is not uncommon to see small masses in adjacent lung tissue in as many as 50 percent of people scanned. The vast majority of these are benign—scars from prior viral or fungal infections, etc.—with less than 1 percent representing early cancer. As a practical matter, any mass less than 4 millimeters in diameter is nearly always benign; a mass larger than 1 centimeter is more likely to represent a cancer.[5] This rule is often ignored, however, and many people are advised to undergo additional testing, such as a full CT scan of the lung (the different settings of this form of scanning expose you to the equivalent of approximately 300 chest x-rays of radiation, compared to 8 to 10 for the screening CT heart scan), or even a lung biopsy. As a result, many people undergo needless testing for benign findings, all in the hopes of identifying the rare early cancer or because of "defensive medicine." While heart scans can be applied in an Undoctored, self-directed mode to create a powerful heart disease prevention effort, they can also be used by imaging centers and doctors to profit from downstream testing. It unfortunately means that just about anything can trigger additional unjustified testing—and the healthcare system profits from the mistake.

Because of the variety of potentially abnormal findings that crop up on screening tests, each instance needs to be considered individually. The key here is to *never* accept advice to undergo additional testing for an unanticipated finding at face value and *always* question why it is necessary and the likelihood of genuinely abnormal findings. More often than not, you will discover that a watch-and-wait approach does just fine.

ESSENTIAL UNDOCTORED
HOME HEALTH TOOLS

In truth, the only truly essential tool you are going to absolutely need to navigate your life Undoctored is information and the Wild, Naked, and Unwashed strategies. But there are a number of tools that can expand your experience, yield new ways to assess and track health measures, and make it easier, more effective, and more fun, especially as your Undoctored ambitions expand over time. These basic tools will be discussed along the way in more detail later in the book. The sky is the limit in this brave new world of consumer health technology, but there are some basic tools that nearly everyone will find helpful.

Digital thermometer—This is not to take your temperature for a suspected fever but to get your basal temperature as a means of assessing thyroid hormone status. We will discuss later how an immediately-upon-arising oral temperature of 97.3°F suggests favorable thyroid status and how lower temperatures suggest common health- and weight loss-impairing hypothyroidism. Kinsa (kinsahealth.com) makes a smartphone-compatible device that allows you to store and track temperatures, although the device costs about twice the price of simple thermometers.

Finger-stick glucose meter and test strips—Even if you do not have diabetes or prediabetes, an inexpensive glucose meter and test strips are powerful tools that can be used to accelerate weight loss, reverse high blood sugars, and craft a more effective diet. You will be stunned, for instance, at the effects of foods that you were advised were healthy, such as steel-cut oatmeal.

that a deficient blood level of vitamin D explains your low bone density allows you to take action and follow the results of your program over time. Tracking triglycerides as you convert from a low-fat, grain-filled diet to an unrestricted-fat, grain-free diet—dropping from, say, an abnormally high 300 mg/dL to a wonderful 40 mg/dL—provides feedback on the effects of your diet. A test called hemoglobin A1c, an index of blood sugar fluctuations over a 3-month period, can track a decline from diabetic range to nondiabetic range or, conversely, show failure to achieve nondiabetic range, prompting you to intensify your efforts. We will discuss the use of selected lab tests as we go along in this book, with resources to obtain such testing—Undoctored—listed in Appendix D.

The world of direct-to-consumer medical imaging services has yet to experience the explosive growth witnessed in other areas, but it already includes self-ordered CT scans, ultrasounds, and MRIs, imaging studies

Nutritional analysis app—The easiest, most efficient way to manage your carbohydrates—the one dietary measure we track—is to have a smartphone app that provides two pieces of information: total carbohydrates and fiber per serving of various foods. (See Chapter 9 for a listing of apps.)

Blood pressure device—If you have struggled with high blood pressure in the past, then you should most definitely have your own device to monitor changes as you proceed through this program. Omron and BD make excellent devices. Look only for devices that take blood pressure on the upper arm, never the finger or wrist, as these are subject to excessive imprecision. Qardio makes a device, QardioArm, that takes upper-arm blood pressure and then transmits the information to your smartphone (getqardio.com). Withings also makes a similar smartphone-compatible device (withings.com). Smartphone-compatible devices also let you store, track, and review your blood pressure history, though they are pricier than standalone monitors.

There are many other new and exciting do-it-yourself health tools that suit specific interests or conditions, such as finger-stick test kits for assessing levels of thyroid hormones and progesterone and testosterone and a variety of biofeedback devices to help you relax or even reduce blood pressure, devices that you can explore but that are not required in this Undoctored approach. Our expanding world of self-directed health is sure to turn up some interesting opportunities to put some of these tools to use in the future.

that were only obtainable with a doctor's order just until a few years ago. As public demand grows, however, more services like these will become available, just like with any other consumer product, and they will most likely be priced far below the costs typically charged to health insurance. Here are some of the tests (with interpretation of results) that are directly available (accessibility varies from state to state depending on local laws).

- CT colonography imaging of the colon using a CT scanner to screen for colon cancer
- CT coronary imaging for calcium scoring that screens for and quantifies coronary artery disease, and CT coronary angiography for additional detail on coronary disease
- CT lung imaging to screen for lung cancer
- Bone density testing via CT, DEXA, and ultrasound

- Carotid, femoral, and abdominal aorta ultrasounds to screen for carotid atherosclerosis, atherosclerosis of the leg arteries (peripheral arterial disease, or PAD), and abdominal aortic aneurysms
- MRI scans of the brain, thorax, abdomen, pelvis, and joints

While you will find most Undoctored strategies straightforward and easy to navigate, direct-to-consumer testing is among the most complex with the greatest need for additional information, as well as guidance to avoid some common pitfalls (see "Car Buying, CT Scans, and Caveat Emptor," page 172).

Imagine your poor grandmother trying to sort through all the new health tools we now have available, compared to the crude methods of her day; she'd throw up her hands in frustration and go back to *Queen for a Day* reruns. Thankfully, most of you reading this book start with a more confident background in technology, online search, and social media, in which case diverting these capabilities into the service of personal health is just a matter of a little direction.

Your imagination in health may have been inspired by images like the tricorder Bones applied in *Star Trek*, the scan-and-heal device of *Elysium*, or maybe just by the prospect of enjoying health without the cold hands and indifference of doctors and the too-eager-to-get-your-health-insurance-card staff. Handheld, miniaturized, self-administered—we all share the same vision of health care as something far reduced in size, intrusiveness, and cost than what we currently have.

Undoctored and Unleashed

You may be Undoctored, but you are not unworthy or unequipped, given the new and extraordinary tools now available to you.

Pursuing Undoctored, self-directed health turns the tables on the healthcare process that formerly made you helpless and dependent on a system that, all too often, failed you, even exploited you. It exploited you because the rules were rigged: You lacked the information, did not have the means to collaborate with crowds of helpful people, did not fully comprehend the incredible power of nutrition and nutritional supplements when used properly, and were unaware of the impressive range of self-testing tools available to you. It was as if you had a wily car mechanic who took advantage of your lack of knowledge and tools at every opportunity—until one day you discovered that you have the entire repair manual to fix your car, dozens of friends willing to help you, and just about every tool you require. Go ahead: Pop the hood.

I hope that, by now, you have a grasp on what is possible in this new Undoctored world. As promised, I am not simply going to set you free to stumble around to learn all the lessons yourself. I am going to distill all the lessons into the Undoctored Wild, Naked, and Unwashed program. This is the part where you may want to sit at your desk unshaven, unshowered, in an untamed frame of mind—but probably wearing something more than a loincloth. After all, we've made *some* progress in a world capable of green tea and urban bike sharing.

Now let's get down to the nuts and bolts, the concrete, step-by-step efforts we take to be Undoctored.

Chapter Summary:
Your Next Steps to Becoming Undoctored

Part of being Undoctored is to be clear on what and how nutritional supplements can help yield health. We don't treat health conditions; we correct the factors that allow health conditions to appear in the first place. While it seems a minor distinction, therein lies huge potential to seize control over health.

The explosion of information and technology have made tools available that we can apply to our Undoctored health efforts, ranging from smartphone health apps to measuring and tracking devices to direct-to-consumer testing. It is no longer necessary to obtain the blessings of the doctor to engage in health; you can do it on your own—with *your* interests in mind.

PART III

Welcome to the world of health. I know that you are just starting out and that you've endured some tough (though I hope enlightening) conversations in the chapters up until this point. After all, you are taking on a new and unique role of healing—the real job of health care, or what it should have been all along. As you now know, you are not replacing the doctor; you are taking on much of the job that she should have been doing all along.

There will be no need for a white lab coat or fancy European car with vanity plates. You are not trying to intimidate, indulge a midlife crisis, or impress anyone. There is no need to learn Latin, as we'll conduct our discussions in plain English. There is also no packed waiting room, no billing department, no hospital-acquired infection here. There is only a desire to heal and to prevent future health issues.

You now know about all the moving parts that are going to go into this process. Let's now let the wheels hit the ground and gain some traction in this real world of Undoctoring, delivered to you as a 6-week program, the amount of time required to undergo some astounding transformations in personal health. Because so much of the Undoctored approach is built around nutrition, let's begin with food while weaving many of the other health-empowering strategies around this starting point.

After the discussion on food, I will detail the other strategies to follow, starting with how to restore healthy bowel flora and then going into the nutritional supplements that fit nicely into our natural framework to provide outsize benefits—altogether creating a level of health that you probably did not know was possible.

The 6-week, start-with-the-solutions-first Undoctored approach can reverse a long list of health conditions. Most people can engage in the basic Undoctored strategies and enjoy a life marvelously free of health problems, or at least with problems dramatically minimized. But some people will encounter only a partial response or have a condition that falls outside of the ones addressed by the Undoctored program, such as calcium oxalate kidney stones or a stubborn weight-loss plateau that refuses to break with even the most serious effort. I will address some of these issues in coming chapters, and there is an appendix that includes a list of Undoctored protocols, as well. The protocols contain suggested additional strategies outside of the core Undoctored menu to incorporate for each situation. Over time, I will be adding protocols for even more conditions, delivered via undoctoredhealth.com.

It's not about money, it's not about health insurance, it's not about pushing some revenue-raising agenda involving implants, catheters, or prostheses; it's about health. Imagine that.

CHAPTER 9

Eating While Wild, Naked, and Unwashed

Dirt used to be a badge of honor. Dirt used to look like work. But we've scrubbed the dirt off the face of work, and consequently we've created this suspicion of anything that's too dirty.

—Mike Rowe, *Dirty Jobs* on the Discovery Channel

tep into the room. Put the cell phone down; strip off the nice clothes and shoes; forget the advice given to you through TV commercials, dietitians, magazines, and various pyramids and plates; and bare yourself for what you are beneath the social niceties and makeup: You are a member of the species *Homo sapiens,* whose body operates as if you were still a wild-living primate, mostly hairless and unwashed, scrambling for survival. Your eyes and brain may know their way around a touch screen, but your liver and digestive tract have not made any technological leaps, still expecting foods and nutrients to which they have adapted. They are not bargaining for a huge flow of carbonic acid–infused cola with a year's worth of sugar in one gulp. They lack resources to deal with preservatives, herbicides, pesticides, emulsifiers, heavy metals, and industrial chemicals. Nor do your organs know precisely how to handle proteins from seeds of grasses, lacking digestive enzymes to break down unrecognized amino acid sequences.

We therefore eat foods that your body requires and is able to handle, breaking down nutrients into simple components that allow, for instance, the protein from a slice of bacon to be transformed into the proteins, enzymes, and building blocks for muscle and bone your body needs without provoking inflammation, autoimmunity, or damage to your intestinal lining. Eat to build and restore without a health or weight price to pay.

I am a big fan of simplicity, of boiling issues down to their essentials. It makes life easier, less cluttered. You will find that by eliminating wheat and grains, by not limiting fat or calories, by avoiding processed foods, and by gravitating to real, whole foods, many of the elaborate rules advocated in dozens of diets become unnecessary. We will not get bogged down with elaborate swaps, point systems, or dietary phases or other complicated rules. Once you grasp the essentials, everything falls in place. Health, weight loss, and freedom from prescription drugs follow naturally.

We've previously discussed the rationale for food choices. Let's now get down and dirty so that over the next 6 weeks of this program, you can begin shopping, cooking, and eating with Undoctored confidence.

De-Grain the Kitchen

Perhaps you've previously purged ants and cockroaches from kitchen cabinets, creatures that you don't want to discover scurrying in food boxes or underfoot on your nice clean kitchen floor. I'd like you to take the same approach with grains: De-grain the entire place right from the start. Just as you do not want vermin inhabiting your cupboard, you also do not want any seeds of grasses sitting on the shelves. Unlike insecticide you spray to eradicate varmints, there is no such grain killer to fumigate the home; you have to physically examine every item in your kitchen for evidence of grain ingredients, and then dispose of it.

Accomplish this in two steps. First, pitch (or feed to the birds or donate to a food charity) all obvious grain-based foods. They're easy to recognize: wheat-containing products such as pastas, breads, rolls, bagels, bread crumbs, frozen pizza and waffles, breakfast cereals, crackers, and pretzels; rye products such as rye bread or rye crackers; barley pearls or barley flour; corn products such as corn on the cob, corn kernels, grits, taco shells, cornstarch, and cornmeal; rice regardless of whether wild, brown, or white and rice cakes and crackers; and oats in the form of oatmeal, oatmeal cookies, and granola bars. On the small chance you've got any millet, triticale, sorghum, spelt, kamut, or bulgur, those need to go, too.

Second, look for foods with hidden grain ingredients. This is trickier because wheat and corn, in particular, come in some tough-to-recognize names. Panko, textured vegetable protein, and farro are all forms of wheat, and hominy, modified food starch, and zein are all forms of corn. (See Appendix B for a full listing. Don't try to memorize these grain aliases—just be familiar with the items on the list and don't buy a product if you are unsure.) You will be shocked at how many processed food products contain grains—frozen dinners, bottled salad dressings, dry salad dressing mixes, seasoning mixes, canned soups, instant soup mixes, candy bars, licorice— the majority of foods filling the aisles in supermarkets. And, yes, most beers—made from wheat, barley, and other grains—are off the list. (We shall discuss which beers and other alcoholic beverages are safe later.)

This may seem overwhelming, especially when you see the piles of food that need to be discarded, donated to charity, or given away to people you are not too fond of. But it is important to get this behind you without regret, not saving some of these items "just in case." A complete break will—like a cocaine addict no longer having access to her dealer—help free you of wheat and other grains. Remember, grains yield opiates that drive appetite and are responsible for addictive relationships to food. Stop eating zucchini and what happens? Nothing except having one less sliced veggie in a salad. Stop eating portobello mushrooms, pork ribs, or shrimp cocktail and what happens? A few holes in food choices for dinner—but nothing else. Stop eating wheat and grains and what happens? All hell breaks loose for about a week—an opiate withdrawal syndrome causing 5 to 7 days of misery, an issue we shall discuss in detail later. But like a drug addict who will do almost anything for another "hit," having a secret stash of cheesy crackers hidden in the hall closet can, as sure as real cheese does not come whizzing from a can, booby-trap any effort to purge grains from your life. Make the break complete.

The same approach applies to grocery shopping. Avoid obvious sources of wheat and other grains by steering clear of the bread, breakfast cereal, and baking aisles. But you also need to avoid foods that contain hidden grain ingredients. You will discover that most of the safe foods are found in the produce, butcher, and refrigerated dairy areas, sections that are, in most modern supermarkets, on the periphery, while aisle after interior aisle are filled with foods you should avoid.

This can be a costly venture at first as you replace the astounding number of products containing grains, the cheap filler passed off as a healthy staple. And because we gravitate toward higher-quality foods that are often

(continued on page 186)

HANG ON:
IT GETS WORSE BEFORE IT GETS BETTER

If you are like most people, you've been struggling with some combination of acid reflux, bowel urgency or constipation, unexplained fatigue, skin rashes, mood swings, anxiety, and a multitude of other undeserved and unexplainable symptoms, some of which you may "treat" with prescription medications. Remove the cause—wheat and grains—and you typically feel worse, not better, in the beginning. Does this mean that you actually *need* grains?

No, absolutely not. Just like an alcoholic who goes dry and misses his 16 shots of bourbon on Tuesday does not feel healthy and restored by Wednesday afternoon, you will also have to transition through a withdrawal/detoxification process before emerging on the other end.

I won't kid you: While this program is designed to yield the majority of health benefits within a 6-week timeline, the first week—7 days, 168 hours—may be distinctly unpleasant for about half the people engaged in this lifestyle. This is not your imagination; it is not from being "deprived" of carbohydrates or from cutting calories (which we most definitely do *not* do). It is from cutting off *gliadin protein–derived opiates* from wheat and related grains.

Recall that discussion? The gliadin protein of wheat and related grains cannot be completely digested by humans. Instead, gliadin is degraded to small peptides that bind to the human brain and stimulate appetite and provoke other mind effects. Remove it from the diet and an opiate withdrawal syndrome kicks in: nausea, headaches, fatigue, and depression that usually lasts 5 to 7 days, a tumultuous period that will make you question whether it is all worth it. When the process is over, it typically ends with a dramatic and perceptible wave of relief and a surge of energy and optimism.

If you have symptoms of joint pain, migraine headaches, or skin rashes, they can also worsen for the first few days of the detox/withdrawal from grains. Be prepared to take measures to deal with, for example, a flare-up of migraine headaches or joint pain, but understand that this is the process you endure to be freed of the disease-amplifying effects of grains.

There is no way to avoid enduring this process if you are among those destined to experience withdrawal symptoms. Accept it, live with it, but know that, like a bad case of the flu, it won't last forever. It will pass. As with a virus that causes fatigue, a runny nose, and a cough, there are measures you can take to soften the blow. Here's what you can do.

● Choose a low-stress time to begin. Don't begin the process, for instance, when you have an impending work deadline or final exams at school, as your performance will be impaired substantially. On the other hand, don't use this as an excuse to delay going grain-free indefinitely, as no period of life is entirely stress-free.

- Don't exercise. Just as you would not jog 5 miles when you have the flu, don't engage in anything more than casual activity while enduring detox/withdrawal from wheat and grains because you will feel awful. Casual activity is fine, such as a walk or light bike ride. But forget about your exercise routine for the week, and don't feel guilty about skipping it.

- Drink more water than usual. Part of the first week's process is water and salt loss in the urine. Someone who loses, say, 8 pounds during the first week has lost 3 to 4 pounds of water due to inflammation from grains. Fluid lost at this rate can leave you lightheaded. We therefore compensate by drinking more water than usual and by following the next piece of advice.

- Salt your food lightly. Failure to do so can leave you lightheaded upon standing, even cause you to pass out. Unless you have a serious medical reason to limit salt, lightly salt your food with a mineral-rich salt, such as sea salt.

- Pamper yourself. You are going to feel terrible, so get a massage or manicure, soak in the hot tub (but hydrate before and after), watch a funny movie, binge-watch a great serial drama. But don't reward yourself with a new outfit yet, as it is likely that you will be several sizes smaller in the coming weeks.

- Start the process with a spouse or friend. But don't tell people around you why you feel so awful, because they won't believe you. In fact, most people starting this process are skeptical that such a withdrawal syndrome occurs—until it does. But you won't get much sympathy from those around you who have not experienced it themselves. Grin and bear it, and know that it will pass. But it can sure help if you endure this process with a companion.

I cannot stress enough that it is important to recognize that this process is temporary and will not last forever. The unpleasant experience does not mean that you have done something wrong; you have taken steps to reverse a long-standing wrong and make it right. Nutritional supplements will be helpful during this period, also, which we will discuss in Chapter 12.

Another word of caution regarding exercise: You will find that running, biking, swimming, or other activities at high levels will be impaired—less endurance, longer times, slower speed—for another *4 to 6 weeks* after this process—well after the opiate withdrawal process is over. This phase is not due to gliadin-derived opiates. It is a result of the slow conversion from being reliant on liver glycogen (the storage form of sugar) from prior excessive carbohydrate consumption to becoming efficient in mobilizing energy stored in fat. Once this conversion is complete, you will experience a return of performance or even exceed prior levels of performance without carb-loading or sugary drinks or energy bars, because you will be able to draw virtually limitless energy from body fat, even if you are slender.

organic, free-range, or pastured, not bulked up with cheap processed ingredients, you will tend to purchase more costly foods. But don't be frightened by the expense: I will discuss why, for the majority of people, this lifestyle costs no more than your prior unhealthy lifestyle or even yields cost savings after the upfront expense to replenish your kitchen with healthy ingredients is out of the way, not to mention the cost savings from all the drugs you will not be taking.

And don't panic in fear that you will never have a slice of Italian pizza again or a chocolate cupcake or peanut butter cookie or that you will have to forgo birthday cakes for the kids. You *will* have them again, but re-created with healthy, nongrain ingredients and without sugar. There is, in fact, almost nothing we cannot enjoy as a nongrain, nonsugar, healthy counterpart to health-destroying grain- and sugar-containing foods, so we can still keep the kids happy, entertain friends, and continue with traditional dishes at holidays. Yes, you could don a loincloth, hunt and kill your food, dig in the dirt for the roots you need, and ignore modern conveniences—but most of you have no such intentions. Instead, shopping will be selective, and you will identify sources of new baking ingredients, such as almond and coconut flours. You will also learn how to make simple changes in cooking and baking methods, all to accommodate health.

Eat Wild, Naked, and Unwashed

Eat as if you were a wild human maintaining warmth under the skins of animals you've killed, not overly concerned with bathing or the length of your hair or toenails. And that is how your food should be, as well: wild, naked, and unwashed.

Food should be wild, naked, and unwashed in the sense that it should be as unchanged as possible from its natural state. Think eggplant, mesclun, pork chops, and walnuts, rather than boxed, cellophane-wrapped, or canned foods with preservatives, chemicals for color, synthetic flavorings, emulsifiers, and blending agents or foods packed in a foam container handed to you through a drive-thru window. Think avocado, salmon, asparagus, and eggs rather than dried soup mixes, frozen dinners, ramen noodles, or chips. Choose organic or even wild foods whenever possible to avoid herbicides, pesticides, and antibiotic residues that alter bowel flora and introduce hormonal effects that increase risk for breast and colon cancer. The more processed a food is, the less healthy it becomes.

Some forms of food processing are just fine, however. This includes cooking (particularly low-temperature cooking, such as boiling, sautéing, and baking), refrigeration, grinding, adding salt and spices, and fermentation.

Remember: Food tastes better once you undertake the process of grain elimination, so you will appreciate, for example, the rich flavors of beets or walnuts. You will also start to perceive the "off" and peculiar flavors present in processed foods, as well as the excessive sweetness that modern palates have grown to prefer, making it even easier to avoid processed foods containing lots of sugar and high-fructose corn syrup.

It is testimony to how highly processed our lives have become that returning to wild, naked, and unwashed foods seems so bewildering. Pretend you are your great-grandmother, unaccustomed to hand sanitizers and dishwashers, who would just pluck a ripe tomato off the vine and eat it, whose idea of handwashing was a quick wipe of the hands on her apron. Show her a plastic tube of yogurt, brightly colored, pasteurized, sweetened, emulsified, flavored, and she'd have no idea what it was. How about a cured piece of sausage or bacon, still bright red many weeks after it was made? That's the effect of sodium nitrite, a preservative associated with colon cancer. Anyone over the age of 60 would recognize that this is an unnatural condition, maintained only through use of chemicals, most unsafe for human consumption, despite the visual palatability. We therefore choose only uncured meats without sodium nitrite.

Return to the most basic forms of food you can find that avoid processing, pesticides, herbicides, preservatives, artificial colorings, and the rest. If you ate a wild blueberry off the vine, that would qualify as wild, naked, and unwashed. If you dug in the dirt for an edible root, brushed off the dirt, and ate it as is, that too would qualify.

Don't be overly concerned with making everything in your kitchen, such as dishes and utensils, excessively clean by using caustic cleaning agents. Inadequate hygiene was a major health problem until the 20th century when public health efforts such as public sewers and water treatment were introduced, reducing concerns such as cholera and dysentery. But the pendulum has now swung too far in the opposite direction, and we are obsessed with cleanliness. Excessive hygiene is part of the reason that modern humans are more susceptible to infections and experience more allergies and rashes, since we are no longer colonized by a wide variety of protective microorganisms. Excessive handwashing, caustic mouthwashes, hand sanitizers, antibiotics, and home cleaning agents don't just eliminate healthy organisms but also allow undesirable organisms to proliferate in their place.[1] Rinsing organic vegetables and fruits is still necessary, but do not view food as something that should be sterile. Note that including fermented foods in your lifestyle can partially counteract the effects of excessive hygiene by reintroducing healthy organisms, such as lactobacillus and leuconostoc found in sauerkraut and kefir. (We shall discuss the importance of fermented foods later.)

Yes, a life of playing outside, dirt, pets, washing dishes by hand rather than sterilizing them in a dishwasher, and not wiping the house down with chlorine or ammonia adds to health, though it may raise eyebrows among soccer moms bearing boxes of hand wipes. Keep your smartphone, but reject modern food processing and instead return to the wild, naked, and unwashed way your food and life were supposed to be.

Carb Countdown

Our first dietary undertaking, wheat and grain elimination, allows many other issues to fall in place without conscious effort. Most people, for instance, lose their desire for sugary foods and are no longer enticed by carbonated sodas or sweetened yogurt. We will not count calories or fat grams, as they essentially regulate themselves in the absence of the appetite-stimulating effects of grains. We do not resort to processed protein powders (except as an occasional convenience), as more than sufficient protein is obtained through fish, poultry, meats, and eggs.

But there is one component of diet we do count: carbohydrates. Modern dietary habits, flawed dietary advice, and processed food trends have conspired to send the carbohydrate content of modern diets sky-high, leaving the majority of people with various degrees of insulin resistance that leads, over time, to diabetes and other conditions. Carbs come in the form of sugars such as sucrose (table sugar), brown sugar, raw sugar, corn syrup, and high-fructose corn syrup; the amylopectin A of grains; and the amylopectin C of legumes (though a somewhat less efficiently digestible form compared to the form in grains). Carbs also come in forms that are often misleadingly passed off as healthy alternatives, such as honey, maple syrup, agave, and coconut nectar or coconut sugar.

To count carbohydrates, you will need a nutritional analysis app on your phone (see "Smartphone Apps for Undoctored Eating"), a handbook of nutritional analysis (available for around $10 in most bookstores), or one of the many Web sites offering this information to obtain the two pieces of information about any food in question: total carbohydrates and fiber per serving.

To calculate net carbs:

Net carbs = total carbs − fiber

We subtract fiber from total carbs because fiber, though counted as a carbohydrate in nutrition tables, is not metabolized to blood sugar by humans, so we can remove it from the total count. We maintain a net-carb

SMARTPHONE APPS FOR UNDOCTORED EATING

Let's face it: Eating should be low-tech. The healthiest populations on earth know from experience passed on from parents and grandparents what to eat, how to find it, and how to eat it. A member of the Yanomami tribes of South America does not need an app to help him decide how to eat the peccary or tapir he caught, nor does he need a table to tell him how much fat, protein, or carbohydrates to eat. Despite the fact that you are 99.99 percent genetically the same as the Yanomami hunter, the world in which you live is dramatically different. For that reason, you can use technology to navigate food safely.

There are many smartphone apps that serve as a convenient and portable means of looking up foods, all based on the USDA National Nutrient Database. However, we do not want apps that steer us toward low-calorie foods or that offer advice on cutting fat grams or that divert us down other dietary dead ends. The apps listed below provide nothing more than the basic nutrition facts you need, specifically the two values required to manage your carbohydrate intake: total carbs and fiber.

I also only list apps that allow you to vary serving size. For example, these apps allow you to change from 100-gram portions to 1 cup or other measures that suit your needs. All are also free downloads.

Nutrition Lookup by SparkPeople

Food Facts by FatSecret Platform API

Daily Carb by Maxwell Software

Calorie Counter and Diet Tracker by MyFitnessPal

There are also apps to help navigate restaurant food—such as Super Size Me by Morgan Spurlock (the same Spurlock who produced the documentary film *Super Size Me*) and HealthyOut (Rise Labs, Inc.)—that provide analyses of foods from hundreds of chain restaurants, from Au Bon Pain to Wings To Go. If you are trapped in the asphalt jungle one day or traveling and hope to stay on course, you might find one of these apps useful.

exposure of no more than 15 grams per meal. By not exceeding this threshold, you will have a greater chance of reversing insulin resistance, diabetes (type 2) or prediabetes, and inflammatory phenomena faster and enjoying faster and greater amounts of weight loss.

To illustrate, let's calculate net carbs for a medium-size Red Delicious apple. Look up total carbs and fiber in your app, handbook, or Web site and plug the values into the formula.

22 grams – 5 grams = 17 grams net carbs

Even if you ate only the apple and nothing else, you have exceeded the 15-gram-net-carb cutoff by a bit—but just enough to stall weight-loss efforts and raise blood sugar modestly. So eat only half, or buy smaller apples.

You will find that a net-carb calculation is not necessary for foods such as meats, poultry, fish, eggs, green vegetables, mushrooms, or full-fat cheeses, but it will be necessary for starchy vegetables, legumes, fruit (except avocado), nuts, and seeds.

Don't be intimidated by this effort. After calculating net carbs for a handful of foods over your 6-week program, you'll get the hang of it and soon know which foods are safe, which are not, without even having to make the calculation. You will identify what foods and how much fit into your lifestyle, while also realizing that you can consume unlimited amounts of foods with zero or low net-carb counts. Unlike the misguided glycemic index and glycemic load, managing your net carbs will give you extraordinary control over your metabolic fate.

Fat Makes the World Go 'Round

For the first 70,000 or so generations of human time on earth, nobody worried about eating fat on meat or organs. We ate it, we enjoyed it, and we saved it to cook other foods. And evidence of heart disease was rare.[2]

Then something caused us to veer off course in the 1960s, complete with terrifying catchphrases like "artery-clogging saturated fats." Saturated fats were replaced by polyunsaturated fats. Sales of margarine and corn and "vegetable" (a catch-all term usually referring to corn, sunflower, safflower, canola, or soybean) oils skyrocketed. We've since learned that margarines—polyunsaturated oils made solid by the process of hydrogenation—are the worst, yielding "trans" fatty acids that we need to avoid completely; absolutely no margarine fits into this lifestyle, regardless of claims such as "heart healthy" or "part of a balanced diet." Oils like corn and vegetable are hexane-extracted, mass-produced, obtained from suspect sources, and overly rich in the oxidation-prone omega-6 fraction of oils and should also not find a way into your cupboard. While consumption of seed oils until 1950 had been negligible, soybean oil consumption alone increased one-thousand-fold—a very unnatural situation.

OMEGA-6 FATTY ACIDS: TOO MUCH OR TOO LITTLE?

Foods containing plentiful corn oil, canola oil, soybean oil, and other seed oils send omega-6 (linoleic acid) intake ten- or twentyfold higher than it should be. Such high intakes of omega-6 fatty acids contribute to inflammation, depression, heart disease risk, and developmental defects in children, particularly if combined with low levels of omega-3 fatty acids, EPA and DHA, and linolenic acid—a common situation. Intake of such oils has increased so much that the linoleic acid content of fat cells has tripled.[3]

Avoiding processed seed oils helps bring omega-6 intake down while you restore omega-3 fatty acids with fish consumption and fish oil supplements and include some linolenic acid–rich foods, such as walnuts, chia seeds, flaxseed, and pasture-fed meats. Unfortunately, some people have interpreted this advice to mean *absolute avoidance* of omega-6 fatty acids—but that is flat wrong. In fact, if you were to engage in complete avoidance of omega-6 fatty acids, you would get ill and eventually die. This is because omega-6 fatty acids are *essential* (the human body cannot make omega-6 fatty acids). Lack of omega-6 leads to skin rashes, impaired immunity, and impaired growth in children because they are needed to perform critical physiological processes. So it is foolhardy to avoid all omega-6 fatty acids.

So we don't want omega-6 *overload*, but we also don't want omega-6 *deficiency*. Once omega-6-heavy seed oils are avoided, modest consumption of the seeds themselves, such as sunflower or pumpkin; walnuts and other nuts; chia seeds; flaxseed; and meats provides a healthy intake of omega-6 fatty acids while not tilting the scales toward overload (just as humans have done it all along). Consume no grains and no processed seed oils while eating whole foods like nuts, meats, and vegetables and you do not have to count omega-6 fat grams or any other measure, as it simply takes care of itself.

Down the road, if you are not confident that you are maintaining a healthy balance of omega-6 and omega-3 fatty acids, you can measure your own omega-6:omega-3 index with a finger-stick blood test that you can do yourself at home, such as the one by OmegaQuant (omegaquant.com/omega-3-index/). An ideal omega-6:omega-3 index is 2:1 or less.

We are going to embrace fat again and completely ignore any concerns over total fat or saturated fat content—absolutely avoiding any food labeled "low-fat." The fats that we are going to embrace are the fats that grandma and her predecessors would have enjoyed. We will choose fats such as lard and tallow (provided they are not hydrogenated, if store-bought), coconut oil, palm oil (look for sustainably produced brands), extra-virgin olive oil, avocado oil, cocoa butter, and organic butter and ghee. We will avoid corn, sunflower, safflower, cottonseed, rice bran, grapeseed, canola, peanut, soybean, and "vegetable" oils. We will also avoid any oil that is hydrogenated or partially hydrogenated, as well as margarine. Linolenic acid–rich oils, such as flaxseed and walnut, are somewhere in between—use them, but don't rely on them excessively (as they also contain substantial omega-6 oils).

Eat Until You're Satisfied

That's a bold statement—eat until you're satisfied—in a world in which just about every nutritional authority tells you the opposite. But conventional advice was created by the uninformed to deal with appetite-stimulating opiate effects from wheat and grains. Minus wheat and grains, appetite recedes dramatically, and calorie intake drops off without effort. There will be no mad scrambles for food due to overwhelming hunger, no sneaking ice cream in the middle of the night, no hidden snacks around the house. No one will be anxiously counting minutes until lunch or dinner. There will be no rolling, rumbling stomach growling and gnawing at your resolve. You will be largely indifferent to food, hunger nothing more than a gentle reminder that it might be time to eat something. You will even forget to eat at times, unconcerned if you miss a meal. You'll find the previously daunting prospect of fasting—not eating at all—effortless. (You will also begin to recognize the manipulative nature of the constant barrage of food advertising, all meant to further fuel the insatiable appetite created by wheat and grains, advertising that you will increasingly find incomprehensible.)

Compound this with the appetite-satiating effects of unrestricted fat intake, and you will find that you feel satisfied even without trying. Eat fat on pork, purchase high-fat ground meat (never lean), cook with lard or bacon grease saved from breakfast, eat egg yolks with the whites, and add organic butter and coconut oil to anything and everything, from morning coffee (whipped with an immersion blender) to smoothies. And while everyone else at the office nervously eyes the clock for lunchtime, you decide to go for a walk. They shamelessly pounce on the bagels and doughnuts while you walk right past them to enjoy the fresh air, trees, and birds.

Many people, so accustomed to *not* following dietary rules, ask questions like "How much fat can I eat?" or "How much food intake should be protein?" You are going to find that these are unnecessary concerns. Banish all wheat and grains, avoid added sugars, manage carbs, don't limit fat, eat unprocessed food, and everything else falls in place.

The key factor here is to not just *not limit* healthy fats and oils but also consume *more* fats and oils. The greater your fat and oil intake, the more appetite is suppressed, the more blood sugar drops, the more insulin resistance reverses, the more weight is lost—and, no, you do not develop heart disease.

You will find that if there is a struggle here, it is to get the fat you need in a world focused on cutting fat, with restaurants, for instance, serving lean cuts of meat and low-fat dairy products. I had dinner with my daughter, a tennis pro, recently while she was on the road for a tournament. I suggested she order the rib eye steak as the fattiest cut of meat on the menu, typically a well-marbled cut. When the steak arrived, the chef had cut it into cubes and trimmed off all the fat, essentially removing the healthiest part of the meat. Make it a point to get the fat, and don't let them cut it off or use low-fat replacements.

Don't worry: You cannot overdo healthy fats. Understand that the widespread advice to cut dietary fat sets you up for health and weight-loss failure. Just give it a try: Eat a fatty cut of beef or pork, fattier than usual, and see what happens to hunger. I'd be shocked if you had room for dessert. I'll bet your first response to hearing the details of this lifestyle was to declare something like "I can't do this. I can't just cut out entire food groups!" I hope that you now appreciate that, first of all, they weren't meant to be food groups for humans in the first place. Second, cutting out fats that satiate sets you up for health and weight failure. Go completely against—yes, the grain—of conventional health advice, and you will be empowered in extraordinary ways.

Hors D'oeuvres Are Served

Here we go, now serving little bits and pieces of nutritional wisdom to help you navigate modern nutritional choices.

(continued on page 196)

DRUNKEN MONKEYS:
ALCOHOLIC BEVERAGES AND HUMANS

Robert Dudley, PhD, a professor of integrative biology at the University of California, Berkeley, has observed numerous examples of "inebriated baboons" and "sozzled chimps" drunk from consuming fermented fruit. He measured alcohol content of overripe fruit in the wild, finding levels as high as 8 percent (alcohol by volume), similar to levels in beer and some wines.[4]

So humans are not alone in enjoying a cold beer or margarita. Alcohol consumption among baboons and chimps reflects a universal phenomenon among large primates, exposed to alcohol whenever ripe or overripe fruit comes within reach. Putting alcohol-avoiding Mormons, Muslims, and fundamentalist Christians aside, alcohol consumption is found in virtually all cultures, dating from times that precede humans walking upright. Bolstering the alcohol-as-natural for primates argument is the recent discovery that the common ancestor of gorillas, chimps, and humans developed a gene mutation (ADH4) 10 million years ago that increased the ability to metabolize alcohol.[5]

Alcohol consumption is therefore programmed into human physiology, and having a glass of wine or cognac fits into the Undoctored back-to-our-roots lifestyle. But because modern alcoholic beverages come from a variety of sources and many are considerably altered from their original state, you will have to be selective. Poor choices can have real consequences, such as provoking return of an autoimmune condition or sending blood sugars sky-high. Recognize that any amount of alcohol over a single serving can also stall weight loss.

Of all alcoholic beverage choices, wine fits most naturally into our lifestyle. As fermented foods are the product of bacterial fermentation to lactic acid, wines are the product of yeast fermentation of fruit sugars to ethanol (alcohol), a process as natural as overripe fruit. The driest (least sweet) are the best: dry reds such as pinot noir, malbec, merlot, and cabernet sauvignon and dry whites such as pinot gris, chardonnay, and sauvignon blanc. Be very careful with sweet wines, such as sauternes; ice or dessert wines; and sweet ports, as more than a sip or two and you will be tangling with messy blood sugar issues.

The majority of ales, beers, malt liquors, and lagers are brewed from grains and contain measurable grain protein residues, generally 1 to 2 grams per 12 ounces—not a lot, but enough to provoke effects such as stimulating appetite and inflammation and initiating autoimmunity. People with celiac disease or the most extreme forms of gluten sensitivity should avoid beers except those designated gluten-free. Likewise, those of us trying to escape the health effects of grains should also avoid these beers. Gluten-free beers made from sorghum, rice, buckwheat, millet, or chicory are available but tend to be moderate to high in carbohydrate content; more than a single bottle or serving and you exceed the net-carb cutoff. While sorghum, rice, and millet are grains (buckwheat and chicory are not), the low quantity of proteins seems to not provoke reactions in people without extreme gluten sensitivity. Among alcoholic beverages, beer is the most hazardous, so be careful. If you must have a beer, here are some of the least problematic ones.

Bud Light—Anheuser-Busch Bud Light is brewed from rice but also contains barley malt. So the most severely gluten-sensitive should not indulge because of the gluten content. But most of us just avoiding grains without a gluten sensitivity can safely consume these beers without exposing ourselves to the undesirable effects of grains. One 12-ounce bottle of Bud Light contains 6.6 grams of carbohydrates.

Redbridge—Redbridge—brewed from sorghum and not with wheat or barley—is gluten-free, though still brewed from a grain. Carbohydrate content is high at 16.4 grams per bottle; just one and you have exceeded the carb cutoff. Go carefully with this one.

Bard's—Brewed from sorghum without barley, this beer is also gluten-free. It contains 14.2 grams of carbohydrates per 12-ounce bottle, so more than one and you exceed our net-carb cutoff.

Green's—Green's, a UK brewer, provides several gluten-free choices made from sorghum, millet, buckwheat, brown rice, and "deglutenized" barley malt. They are not grain-free and thereby have low quantities of grain proteins. So go carefully here, also, and make judgments based on individual experience. Carbohydrate content of these beers is a bit less than most others, ranging from 10 to 14 grams per 330-milliliter bottle.

Glutenator—From the Epic Brewing Company in Salt Lake City, Utah, this beer is gluten-free, brewed from sweet potatoes and molasses, with 16 grams of net carbs per 11 ounces. My unskilled beer palate detected just a hint of the sweet potato coming through, but it still tasted much like conventional beer in flavor, similar to what I remember ales to be like.

Omission—These beers are brewed from malted barley with the gluten removed and are available in an IPA, a lager, and an ale. I tasted the IPA and thought it was too syrupy, but perhaps those of you looking for a heavy-bodied beer might like these.

SPIRITS

Spirits are a mixed bag, but you are likely to find at least several that you can enjoy without provoking health problems. Beware of flavored varieties of vodka or rum, as they are loaded with sugar and/or high-fructose corn syrup. In general, simple unflavored spirits are safest.

Vodkas brewed from nongrain sources, including Chopin (potatoes; outside of North America you will have to ask or examine the bottle for the source as there are also wheat and rye vodkas from Chopin) and Cîroc (grapes), are safe. Recently, many more vodkas are appearing on the market brewed from grapes, quinoa (not a grain), potatoes, and other sources, though not always nationally distributed.

Brandies and cognacs are generally safe since they are distilled from wine. Safe brands include Grand Marnier, Courvoisier, and Rémy Martin. There are exceptions, such as Martell, that add caramel coloring (a potential grain exposure).

(continued)

DRUNKEN MONKEYS:
ALCOHOLIC BEVERAGES AND HUMANS *(CONT.)*

Gins are likewise safe, brewed from juniper and other herbs.

Rum is distilled from sugarcane and therefore does not contain residues of grain proteins (and the sugar is fermented to alcohol).

Whiskeys and bourbons are, like most beers, distilled from rye, barley, wheat, and corn and thereby potential problem sources. However, given the distillation process, whiskeys typically test below the 20-parts-per-million limit for gluten that the FDA set as the safe threshold for people with celiac disease and gluten sensitivity. Nonetheless, some people still seem to react to whiskeys distilled from grains. It means that many popular whiskeys— such as Jack Daniels (barley, rye, corn), Jameson (barley), and Bushmills (barley)—can potentially cause a gluten (gliadin) reaction. People without extreme sensitivities are likely safe, though, given the very low quantity of grain proteins.

Liqueurs that are safe include Kahlúa (dairy), fruit liqueurs like triple sec and Cherry Kijafa, Disaronno (amaretto-flavored), and Baileys Irish Cream (dairy). The most gluten-sensitive may need to avoid liqueurs blended with whiskey. Also, liqueurs tend to be high in sugar, so small servings are key.

Avoid Processed Meats

Sausage, pepperoni, bacon, salami, ham, and deli meats contain the preservative sodium nitrite that upon cooking reacts with proteins in meat, yielding nitrosamines that have been linked to gastrointestinal cancers.[6, 7] This is a confusing issue that is often misinterpreted. For instance, nitrates, a closely related compound, occur in green vegetables and are converted into nitrites, or NO_2, in the body to nitric oxide, a beneficial compound that reduces blood pressure and yields other health benefits. This has caused some to dismiss the issue of nitrates and nitrites. The problem is not the direct ingestion of nitrites or nitrates but when the heat of cooking causes nitrites to *react with the meat* yielding nitrosamines, such as N-nitrosoproline and N-nitrosothiazolidine, and other compounds that cause gastrointestinal cancers in experimental models and are associated with cancers in humans.[8, 9] Nitrosamine exposure also occurs with cigarette smoking and is responsible for effects such as insulin resistance and nervous system damage.

Choose meats that are processed naturally without sodium nitrite, often containing nitrates that do not react to form nitrosamines in meat. Also avoid meats (particularly sausage and deli meats) that contain wheat, corn-starch, and other hidden grain ingredients.

No Sacred Cows

We discussed in Chapter 7 how the products of the mammary glands of cows—dairy products—have issues and that the choice to include them in limited quantities or exclude them should be made on an individual basis, since some people can consume dairy in limited quantities without any speed bumps along the way, while others develop serious, even irreversible, health problems. Understand the issues we've discussed and be empowered to make the right choice, but understand that it has *nothing* to do with fat or other common dietary concerns.

Should you choose to keep dairy products in your life, be sure to choose organic whenever possible, as organic dairy products have reduced estrogen content, don't contain bovine growth hormone, and are less likely to contain antibiotic residues. Also, fermented dairy products—such as cheese, yogurt, and kefir—are safer due to the process of fermentation, which modifies (denatures) casein structure and, at least in cheese and Greek yogurt, reduces whey and lactose sugar content. Readers living in Australia or New Zealand have the added choice of dairy products with A2 beta-casein (A2 dairy), a less harmful form of casein. Yogurt, kefir, and cheese can also serve as healthy sources of probiotic organisms for bowel health.

Sweeten Food Naturally and Safely

We avoid sweeteners with unhealthy consequences: sucrose (table sugar) and fructose-containing sweeteners including corn syrup, high-fructose corn syrup, and agave. And we minimize honey and maple syrup, as well as raw sugar, coconut nectar, and other sugar products meant to conceal the fact that they are still sugar.

We obtain sweetness by using safe *natural* sweeteners that have little to no downsides. Our choices of safe sweeteners are pure liquid or powdered stevia (avoid those bulked up with maltodextrin, which is essentially sugar under a different name), monk fruit (also known as lo han guo), inulin (which also has the benefit of prebiotic properties, to be discussed later), erythritol, and xylitol (be careful around dogs with xylitol, as it is toxic to them). The *Wheat Belly Cookbook*, the *Wheat Belly 30-Minute (or Less!)*

Cookbook, and the *Wheat Belly Blog* (wheatbellyblog.com) are all sources of plenty of grain-free recipes that put such sweeteners to work when needed. These natural sweeteners allow us to re-create foods such as cookies, muffins, cakes, and other goodies to serve during holidays, when entertaining, and to kids. Conversions to equivalent quantities of sugar vary widely with each sweetener and brand, so consult the label on your choice of sweetener to calculate a sugar-equivalent conversion. Note that an occasional person experiences a "sweet tooth" effect (i.e., driving appetite for sweets) even with these natural sweeteners, but it is uncommon. If you are among the few who do, then find solace in the satisfaction provided by fats and oils, not sweeteners.

Salt Your Food

You should no longer be surprised that "official" advice is not just ineffective but actually *causes* health problems. Advice to strictly limit salt is no different. In a surprising turnaround, that advice has recently been retracted in light of clinical studies demonstrating *increased cardiovascular death* with sodium restriction to levels below 1,500 milligrams per day (yes, another example of conventional dietary advice being no different than something like, "Smoke a pack of cigarettes a day for lung health"). Nonetheless, the Institute of Medicine stands by its advice to limit sodium to no more than 2,300 milligrams, or about 1 teaspoon, per day, advice meant to avoid water retention caused by too much salt.

Average sodium intake in the United States is 3,400 milligrams, which is a perfectly fine level for those of us following a wheat- and grain-free lifestyle—not too high, not too low. You will likely observe, for instance, during your first week of beginning this lifestyle that weight drops and leg and facial edema reverses—reflecting loss of excess water caused by prior grain consumption, as well as fat. If you *fail* to lightly salt your food, you can become lightheaded, even passing out upon standing. We therefore break the "rules," rules that are different for those of us engaged in this lifestyle. Advice to strictly limit salt is useless, outdated, and dangerous, and advice to limit salt to 1 teaspoon per day is also unnecessary and counterproductive. We simply follow a commonsense rule: Lightly salt your food. Light to moderate use of the salt shaker to sprinkle mineral-rich forms of salt, such as sea salt, is actually healthier than severely restricting salt, particularly when combined with healthy foods rich in potassium (vegetables, avocados, coconut). Begin this habit during your initial detox/withdrawal experience and continue for a lifetime.

There are problems, however, with unlimited salt use, as in eating heavily salted foods and foods from fast-food restaurants and drinking some carbonated soft drinks; salt intakes as high as 10,000 milligrams or more per day are associated with adverse cardiovascular and bone health effects. Also, there is a minority of people who have sensitivities to salt and should

IF YOU START WITH DIABETES OR HIGH BLOOD PRESSURE . . .

The Undoctored nutritional program is so effective at reducing blood sugars and blood pressure that anyone with diabetes (both type 1 and type 2) will have to reduce their insulin or oral medication *immediately* upon starting, as you want to avoid hypoglycemia at all costs. High blood sugars are a long-term threat, but low blood sugars, or hypoglycemia, are an acute danger, so we avoid episodes altogether. Cutting insulin in half in the first 24 hours is a common way to avoid hypoglycemia. The oral drugs glipizide, glyburide, and glimepiride, in particular, are oral agents that are most likely to result in hypoglycemia; doses will need to be reduced, preferably even before you begin to make dietary changes (since the drugs can exert effects for many hours). If you take multiple diabetes drugs, the combination can also result in hypoglycemia if you do not reduce doses.

Likewise, people with high blood pressure can experience lightheadedness, even passing out, if the doses of their blood pressure medications are not reduced right away. Some drugs—such as the beta-blocker class that includes metoprolol, carvedilol, propranolol, and nadolol as well as the drug clonidine—cannot be stopped but must be "weaned," or reduced gradually, to avoid a withdrawal process. Other drugs can be reduced or eliminated (typically one at a time) without a weaning process.

In either situation, you will need to work with your doctor to reduce or eliminate medications and do so safely. Don't be surprised if you encounter resistance or are advised that what you are doing is silly or dangerous; after all, the doctor was likely the one who prescribed the drugs in the first place, entirely unaware of the power of the Undoctored strategies. If your doctor refuses to work with you, find one who will.

Also, note that the other strategies that I will be discussing further reduce blood sugars and blood pressure, and additional reductions in dosages or elimination of prescription medications will be required. This is the process you must go through to undo the unnecessary doctoring in your life, another big step toward your life Undoctored.

not engage in unrestricted salt intake, such as people with kidney disease or heart failure. In these situations, a sodium prescription should come from your doctor (though you may have to educate her about the revised sodium guidelines).

Consider Fermented Foods

Fermented radishes, cucumbers, and onions are among the many delicious and healthy ways to add some exotic spice to your vegetables while obtaining healthy quantities of bacteria, such as *Lactobacillus plantarum*, that benefit bowel health. (Fermented foods are wonderfully easy to make yourself; see Appendix C.) Fermented foods can be eaten as is, added to salads, or dipped into hummus or salsa. Fermented milk or coconut milk as yogurt and kefir provide delicious variations for breakfast, desserts, or snacks. Given the constant onslaught of factors that can distort bowel flora, fermented foods provide a "reseeding" effect for healthy bowel flora species. Eating a fermented food at least once per day is a terrific habit to develop, and it introduces no additional cost since you make them yourself.

There Are 6 Weeks between You and Being Undoctored

Six weeks, or 42 days, is what it takes to be confidently on the path to being Undoctored while you release your wild inner primate. As you now understand, some peculiar things happen in the first week, with additional changes unfolding in the ensuing days and weeks. But 6 weeks will pass before you confidently look in the mirror and declare, "I'm not the same person I used to be" or "The health problems I had 6 weeks ago are almost completely gone" (although, for some people, that statement can be made even within the first few days).

Besides the initial week or so of detoxification/withdrawal we've discussed, the timeline of the Undoctored experience plays out something like this.

WEEK 1: Weight loss begins within the first 48 hours for the majority, a combination of fat loss and diuresis (i.e., loss of water previously retained because of inflammation). Symptoms of acid reflux/esophagitis, the bowel urgency of irritable bowel syndrome, and sleep improve by the end of week 1. Joint pain in the fingers, wrists, and elbows also commonly improve in this early period. People with mood problems—such as depression, irritability, anxiety, and suicidal thoughts—will usually find partial or total relief by the end of the first week. Appetite drops over the week due to the removal of gliadin protein–derived peptides.

WEEKS 2 THROUGH 4: Many inflammatory phenomena recede during this period, such as joint pain in the knees and hips, asthma, and skin rashes, especially eczema and seborrhea. Energy ramps up during this period (although exercise capacity for serious athletes will not return until 4 to 6 weeks have passed). Migraine headaches and severe premenstrual syndrome pain and bloating typically start to recede in this period. People with severe chronic constipation (obstipation) will also generally begin to experience more normal bowel movements (when combined with efforts to restore healthy bowel flora, to be discussed later). People with autoimmune conditions—such as ulcerative colitis, Crohn's disease, celiac disease, rheumatoid arthritis, and psoriasis—typically start to experience improvements during this period and onward.

WEEKS 5 THROUGH 6: It takes this long for the human body to regain its full capacity to draw energy from fat stores, rather than from the limited sugar energy stored in the liver as glycogen from prior excessive carbohydrate intake. Athletes can resume high levels of exercise after this period and will commonly experience higher levels of performance—faster running and biking times, greater weight handled, etc. Improvements in autoimmune disease symptoms continue and will likely proceed further even beyond the 6-week period of this program. Most people with type 2 diabetes and hypertension will be on far fewer medications at lower doses at this point, most on their way to becoming free of these conditions.

While most autoimmune issues begin to respond in the first several weeks of this program, improvement generally continues over a more extended period of months, sometimes years, with additional relief compounded by efforts including vitamin D restoration and cultivation of bowel flora. Neurological conditions, such as multiple sclerosis and peripheral neuropathy, are the slowest to respond, as nervous system tissue is slow to heal. Timelines for response of neurological conditions can extend to years, so patience and continued commitment are key.

Experiences vary, of course, based on age, severity of health conditions at the start, genetic factors, commitment—but know that by drawing from the wisdom of primitive but time-tested experiences, wonderful things can happen in your life.

MIKE IS UNDOCTORED

St. Paul, Minnesota

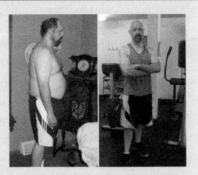

This has made a huge difference in my life.

After severely injuring my back in December 2013, I ballooned up to 299 pounds from an already heavy 265 pounds by April 2014. I decided I had to do something and dropped 50 pounds the "old-fashioned way"— lots of small meals, plenty of whole grains, and *tons* of willpower. Of course, like many times before, I could only keep this up for so long, and the weight started coming back.

After gaining back 8 pounds, I happened to see you on TV. After 5 minutes, you had me convinced. I lost 100 pounds in 361 days and 117 pounds overall. I have kept it off over a year with the exception of the 8 pounds of muscle I've gained by adding some weight training. Also, I am off acid reflux and cholesterol medications. I've avoided fusion surgery on my back from weight loss and health gains. I still have pain, but it's manageable and no surgery.

Thank you, Dr. Davis, for teaching the truth about what it truly means to be healthy!

You Can Put Away Your Ax

If you're like me, the experience to draw a knife across the throat of an animal to eat its organs and muscle seems foreign and grotesque, and most of us would not look forward to rising in the morning then digging up the bulbous root of a plant to bite into. There are indeed people who recognize how perverse modern living and diets have become and take to the wild to hunt and forage. But I imagine that the majority of Undoctored readers prefer the comfort and safety of modern life, have families and careers that they wish to maintain, and have no interest in a *Return to the Wild* adventure. Then how do we re-create this primitive but essential need called "diet" in a world of brightly lit supermarkets, trendy restaurants, and Internet groceries?

We tackle that question next, followed by recipes with ingredients that provide tasty foods—like pizza, muffins, and cookies—with no health downsides.

Chapter Summary:
Your Next Steps to Becoming Undoctored

In order to organize your kitchen and eating habits to follow the Undoctored lifestyle, start by doing the following:

- De-grain your kitchen of both obvious and hidden sources of wheat, rye, barley, corn, oats, and other grains.
- Eat real, whole foods—what I call eating Wild, Naked, and Unwashed.
- Limit net carbs to no more than 15 grams per meal. Use a smartphone app, a nutritional analysis Web site, or an old-fashioned carb-counting handbook to manage your carb intake.
- Embrace fats. Get over your fat phobia instilled by decades of useless dietary advice.
- Eat until you're satisfied—because we *never* limit calories.
- Choose alcoholic beverages that fit into the Undoctored lifestyle if you are going to indulge in a drink. Use the list provided in this chapter to avoid backpedaling on the health progress you make with these changes.

And don't forget that the first week of living the Undoctored lifestyle can be unpleasant, given the opiate withdrawal/detoxification process many people have to endure before they start feeling fabulous.

CHAPTER 10

Wild, Naked, and Unwashed: 6 Weeks of Recipes

H ere are recipes that you can use to help fill 6 weeks of breakfasts, lunches, dinners, and snacks—recipes for filling, tasty, and healthy dishes that you can mix and match to fill out the 42 days of this process.

Don't think of this section as a comprehensive, every-recipe-you'll-ever-need kind of cookbook; think of it as a collection of recipes that illustrate how to incorporate useful health practices into your cooking. I call these "prototype recipes" because they illustrate a method that you can then adapt to suit your own tastes and needs. For example, the Pesto Noodles (page 231) includes noodles made from spiral-cut zucchini, demonstrating how to re-create a pasta dish with none of the health problems of wheat- or other grain-based pasta. Once you are comfortable with making noodles from spiral-cut zucchini, this can serve as the starting point for dozens of other recipes. Likewise, the Sausage "Rice" Skillet recipe (page 216) illustrates how we use riced cauliflower as a substitute for all forms of rice without sacrificing taste or texture. Not all recipes, of course, serve to re-create grain-based recipes, but such dishes can serve you well at holidays, while entertaining, and keeping the kids and spouse happy. They complement the real, whole foods that should comprise the majority of your meals.

I've broken the recipes down into common staples, breakfasts, lunches/ side dishes, main dishes, and desserts and snacks that you can pick and choose from each day. The net-carb cutoff of no more than 15 grams per meal is built into each recipe so that you do not need to make the calculation if you eat a single serving.

I've also kept the recipes simple so that your transition to this lifestyle is as easy as possible. You'll find additional recipes at undoctoredhealth.com that are downloadable upon providing your e-mail address.

Basic Recipes

Here is a collection of basic recipes that allow you to make, for example, healthy grain-free and otherwise problem-free breads, mayonnaise, salad dressings, and jams—the staples of everyday life that can be tough, sometimes impossible, to purchase without the ingredients we are trying to avoid.

All-Purpose Baking Mix

This is the All-Purpose Baking Mix I shared with Wheat Belly readers that has stood the test of time, yielding breads, muffins, cupcakes, and other baked products without the problems of grains.

MAKES 5 CUPS

> 4 cups almond meal/flour
> 1 cup ground golden flaxseed
> ¼ cup coconut flour
> 3 teaspoons baking soda
> 1 teaspoon ground psyllium seed

In a large bowl, mix together the almond meal/flour, flaxseed, coconut flour, baking soda, and psyllium seed. Store in an airtight container, preferably in the refrigerator, for up to 1 month.

Basic Mini Sandwich Bread

This virtually foolproof way to make bread for mini sandwiches uses a whoopie baking pan as the mold.

MAKES 8

> 1½ cups All-Purpose Baking Mix (page 205)
>
> ¾ teaspoon sea salt
>
> 4 tablespoons extra-virgin olive oil or avocado oil
>
> 1 egg
>
> 1½ tablespoons water + additional water if needed

Preheat the oven to 350°F. Lightly grease 8 wells of a whoopie baking pan.

In a medium bowl, combine the baking mix, salt, oil, egg, and water and mix thoroughly. Add more water, 1 teaspoon at a time, to thin to the consistency of thick pancake batter. Divide the dough into the 8 wells of the baking pan, spread, and flatten.

Bake for 18 minutes, or until the edges just begin to brown. Allow to cool for several minutes before removing from the pan.

Basic Focaccia Bread

One of the challenges with grain-free baking is generating "rise" in breads, so it is a real challenge to make breads suitable for sandwiches. One easy workaround is to make flatbread, or focaccia, which can be every bit as tasty and versatile, though heavier in texture.

You can liven up this tasty recipe by adding sliced kalamata olives, tapenades, sun-dried tomatoes, or other herbs and spices.

If you plan to use these breads for nonsavory sandwiches, such as peanut butter and "jelly" (see the Strawberry Jam recipe on page 210 or use pureed fruit sweetened with stevia or other benign sweetener from our list on page 352), omit the rosemary, oregano, and onion powder.

MAKES 15 SLICES (2½" x 4")

> 6 cups All-Purpose Baking Mix (page 205) or almond meal/flour
> ¼ cup ground psyllium seed (omit if using the baking mix recipe)
> 2 teaspoons dried rosemary, crushed
> 2 teaspoons dried oregano
> 2 teaspoons onion powder
> 2 teaspoons sea salt
> 5 medium to large eggs, separated
> 1 cup warm water
> ½ cup extra-virgin olive oil, avocado oil, coconut oil, or butter

Preheat the oven to 375°F. Grease an 11" x 17" shallow baking pan.

In a large bowl, combine the baking mix or almond flour/meal, psyllium seed (if not using the baking mix), rosemary, oregano, onion powder, and salt.

In a medium bowl, whisk the egg yolks, water, and oil or butter to combine.

Whip the egg whites in an electric mixer until frothy and stiff.

Pour both the egg yolk mixture and whipped egg whites into the flour mixture and combine thoroughly to create the dough. Transfer the dough to the baking pan and spread with a spoon or by hand to fill the pan edge-to-edge.

Bake for 18 minutes. Using a knife or pizza cutter, cut lengthwise into 3 lengths and then horizontally into 5 to yield 15 slices, or cut into the sizes you desire.

Mayonnaise

Most store-bought mayonnaises are made with unhealthy oils that we avoid, such as soybean oil or safflower oil. Making mayonnaise yourself can sometimes be tricky, but here is an easy version made with an immersion blender. The same process can be followed with a regular blender or food processor. I specify extra-light olive oil to avoid the vegetal flavors of extra-virgin, but if you don't mind such flavors, extra-virgin works fine.

All the ingredients must be at room temperature. If the ingredients are refrigerated, wait at least 2 hours while the ingredients warm to room temperature before blending, otherwise your ingredients will not blend properly.

MAKES 1½ CUPS

> **2 egg yolks**
>
> **2 tablespoons white wine vinegar**
>
> **1 cup extra-light olive oil or avocado oil**
>
> **½ teaspoon sea salt**

In a tall, narrow jar that accommodates an immersion blender, blend the egg yolks and vinegar for 15 to 20 seconds, or until frothy. Pour in ¼ to ⅓ cup of the oil very slowly over 2 to 3 minutes. As the mixture thickens, pour in the rest of the oil more rapidly over 1 to 2 minutes. Add the salt while continuing to blend.

Cover and store. Mayonnaise will keep in the refrigerator for up to 1 week.

Ketchup

No high-fructose corn syrup or added sugars in this ketchup!

MAKES ABOUT 1 CUP

> **1 can (6 ounces) tomato paste**
>
> **¼ cup apple cider vinegar or white wine vinegar**
>
> **¼ cup water**
>
> **1½ teaspoons onion powder**
>
> **1 teaspoon garlic powder**
>
> **¼ teaspoon sea salt**

In a small saucepan over low heat, cook the tomato paste, vinegar, water, onion powder, garlic powder, and salt, stirring occasionally, for 20 minutes.

Cool and store in an airtight container in the refrigerator for up to 2 weeks.

Strawberry Jam

Here is a basic method to convert fruit to a spreadable jam using chia seeds. While this recipe calls for strawberries, it can easily be modified to use other berries, apricots, plums, or other fruit.

MAKES 2 CUPS

> **2 cups fresh strawberries**
> **¼ cup whole chia seeds**
> **Sweetener equivalent to ¾ cup sugar**
> **1 tablespoon lemon juice**

In a food processor or food chopper, pulse the strawberries to a puree.

In a small saucepan over low heat, cook the processed strawberries, chia seeds, and sweetener, stirring frequently, for 5 minutes, or until the mixture thickens.

Allow to cool for several minutes, and then stir in the lemon juice. Store in the refrigerator, covered, for up to 1 week.

Salad Dressings

If you've become accustomed to premade, store-bought salad dressings, then you are going to love the fresher, sharper flavors when you make the real thing—with none of the health problems.

Spicy Curry Dressing

This is a two-birds, one-stone salad dressing: Not only is it healthy, but it also provides prebiotic fibers to add to your efforts to cultivate healthy bowel flora by including hummus, a source of the galactooligosaccharide, GOS, variety of prebiotic fibers.

The exotic combination of flavors in garam masala—cinnamon, nutmeg, cloves, cardamom, cumin—blend with those of red curry to make a delicious salad dressing or sauce for meats and other dishes. This dressing is best prepared and consumed on the same day, as the spices of the garam masala tend to lose their flavors rapidly.

If used as a sauce on a hot dish, such as baked chicken or fish, add only during the last few moments of cooking to avoid excessive heating that can degrade the GOS prebiotic fibers into sugars.

MAKES 1½ CUPS

> ½ cup hummus
> ½ cup extra-virgin olive oil
> ¼ cup red curry paste
> 2 tablespoons apple cider vinegar
> 2 tablespoons water
> 1 teaspoon garam masala
> 1 teaspoon red-pepper flakes

In a small bowl, combine the hummus, oil, curry paste, vinegar, water, garam masala, and red-pepper flakes and mix thoroughly. Store in an airtight container in the refrigerator for no longer than 2 weeks.

Italian Tomato-Basil Vinaigrette

You can be confident that your Italian Tomato-Basil Vinaigrette contains no grains or added sugar but loses nothing in flavor for topping salads or as a sauce or marinade for meats, poultry, or fish.

MAKES 2½ CUPS

   ½ cup oil-packed sun-dried tomatoes

   ½ cup coarsely chopped fresh basil

   2 cloves garlic, minced

   1 cup extra-virgin olive oil

   ¼ cup tomato paste or ½ cup tomato sauce

   ½ cup apple cider vinegar, white wine vinegar, or red wine vinegar

   ½ teaspoon sea salt, or to taste

In a food processor or food chopper, combine the tomatoes, basil, garlic, oil, tomato paste or sauce, vinegar, and salt. Pulse until pureed.

Store in an airtight container in the refrigerator for up to 1 week.

French Dressing

If you have made the healthy Ketchup and Mayonnaise recipes, then this French Dressing is just a handful of ingredients away. I predict that this salad dressing, more than the others, will turn you away from the store-bought stuff forever.

MAKES 2 CUP3

> ½ cup extra-virgin olive oil or avocado oil
>
> ½ cup Ketchup (page 209)
>
> ½ cup Mayonnaise (page 208)
>
> ⅓ cup white wine vinegar or apple cider vinegar
>
> 1 small onion, chopped
>
> Sweetener equivalent to ¼ cup sugar
>
> 1 teaspoon paprika
>
> ½ teaspoon sea salt

In a blender, combine the oil, ketchup, mayonnaise, vinegar, onion, sweetener, paprika, and salt. Blend until mixed well.

Store in an airtight container for up to 1 week.

Breakfasts

Huevos Rancheros

Jazz up your eggs with this quick and easy version of huevos rancheros that does not end up being a carb-fest like standard recipes for this dish. I serve the sauce and fixings over fried eggs, but any form of cooked eggs will do. This simple recipe yields more sauce than most people will need for a single breakfast, so store the remainder covered in the refrigerator to enjoy on another day.

For convenience, this recipe uses store-bought tomato sauce. Choose bottled over canned with the least carbohydrates/sugars (no more than 6 grams net carbs per ½ cup) and, of course, no high-fructose corn syrup.

For a deeper, richer flavor, add sun-dried tomato tapenade to the sauce.

MAKES 8 SERVINGS OF SAUCE

¼ cup extra-virgin olive oil

1 yellow onion, chopped

2 cloves garlic, minced

1 small green bell, poblano, or Anaheim pepper, seeded and chopped

3 cups tomato sauce

¼ cup sun-dried tomato tapenade (optional)

1 tablespoon chili powder

Sea salt and ground black pepper, to taste

¼ cup chopped fresh cilantro

1 cup shredded Cheddar cheese (optional)

In a medium saucepan over medium heat, warm the oil. Add the onion, garlic, and bell, poblano, or Anaheim pepper and cook, stirring occasionally, for 3 to 5 minutes, or until the onion and pepper are softened and the onion is translucent.

Add the tomato sauce, tomato tapenade (if using), and chili powder and simmer, stirring occasionally, for 5 minutes. (Reduce the heat if the sauce boils.) Add the salt and black pepper.

Serve over fried eggs and top with the cilantro and cheese (if using).

Italian Sausage and Brussels Sprouts Breakfast Skillet

This is one of those breakfast recipes that will keep you in breakfasts for another 2 or 3 days after making it. It's also filling enough to make you lose interest in lunch.

I include turnips to provide a modest quantity of prebiotic fibers and, if cooked sufficiently, to replace the role of potatoes in a skillet without the huge carbohydrate burden.

MAKES 6 SERVINGS

> ¼ cup extra-virgin olive oil or butter
>
> 1 yellow onion, chopped
>
> 2 cloves garlic, minced
>
> 1 pound ground Italian sausage
>
> 2 tablespoons chicken broth or beef broth or water
>
> 1 pound Brussels sprouts, halved
>
> 1 turnip, cut into ½" cubes
>
> 2 red or yellow bell peppers, seeded and sliced
>
> 4 ounces button or portobello mushrooms, sliced
>
> Sea salt and ground black pepper, to taste
>
> 6 eggs

Preheat the oven to 350°F.

In a large ovenproof skillet over medium-high heat, warm the oil or butter. Cook the onion and garlic for 3 to 5 minutes, or until the onion is softened and translucent.

Add the sausage, breaking it up as it heats, and cook for 5 minutes, or until lightly browned and no longer pink.

Add the broth or water, Brussels sprouts, turnip, bell peppers, and mushrooms. Reduce the heat to medium, cover, and cook, stirring occasionally, for 10 minutes, or until the sausage is cooked through and the Brussels sprouts and bell peppers start to soften. Add the salt and black pepper.

Remove the cover and create 6 indentations in the top of the mix with a large spoon and drop an egg into each. (Alternatively, make the eggs any way you want separately, and top the finished skillet mixture with them.)

Bake for 12 to 15 minutes, or until the eggs are set. Remove (careful: use oven mitts!) and serve.

Sausage "Rice" Skillet

I put this skillet recipe in the breakfast section, but it could easily serve as a main or side dish. The flavors will be dominated by the sausage, so choose one you and your family really like. I specified Andouille sausage, but you can easily substitute your favorite.

MAKES 4 SERVINGS

> 1 large cauliflower, broken into florets
>
> ¼ cup olive oil
>
> 1 yellow onion, chopped
>
> 1 green bell pepper, seeded and chopped
>
> 2 carrots, sliced
>
> 1 pound andouille sausage, sliced
>
> 2 tablespoons chicken broth
>
> Sea salt and ground black pepper, to taste

In a food processor or food chopper, pulse the cauliflower (in batches, if necessary) until reduced to rice-size granules. Set aside.

In a medium to large skillet over medium-high heat, warm the oil. Cook the onion, bell pepper, and carrots for 3 to 5 minutes, or until the onion is softened and translucent. Add the sausage. Reduce the heat to medium, cover, and cook, stirring occasionally, for 10 minutes, or until the sausage is cooked through.

Add the broth and reserved cauliflower, cover, and cook, stirring occasionally, for 10 minutes, or until the cauliflower is softened. Add the salt and black pepper.

Apple Cinnamon "Granola"

When you need some crunch in your breakfast, this is the way to go. Mix up a batch on, say, Sunday, save in an airtight container (refrigeration optional), and then eat with breakfast over the course of several days.

The dried apple in this recipe can be replaced with dried peaches, strawberries, raspberries, or any other dried fruit you have available. Just be sure to use unsweetened dried fruit. Even better, save money by dehydrating the fruit yourself (that way you know there will be no added sugar). The fruit is added after baking, as it tends to burn, even at low temperatures.

MAKES 10 SERVINGS

> **4 cups unsweetened coconut flakes**
>
> **2 cups sliced almonds**
>
> **1 cup raw pumpkin seeds**
>
> **1 cup raw sunflower seeds**
>
> **¼ cup whole chia seeds**
>
> **1 tablespoon ground cinnamon**
>
> **Sweetener equivalent to ¾ cup sugar**
>
> **½ cup avocado oil or extra-light olive oil**
>
> **2 teaspoons vanilla extract**
>
> **1½ cups unsweetened dehydrated apples, broken up into small pieces or chopped (see note)**

Preheat the oven to 300°F.

In a large bowl, mix together the coconut, almonds, pumpkin seeds, sunflower seeds, chia seeds, cinnamon, and sweetener.

Add the oil and vanilla and mix thoroughly.

Spread the mixture on a large, shallow baking pan and transfer to the oven. Remove every 4 to 5 minutes and turn over with a spoon. Repeat once or twice until the mixture is very lightly browned. Remove and cool for 10 minutes.

Transfer the mixture to a large bowl. Mix in the apples. Cover the mixture and store. (Refrigeration is not necessary if the mixture will be consumed over the next several days.)

Note: Dehydrated fruit often comes in a pouch that you can roll a heavy glass or jar or rolling pin over while still sealed to break up the fruit.

Asparagus-Tomato Frittata

Frittatas are essentially quiches without the crust. (This recipe can be readily converted to a quiche by simply adding an almond meal/flour, walnut meal, or pecan meal crust. See the recipe for Strawberry Cheesecake on page 247 for details.) Frittatas require a bit of preparation, so consider preparing it ahead of time on, say, the weekend to eat slice by slice over the work or school week.

MAKES 6 SERVINGS

8 eggs

3 tablespoons extra-virgin olive oil, divided

½ yellow onion, chopped

2 cloves garlic, minced

8 asparagus spears, cut into 1" pieces

1 tomato, cut into ½" cubes

½ cup oil-packed sun-dried tomatoes

¼ cup finely chopped fresh basil

½ teaspoon sea salt

½ teaspoon ground black pepper

¼ cup grated Romano cheese

Preheat the oven to 350°F.

In a medium bowl, whisk the eggs. Stir in 2 tablespoons of the oil. Set aside.

In an ovenproof skillet over medium heat, warm the remaining 1 tablespoon oil. Cook the onion and garlic for 3 to 5 minutes, or until softened and translucent. Add the asparagus, tomatoes, basil, salt, and pepper and cook for 3 minutes.

Pour in the reserved egg mixture and mix together. Cover and cook at low to medium heat for 3 minutes.

Remove the cover and top with the cheese. Bake for 15 minutes.

Remove (Careful: Use oven mitts!) and cool for 5 minutes. Using a spatula, release the frittata around the edges and under the bottom. Slice and serve.

Maple-Cinnamon Quick Muffin

Here is a representative recipe for a quick muffin, a 90-second or so muffin-in-a-mug that provides a filing breakfast. For other variations, replace the ground cinnamon and maple extract with unsweetened cocoa powder or ¼ cup fresh or frozen berries.

MAKES 1

> **½ cup almond meal/flour**
>
> **2 tablespoons ground golden flaxseed**
>
> **Sweetener equivalent to 1½ tablespoons sugar**
>
> **¾ teaspoon ground cinnamon**
>
> **2 eggs**
>
> **1 tablespoon coconut oil or butter, melted**
>
> **¾ teaspoon natural maple extract**

In a large mug, combine the almond meal/flour, flaxseed, sweetener, and cinnamon and mix thoroughly.

Stir in the eggs, oil or butter, and maple extract. Microwave on high power for 90 to 120 seconds, or until a wooden pick withdraws dry.

Main Dishes

Pepperoni and Poblano Pepper Pizza

I think there's something magical in the combined flavors of pepperoni, lightly hot poblano peppers, mozzarella cheese, and tomato sauce in this simple pizza recipe.

For convenience, this recipe uses store-bought pizza sauce, so choose a brand with little or no added sugars, preferably no more than 6 or 7 net carbs per ½ cup. If you buy preshredded cheese, examine the label to avoid those containing cornstarch or rice starch as an anti-clumping ingredient. (Cellulose or nothing at all is a safe alternative.)

Also, note that the order of toppings is important; not spreading the pizza sauce onto the partially baked crust first is a way to avoid making the crust soggy. If your crust becomes soggy, all it means is that you will need to eat your pizza with a fork, rather than picking it up by hand. If you follow the sequence below and top the pizza with the sauce nearly last, then you are likely to have a sturdy pizza that you can indeed eat by hand.

MAKES 6 SERVINGS

- **3 cups almond meal/flour**
- **¼ cup ground psyllium seed**
- **2 cups shredded mozzarella cheese, divided**
- **½ teaspoon sea salt**
- **2 medium eggs**
- **½ cup extra-virgin olive oil, divided**
- **½ cup water**
- **2–3 poblano peppers, seeded and sliced**
- **1 onion, chopped**
- **16 ounces pizza sauce**
- **4 ounces uncured pepperoni, thinly sliced**

Preheat the oven to 350°F. Line a pizza stone or other flat baking sheet with parchment paper.

In a large bowl, combine the almond meal/flour, psyllium seed, 1 cup of the cheese, and the salt and mix thoroughly.

In a small bowl, combine the eggs, ¼ cup of the oil, and the water. Add to the almond meal/flour mixture and mix thoroughly.

On the pizza stone or baking sheet, spread the dough out by hand into a circular shape until approximately 12" wide and ½" thick, creating a lip at the edges. Bake for 15 minutes, or until just lightly browned.

Remove from the oven and spread the remaining 1 cup cheese, the peppers, and onion on the pizza. Pour on the pizza sauce evenly, spreading with a spoon, followed by the remaining ¼ cup oil. Top with the pepperoni.

Bake for 10 minutes, or until the cheese is melted.

Red Curry Coconut Chicken

The mix of onion, curry, shiitake mushrooms, and coconut makes simple chicken an exotic and flavorful main dish. While many popular chicken recipes use skinless chicken breast to reduce fat, we use chicken thighs (or mixed parts, if you start with the whole chicken) for their greater fat content. It is also less expensive.

This chicken dish can also be converted to a soup simply by adding 4 cups of chicken broth and adjusting seasonings to taste.

MAKES 4 SERVINGS

1½ pounds chicken thighs

¼ cup extra-virgin olive oil or coconut oil

1 yellow onion, chopped

2–3 cloves garlic, minced

2 tablespoons chicken broth

8 ounces shiitake mushrooms, sliced

2 large carrots, sliced

4–5 scallions, sliced

1 can (13.5 ounces) coconut milk

¼ cup red curry paste

Sea salt and ground black pepper, to taste

½ cup chopped fresh cilantro

Preheat the oven to 350°F.

Arrange the chicken on a baking sheet and cook for 35 to 40 minutes, or until cooked through.

Remove from the oven and cool. When cooled enough to handle safely, remove the meat, skin, and fat from the bone and set aside. Save any liquid fats that remain, also. (Remember: Because we never limit fat, we do not want just white meat, but also the dark meat, fat, and skin—all rich in nutrition.)

Meanwhile, in a large skillet over medium-high heat, warm the oil. Cook the onion and garlic for 3 to 5 minutes, or until the onion is softened and translucent. Add the broth, mushrooms, carrots, and scallions, cover, and cook, stirring occasionally, for 5 to 7 minutes, or until the carrots begin to soften. Reduce the heat to low and stir in the coconut milk and curry paste. Sprinkle with the salt and pepper.

Add the reserved chicken (including any liquid oil, fat, and skin) and simmer for 5 minutes before serving. If making soup, add an additional 4 cups chicken broth at the same time as the cooked chicken, increase the heat to medium, and simmer for 5 minutes.

Italian Meat Loaf

Here's a simple but delicious variation on meat loaf, another demonstration of how to use nongrain flours and meals to replace grain flours. While ground golden flaxseed and almond meal/flour are common replacements, in this version I've used coconut flour to provide increased "body," making it easy to slice.

If you use store-bought tomato sauce, be sure to choose a brand with little to no added sugars and no high-fructose corn syrup.

MAKES 6 TO 8 SERVINGS

¾ pound ground beef

¾ pound ground sausage

1 yellow onion, chopped

1 green bell pepper, seeded and chopped

¼ cup oil-packed sun-dried tomatoes, chopped

¼ cup coconut flour

2 tablespoons chopped fresh basil or 2 teaspoons dried

1 teaspoon dried oregano

½ teaspoon sea salt

½ teaspoon ground black pepper

2 eggs

2 cups tomato sauce, divided

2–3 ounces salami slices

Preheat the oven to 350°F.

In a large bowl, combine the beef, sausage, onion, bell pepper, tomatoes, coconut flour, basil, oregano, salt, and black pepper.

In a small bowl, whisk the eggs and 1 cup of the tomato sauce. Add to the meat mixture and mix well by hand.

Press the meat mixture into a 9" x 5" loaf pan. Spread the remaining 1 cup tomato sauce over the top. Arrange the salami slices on top.

Bake for 90 minutes, or until the interior temperature reaches 160°F.

Basil, Lemon, and Olive Oil Spaghetti

This simple recipe demonstrates to those of you unfamiliar with spaghetti squash yet another way to re-create pasta.

You could, of course, top these noodles with a marinara sauce with mushrooms, ground beef, and onions, or you could make meatballs with the marinara sauce. This simple recipe draws from the rich flavors of basil, lemon, and extra-virgin olive oil. Choose the best olive oil that fits in your budget, preferably an artisanal oil that preserves the grassy, peppery flavors (signaling the healthy compounds in olive oil) that are often missing from mass-produced brands.

MAKES 4 SERVINGS

> **1 spaghetti squash**
> **½ cup extra-virgin olive oil**
> **3 tablespoons chopped fresh basil**
> **Juice of 1 lemon**
> **Sea salt, to taste**

Preheat the oven to 350°F.

Pierce the squash in several places with a small sharp knife or fork. Place on a baking sheet and roast, turning once, for 1 hour, or until tender.

Remove from the oven and cool. When cooled enough to handle safely, cut in half lengthwise. Scoop out the seeds and discard. Using a fork, scrape the squash strands into a large bowl.

Add the oil, basil, lemon, and salt and toss.

Lamb Stew

This tasty home-style recipe demonstrates one of the safe ways to thicken a sauce, in this case with coconut flour. (Other safe thickening ingredients include butter; cream; sour cream; pureed squash, eggplant, or mushrooms; and avocado.)

MAKES 4 SERVINGS

¼ cup extra-virgin olive oil, coconut oil, avocado oil, or butter

1 yellow onion, chopped

2 cloves garlic, minced

1½ pounds lamb shoulder or stew meat, cut into 1" cubes

2–3 carrots, chopped

1 head broccoli, broken into florets

1 small head cauliflower, broken into florets

1 cup chicken broth or beef broth

2 tablespoons coconut flour

1 teaspoon dried thyme

1 teaspoon dried oregano

Sea salt and ground black pepper, to taste

In a large skillet over medium-high heat, warm the oil or butter. Cook the onion and garlic for 3 to 5 minutes, or until the onion is translucent.

Add the lamb, cover, and cook, occasionally turning the lamb over to cook all sides, for 8 to 10 minutes. Add the carrots, broccoli, cauliflower, broth, flour, thyme, oregano, and salt and pepper. Cover and cook, stirring occasionally, for 20 minutes, or until the vegetables are softened.

Spicy Pork-Stuffed Peppers

Using riced cauliflower allows you to re-create many rice dishes easily while maintaining a grain-free, low-carb eating style. While you can rice the cauliflower yourself in a food chopper or food processor, food retailers such as Trader Joe's are now selling pre-riced bags for convenience.

Choose your marinara sauce for low sugar/carbohydrate content, ideally no more than 12 grams net carbs per cup (or prepare it yourself, of course). Also choose the roundest bell peppers you can find.

MAKES 4 SERVINGS

¼ cup extra-virgin olive oil, coconut oil, avocado oil, or butter

1 yellow onion, chopped

2 cloves garlic, minced

1 pound ground pork

3–4 cups riced cauliflower

2 cups marinara sauce

¼ cup chopped fresh basil or 1 tablespoon dried

1 tablespoon dried oregano

1 tablespoon red-pepper flakes

Sea salt and ground black pepper, to taste

4 green bell peppers, tops cut off, seeded, and membranes removed

In a large skillet over medium-high heat, warm the oil or butter. Cook the onion and garlic for 3 to 5 minutes, or until the onion is softened.

Add the ground pork and cook, breaking it apart as it cooks, for 8 to 10 minutes, or until no longer pink.

Add the cauliflower, marinara sauce, basil, oregano, red-pepper flakes, and salt and black pepper. Cover and cook, stirring occasionally, for 10 minutes, or until the cauliflower is partially softened.

Preheat the oven to 350°F. Make a shallow horizontal cut across the bottom of each bell pepper to help them stand upright.

When the cauliflower mixture is finished, spoon into each bell pepper. Transfer the stuffed peppers to a shallow baking pan and bake for 45 minutes, or until the peppers are tender.

Fried Curry Shrimp and "Rice"

Cauliflower is a versatile vegetable: mashed, roasted, and riced, here, as part of a flavorful mix of curry and cilantro. You can rice the raw cauliflower yourself or buy it pre-riced (available at Trader Joe's and other retailers).

MAKES 4 SERVINGS

1 large head cauliflower, cut into florets

¼ cup extra-virgin olive oil, coconut oil, avocado oil, or butter

1 yellow onion, chopped

6–8 scallions, chopped

2–3 cloves garlic, minced

2 carrots, chopped or shredded

4 ounces shiitake mushrooms, sliced

¾ pound shrimp, peeled, deveined, and cooked

2 tablespoons curry powder

2–3 tablespoons chicken broth or water, if needed

¼ cup fresh cilantro, chopped

Steam the cauliflower for 20 minutes, or until soft.

Meanwhile, in a large skillet over medium-high heat, warm the oil or butter. Cook the onion, scallions, and garlic for 3 to 5 minutes, or until the onion is translucent. Add the carrots, mushrooms, shrimp, and curry powder. Reduce the heat to medium, cover, and cook, stirring occasionally, for 5 to 7 minutes, or until the carrots are softened.

Transfer the steamed cauliflower to a food processor or food chopper and pulse briefly to rice consistency.

Add the riced cauliflower to the shrimp mixture and stir in. If the mixture is too dry, add the broth or water. Cover and cook, stirring occasionally, for 1 to 2 minutes. Sprinkle cilantro over top and serve.

Cajun-Spiced Mahi Mahi with Rémoulade

You can indeed "bread" meat, fish, and other dishes in a grain-free lifestyle. Here's one of many ways to cover fish, poultry, or other meats with a tasty coating of herbs and coconut flour that makes you forget you ever ate anything breaded with wheat flour. This recipe combines the spicy flavors of the coating with a cool, smooth Louisiana-style sauce.

MAKES 2 SERVINGS

- 2 tablespoons coconut flour
- 1 teaspoon dried oregano
- 1 teaspoon dried thyme
- ½ teaspoon ground red pepper
- ½ teaspoon garlic powder
- ½ teaspoon sea salt
- 2 fillets mahi mahi
- ¼ cup coconut oil, avocado oil, extra-virgin olive oil, or butter
- 2 scallions, coarsely chopped
- 1 clove garlic
- ½ cup Mayonnaise (page 208)
- 1 tablespoon Ketchup (page 209) or hot sauce
- 1 tablespoon stone-ground mustard
- 1 tablespoon lemon juice or white wine vinegar

In a shallow bowl, combine the coconut flour, oregano, thyme, ground red pepper, garlic powder, and salt. Coat each fillet in the mixture.

In a medium skillet over medium-high heat, warm the oil or butter. Cook the fillets for 4 minutes on each side (varying depending on thickness), or until the exterior is lightly browned and the fish becomes flaky.

Meanwhile, to create the rémoulade, in a food processor, food chopper, or blender, combine the scallions, garlic, mayonnaise, ketchup or hot sauce, mustard, and lemon juice or vinegar. Reduce to a puree.

Serve the mahi mahi topped with the sauce.

Chipotle-Breaded Chicken

Here's a tasty way to "bread" chicken or other meats or fish, jazzed up with chipotle and red pepper in this recipe. Be sure to obtain chicken with the skin in place. I like thighs because it's easier to get more fat with this cut, plus they're easy to bread.

MAKES 6 SERVINGS

2 eggs

½ cup grated Parmesan cheese

½ cup coconut flour

2 teaspoons sea salt

1 tablespoon ground chipotle powder

1 teaspoon ground red pepper

1 teaspoon dried oregano

2 pounds chicken (thighs, legs, and breasts, with skin)

Preheat the oven to 350°F.

In a shallow bowl, whisk the eggs.

In another shallow bowl, combine the cheese, flour, salt, chipotle powder, ground red pepper, and oregano.

Roll each piece of chicken in the egg mixture, followed by the cheese mixture. Transfer to a baking pan.

Bake for 40 minutes, or until internal temperature reaches 170°F, turning each piece of chicken halfway through.

Lunches, Simple Main Dishes, or Side Dishes

Tricolor Noodle Salad

Here's a medley of vegetables that is simple to make, aside from the muscle power needed to spiralize your noodles. You will need one of the inexpensive spiral-cutting devices on the market, such as a Veggetti, that makes creating noodles out of vegetables a snap with a few turns of the wrist. The mixture of flavors in this salad makes it a comfortable accompaniment to just about any main course—fish, shellfish, chicken, or beef. The daikon radish also adds a bit of prebiotic fiber to your health effort.

Use your best extra-virgin olive oil, as this simple recipe means that olive oil flavors will show through. The vinegar, even in small quantities, will show, too. I tried a rich and syrupy fig balsamic vinegar, but I thought it overwhelmed the flavors of the root vegetables. I obtained the best results with a bit of simple, plain white wine vinegar—but you be the judge.

This salad is best served immediately, as it will lose its body if stored.

MAKES 4 SERVINGS

> 1 large zucchini, spiral-cut
>
> 1 large daikon radish, spiral-cut
>
> 1 large beet, spiral-cut
>
> ¼ cup extra-virgin olive oil
>
> 2 teaspoons white wine vinegar, apple cider vinegar, or balsamic vinegar
>
> Juice of ½ lemon
>
> 2 tablespoons chopped fresh cilantro

In a large bowl, combine the zucchini, radish, beet, oil, vinegar, and lemon juice and toss together. Top with the cilantro and serve immediately.

Pesto Noodles

These noodles require less than 5 minutes to prepare yet are delicious and filling as either a main or side dish. You will need one of the inexpensive spiral-cutting devices on the market, such as a Veggetti, that make creating noodles out of vegetables a snap with a few turns of the wrist.

MAKES 2 SERVINGS

> **2 medium to large zucchini, spiral-cut**
>
> **½ cup basil pesto**
>
> **2 tablespoons pine nuts**
>
> **4 ounces shaved Parmesan cheese (optional)**

In a large bowl, mix together the zucchini, pesto, and pine nuts. Top with the cheese, if using, and serve.

Ramen Noodles

Though not as quick and easy as tearing open a plastic package with dried seasonings, this healthier version of ramen noodles is still a fairly quick and easy way to enjoy an old favorite.

Look for shirataki noodles in refrigerated sections of the grocery store (they come packed in water), and choose brands made without soy. Upon opening, there will be a fishy odor, which does not suggest spoilage. Rinsing briefly in a colander will remove the odor. Note that shirataki noodles are rich in the glucomannan fiber that has prebiotic properties (discussed in Chapter 11), so this dish is best eaten after the first week of your Undoctored program.

MAKES 2 SERVINGS

> 2 packages (8 ounces each) shirataki spaghetti noodles
> 2 cups chicken broth
> 2 tablespoons toasted sesame oil
> 1½ tablespoons gluten-free soy sauce, tamari sauce, or coconut aminos
> 2 scallions, finely chopped
> 2 tablespoons sesame seeds
> 2 teaspoons onion powder
> 1 teaspoon garlic powder

Drain the shirataki noodles in a colander and rinse with cold water for about 20 seconds.

In a medium saucepan over medium-high heat, combine the noodles and broth. Add the oil, soy sauce or tamari or aminos, scallions, sesame seeds, onion powder, and garlic powder and stir together. Cover and bring to a boil, stirring occasionally. Reduce the heat to medium, cover, and cook for 2 to 3 minutes.

Reuben Sandwich

You likely don't need a recipe for a Reuben—or a peanut butter and jelly or a BLT. But I provided this recipe mostly to remind you that the Basic Focaccia Bread recipe on page 207 can be used to re-create all your favorite sandwiches. To re-create a Reuben, just use the standard ingredients you would have otherwise used in your grain-consuming days. Choose uncured meats, of course, without sodium nitrite. Even better, make your own fermented sauerkraut for added probiotic punch (see page 352). Eat your sandwich cold or as an open-faced sandwich, heated to melt the cheese.

MAKES 1

> **2 slices Basic Focaccia Bread (page 207)**
>
> **4–6 ounces sliced corned beef or pastrami**
>
> **¼ cup sauerkraut, well drained**
>
> **2 tablespoons Thousand Island or Russian dressing or the Spicy Curry Dressing (page 211)**
>
> **2 slices Swiss or Gruyère cheese**

On one slice of the bread, layer the meat, sauerkraut, dressing, and cheese, followed by the second slice of the bread.

Greek Salad

Everybody knows how to make a Greek salad. But in this version, I introduce a couple of unique variations for added health benefits, such as the option of adding the delicious flavors of fermented onions and cucumber (best fermented with fresh dill and garlic), a source of supplemental probiotic flora. (Of course, you will need to start fermenting the vegetables several days before you serve this salad. Alternatively, keep an ongoing supply of your favorite veggies fermenting for use as needed. See Appendix C for instructions on basic fermentation.) I also used dandelion greens in this version to amp up the nutritional profile of the salad and to provide a means for those who forage some of their food to put their dandelions to use. (For those of you inclined to harvest foods from the garden or yard, dandelion roots are also rich in prebiotic fibers.) Dandelion greens can easily be replaced by other green leafy veggies, such as fresh spinach or red leaf lettuce, or just leave it out altogether, as in traditional Greek salads.

Because this salad is relatively spare in ingredients, choose the juiciest tomatoes, the best kalamata olives, and the highest quality extra-virgin olive oil for the richest flavors, as well as the greatest health benefits.

MAKES 4 SERVINGS

3–4 cups dandelion greens, chopped

1 red onion, fermented (if desired), halved, and sliced

1 cucumber, fermented (if desired) and sliced or spiral-cut

1 cup pitted kalamata olives

1½ cups cherry tomatoes

4 ounces crumbled feta cheese

4 tablespoons extra-virgin olive oil

1 tablespoon red wine vinegar

Juice of ½ lemon

Dash of sea salt

In a large salad bowl, combine the dandelion greens, onion, cucumber, olives, tomatoes, and cheese.

In a small bowl or cup, whisk together the oil, vinegar, lemon juice, and salt. Pour into the salad and toss just before serving.

Italian "Pasta" Salad

Here's another way to use fermented foods, red onion in this case. If desired, you can even used fermented cucumber (best fermented with fresh dill and garlic).

MAKES 8 SERVINGS

> 1 pound zucchini, spiral-cut with short strokes
>
> 1 cup cherry tomatoes, halved
>
> 1 cucumber, quartered and sliced
>
> 1 green bell pepper, seeded and chopped
>
> 1 red onion, fermented, halved, and sliced
>
> ½ cup pitted black or kalamata olives, halved or sliced
>
> 8 ounces pepperoni, quartered and sliced
>
> 2 tablespoons chopped fresh basil or 2 teaspoons dried
>
> 1 tablespoon chopped fresh oregano or 1 teaspoon dried
>
> ¼ cup white vinegar
>
> ¼ cup extra-virgin olive oil
>
> ¼ cup grated Parmesan or Romano cheese (optional)

In a large bowl, combine the zucchini noodles, tomatoes, cucumber, pepper, onion, olives, pepperoni, basil, oregano, vinegar, and oil and toss until well mixed. Top with the cheese, if using.

Tomato-Lentil Soup

Along with the rich flavors of poblano peppers and chorizo sausage, this dish packs a prebiotic bowel flora wallop by including lentils, a source of galactooligosaccharide prebiotic fibers.

MAKES 8 SERVINGS

¼ cup extra-virgin olive oil

1 yellow onion, chopped

2 cloves garlic, minced

2 poblano peppers, seeded and chopped

12 ounces chorizo sausage, sliced

6 cups chicken broth or water

3 carrots, sliced

2 stalks celery, sliced

1 cup dried lentils

1 can (14.5 ounces) diced tomatoes (I use the Muir Glen brand with the BPA-free can)

1 tablespoon hot sauce

Sea salt and ground black pepper, to taste

In a large saucepan over medium-high heat, warm the oil. Add the onion, garlic, poblano peppers, and sausage, cover, and cook, stirring frequently, for 7 to 8 minutes, or until the sausage is cooked and the onion is translucent.

In a large stockpot over high heat, add the cooked sausage mixture, broth or water, carrots, celery, lentils, tomatoes, hot sauce, and salt and black pepper and bring to a boil. Reduce the heat to low, cover, and simmer for 30 minutes, or until the lentils have softened.

Shredded Cabbage and Bacon Skillet

Here's a celebration of veggies and bacon fat! As you know, we don't engage in silly behaviors like choosing lean cuts of meat or pouring off bacon fat—the fat is the best part.

Remember: Fat is satiating. While this simple skillet is in the side-dish section, you could easily have this skillet serve as a main dish.

MAKES 4 SERVINGS

> **2 tablespoons butter, coconut oil, or extra-virgin olive oil**
>
> **1 yellow onion, chopped**
>
> **2 cloves garlic, minced**
>
> **8 strips bacon**
>
> **½ head green cabbage, shredded, or 16 ounces preshredded**
>
> **8 ounces Brussels sprouts, halved**
>
> **1 carrot, sliced**
>
> **¼ cup chicken broth**
>
> **Sea salt and ground black pepper, to taste**

In a large skillet over medium heat, warm the butter or oil. Cook the onion and garlic in one half of the skillet and the bacon in the other half for 5 to 7 minutes, or until the onion is translucent and the bacon is cooked through. Transfer the bacon to a plate and set aside.

In the same skillet, add the cabbage, Brussels sprouts, carrot, and broth, cover, and cook, stirring occasionally, for 10 minutes, or until the cabbage and Brussels sprouts are softened. Add the salt and pepper. Transfer the reserved bacon back to the skillet, cover, and cook for 1 to 2 minutes.

Bacon Mashed "Potatoes"

Our replacement for mashed potatoes is mashed cauliflower, a delicious substitute that tastes every bit as good without the excessive carbohydrate load of potatoes.

MAKES 4 SERVINGS

> **1 large head cauliflower, cut into florets**
>
> **6 ounces bacon**
>
> **Sea salt and ground black pepper, to taste**

Steam the cauliflower for 20 minutes, or until softened. Transfer to a food chopper or food processor and pulse down to a puree.

Meanwhile, in a medium skillet over medium-high heat, cook the bacon for 5 to 7 minutes, or until cooked through. Remove from the skillet and cut into small pieces. Do not discard the grease.

In a large bowl, combine the pureed cauliflower, bacon, and at least ¼ cup of the bacon grease. Sprinkle with the salt and pepper.

Ratatouille

Ratatouille is a celebration of vegetables in a tasty mélange, recently in the spotlight with a wanna-be chef/rat in the animated movie by the same name. Use your best extra-virgin olive oil for the best results. Optionally, add some olive oil during the last moment of cooking to gain more of its flavors and health benefits, which are reduced with cooking.

MAKES 6 SERVINGS

¼ cup extra-virgin olive oil

2 cloves garlic, minced

1 yellow onion, chopped

1 eggplant, cut into ½" squares

½ teaspoon sea salt

½ teaspoon ground black pepper

½ teaspoon red-pepper flakes

2 zucchini, sliced

1 green bell pepper, seeded and chopped

In a large skillet over medium-high heat, warm the oil. Cook the garlic and onion for 3 to 5 minutes, or until the onion is translucent. Reduce the heat to medium and add the eggplant, salt, black pepper, and red-pepper flakes, cover, and cook, stirring occasionally, for 8 to 10 minutes, or until the eggplant softens.

Add the zucchini and bell pepper, cover, and cook, stirring occasionally, for 8 to 10 minutes, or until the zucchini and bell pepper soften.

Avocado Salad

In addition to the healthy fats and flavors of avocado and extra-virgin olive oil (use your best for this one, as the flavors will show through), I include white beans for their rich prebiotic fiber content, the richest among legumes. While rich in carbs (as much as 28 grams net carbs per cup), as well, they are distributed among 4 servings, keeping it manageable and below our net-carb cutoff. Use canned (or in the cartons or pouches now being used by some manufacturers) precooked white beans for convenience.

MAKES 4 SERVINGS

> 1 medium to large avocado, cubed
>
> 1 large cucumber, cubed
>
> 2 cups cherry tomatoes, halved
>
> 1 red onion, chopped
>
> 1 cup precooked white beans
>
> ¼ cup extra-virgin olive oil
>
> 2 tablespoons white wine vinegar

In a large bowl, combine the avocado, cucumber, tomatoes, onion, and beans. Add the oil and vinegar and toss to mix.

Desserts and Snacks

Double Chocolate Chip–
Walnut Cookies

Everyone loves chocolate chip cookies! Here's a double-chocolate version that combines cocoa and dark chocolate chips.

Choose the darkest chocolate chips you can find, with no more than 5 net carbs per 40-gram serving. Lately, manufacturers have been putting out lower-carb options, including chips sweetened with stevia and erythritol, which can further reduce carb/sugar exposure, allowing you to be more generous with your chocolate chips.

MAKES 32

> 4 cups almond flour or All-Purpose Baking Mix (page 205)
>
> 1 cup chopped walnuts
>
> 4 ounces dark chocolate chips
>
> ¾ cup unsweetened cocoa powder
>
> Sweetener equivalent to 1¼ cups sugar
>
> 3 eggs
>
> ½ cup butter or coconut oil, melted
>
> ½ cup water
>
> 1 teaspoon vanilla extract

Preheat the oven to 350°F. Line a baking sheet with parchment paper.

In a large bowl, combine the flour or baking mix, walnuts, chocolate chips, cocoa powder, and sweetener and mix thoroughly.

In a small to medium bowl, whisk together the eggs, butter or oil, water, and vanilla. Pour into the flour mixture and mix thoroughly.

On the baking sheet, place approximately 1" wide balls of the dough and flatten to yield 32 cookies, in separate batches, if necessary. Bake for 18 minutes, or until the edges are crisp.

Mango-Coconut Macaroons

Here's a tasty slice of the tropics in bite-size macaroons. A growing number of supermarkets and specialty stores are stocking unsweetened dried fruit: mango, strawberries, blueberries, apples, etc., leaving you with plenty of options for variations on these macaroons. You could also, of course, save money and dehydrate your own fruit.

MAKES 16

> **3 egg whites**
>
> **1 cup unsweetened dried mango**
>
> **2 cups unsweetened shredded coconut**
>
> **Sweetener equivalent to ½ cup sugar**

Preheat the oven to 350°F. Line a baking sheet with parchment paper.

With an electric or handheld mixer, whip the egg whites until stiff.

Meanwhile, in a food chopper or food processor, pulse the dried mango until reduced to a powder. Add to the whipped egg whites, followed by the coconut and sweetener.

Using a 1" ice cream scooper or large spoon, create 16 mounds. Bake for 12 to 15 minutes, or until just starting to brown.

Chocolate-Mint Ice Cream

Store-bought no-added-sugar ice cream is a landmine of sorbitol, maltitol, and other unhealthy sweeteners that not only act much like sugar but also provoke loose stools. Here's a way to make your own thick, rich ice cream without problem sweeteners and without having to endure gas and diarrhea.

If you have a dairy sensitivity in some form or you are among the people whose weight loss is stalled or prevented by dairy products (due to the insulin-provoking action of the whey fraction of protein in dairy products), replace the whipping cream with canned coconut milk. The additional custard step using egg yolks ensures a creamy texture even with coconut milk.

Creating the egg yolk custard is key, and here I use a simplified method directly on the stove. Because we avoid using emulsifying agents (due to their disruptive effects on bowel flora), there is one downside: This ice cream is best consumed right away, as it does not freeze well and becomes icy. You can indeed store it in the freezer, but you will have to wait for it to partially defrost first.

This basic recipe can be altered in an unlimited number of ways. For example, you can leave out the cocoa and replace it with 1 cup fresh or frozen mixed berries, 1 cup wild blueberries, 4 ounces dark chocolate chunks with or without peppermint extract, 1 cup bing cherries, 1 cup pistachios, etc.

MAKES 4 SERVINGS

> **4 egg yolks (preferably large or jumbo eggs, or 5 small to medium)**
>
> **1½ cups heavy whipping cream, preferably organic,
> or 1 can (13.5 ounces) coconut milk**
>
> **Sweetener equivalent to ¾ cup sugar**
>
> **½ cup unsweetened cocoa powder**
>
> **½ teaspoon sea salt**
>
> **1 teaspoon vanilla extract**
>
> **½ teaspoon peppermint extract**

In a small saucepan over low heat, warm the eggs yolks. With an electric or hand mixer, beat the yolks while on the heat for 3 to 4 minutes, or until creamy and smooth. Keep the heat low enough so that the yolks do not scramble or coagulate but are warm to the touch.

Add the cream or coconut milk, sweetener, cocoa powder, salt, vanilla, and peppermint extract and blend until mixed thoroughly.

Pour the entire mixture into an ice cream maker and follow the manufacturer's directions. (My device required 25 minutes to convert to a thick custard texture.)

Peanut Butter Cup Cookies

There's something magical about the flavor combination of peanut butter and chocolate, here combined into a chewy cookie that kids will love. Just don't tell them they're healthy!

MAKES 16

3½ cups All-Purpose Baking Mix (page 205)

2 tablespoons coconut flour

Sweetener equivalent to ½ cup sugar

½ teaspoon sea salt

2 eggs

½ cup peanut butter, at room temperature

½ cup coconut oil, melted

½ cup water

4-ounce bar 85–90% cocoa chocolate

Preheat the oven to 350°F. Line a baking sheet with parchment paper.

In a large bowl, combine the baking mix, flour, sweetener, and salt and mix thoroughly.

In a small bowl, whisk the eggs. Whisk in the peanut butter, oil, and water. Add to the dry mixture and mix until dough forms. Dispense the dough into approximately 16 mounds, flattening by hand or with a large spoon. Bake for 20 minutes, or until a wooden pick withdraws dry.

Meanwhile, melt the dark chocolate in a microwave on high power in 20-second increments or in a double-boiler setup. Transfer to a shallow bowl.

Remove the cookies from the oven and cool for 10 minutes. Then immerse the top half of each cookie into the chocolate and set aside to cool. If any chocolate remains after dipping each cookie, cool the cookies in the freezer for 5 to 10 minutes and then dip in the remaining chocolate for an extra-thick layer.

Blueberry Cream Pie

This recipe includes an easy method of creating a piecrust without wheat or grains and a tasty no-bake filling using gelatin. This version is also dairy-free.

MAKES 8 SERVINGS

1½ cups ground nuts (pecans, walnuts, almonds, or macadamia nuts)

⅔ cup ground golden flaxseed

2 teaspoons ground cinnamon

6 tablespoons butter

1½ cups fresh or frozen blueberries

2 cans (13.5 ounces each) coconut milk

Sweetener equivalent to ½ cup sugar

1 tablespoon or 1 packet unflavored gelatin

Whipped cream (optional)

Preheat the oven to 350°F.

In a large bowl, combine the nuts, flaxseed, cinnamon, and butter until mixed well. Press the mixture into a 9" pie plate, pressing at least halfway up the sides.

Cover the piecrust with foil and bake for 15 minutes. Remove the foil and bake for 10 minutes, or until the crust is golden and no longer moist to the touch.

Meanwhile, in a food chopper, food processor, or blender, reduce the blueberries to a puree.

In a medium saucepan over low heat, warm the coconut milk, blueberries, and sweetener, stirring frequently, for 5 minutes, or until warm to the touch. Slowly add the gelatin while stirring. Leave on the heat, stirring frequently, for 2 to 3 minutes, or until all the gelatin is dissolved. Remove from the heat and cool for 30 minutes.

Add the blueberry mixture to the finished piecrust. Transfer to the refrigerator and cool for at least 2 hours before serving. Serve with the whipped cream, if using.

Spicy Nut Mix

If you are in the mood for a savory, spicy snack, rather than potato chips or crackers, reach for this Spicy Nut Mix. As with many other recipes here, this basic recipe can serve as the prototype for many variations, both savory and sweet. These nuts are a great travel snack, as well.

MAKES 4 CUPS

> **1 cup each of your choice of 4 nuts/seeds (total 4 cups): raw pumpkin seeds, raw sunflower seeds, raw walnut halves, or raw pecan halves or pieces**
>
> **½ cup coconut oil, melted**
>
> **2 tablespoons grated Parmesan cheese**
>
> **2 teaspoons onion powder**
>
> **1 teaspoon garlic powder**
>
> **1 teaspoon ground red pepper**
>
> **1 teaspoon sea salt**

Preheat the oven to 275°F.

In a large bowl, combine the nuts/seeds, oil, cheese, onion powder, garlic powder, ground red pepper, and salt and toss to mix thoroughly.

Spread the mixture on a large baking sheet. Bake for 10 minutes, stirring once halfway through. Remove and cool.

Strawberry Cheesecake

Admittedly, this cheesecake recipe is loaded with dairy. I provide it here not to encourage you to eat dairy but to let you know that if the need arises (entertaining, holidays), you can re-create a delicious cheesecake without grains or sugar. Whenever possible, choose organic cream cheese and sour cream to reduce some of the problems associated with dairy products.

MAKES 8 SERVINGS

> **1½ cups ground pecans**
>
> **⅔ cup ground golden flaxseed**
>
> **2 teaspoons ground cinnamon**
>
> **6 tablespoons butter or coconut oil, melted**
>
> **16 ounces fresh or frozen strawberries**
>
> **16 ounces cream cheese, at room temperature**
>
> **1 cup sour cream**
>
> **2 eggs**
>
> **2 teaspoons vanilla extract**
>
> **Sweetener equivalent to ½ cup sugar**

Preheat the oven to 275°F.

In a medium bowl, combine the pecans, flaxseed, and cinnamon and mix thoroughly. Pour in the butter or oil and mix until dough forms. Press the dough into a 9" pie plate, pushing up the sides. Bake for 10 minutes.

Reserve 4 to 5 strawberries. In a food chopper or food processor, reduce the remaining strawberries to a puree.

In a large bowl, combine the cream cheese, sour cream, eggs, pureed strawberries, vanilla, and sweetener. Using an electric mixer on medium speed, beat until smooth. Pour into the piecrust and bake for 40 minutes, or until a knife or wooden pick withdraws clean. Cool on a rack and then refrigerate until ready to serve.

CHAPTER 11

Wild, Naked, and Unwashed: Cultivate Your Bowel Flora Garden

The destruction of our inner ecosystem surely deserves more attention as global populations run gut-first into the buzz saw of globalization and its microbial scrubbing diet.

—Jeff D. Leach, founder, Human Food Project: Anthropology of Microbes

Every health strategy I introduce in *Undoctored* is consistent with the way humans have survived on this planet since before Lucy had some splainin' to do to Ricky, before Antony and Cleopatra became tragic lovers, before we even had a notion of art or language. All of these Undoctored efforts make evolutionary sense and provide magnificent, outsize, often unexpected benefits, frequently life-changing, even during the initial 6 weeks—nothing unrecognized, nothing foreign, nothing "medical."

Removing wheat and grains from the diet yields extraordinary benefits because that's how humans ate for 99.6 percent of our time on earth, the chronic diseases from grain consumption only appearing in the last 0.4 percent of the time since we were fooled into thinking that breads, corn, and oats were healthy, tasty sources of calories, unaware of their potential for chronic disease.

Likewise, all the other strategies I am going to discuss in this and the next chapter yield substantial benefits because they belong in the human experience, suiting needs your body developed over eons of adaptation. And when these seemingly unconnected strategies are combined, a powerful synergy of benefits emerge, strong enough to reverse numerous health conditions.

Let's begin with what is probably the most challenging but also among the most exciting areas of health to restore, the microcosm of organisms dwelling in your intestines. By restoring healthy bowel microorganisms alone, you can obtain some pretty impressive health benefits. But restore healthy bowel flora in the context of the entire menu of Undoctored strategies, and even bigger and better things happen.

Work on Your Brown Thumb

Below the diaphragm, housed within the privacy of your bowels, is an entire universe of microorganisms that interact vigorously with their environment—and that environment is *you*. You may not be aware of the bacterial hubbub, but this 3- or 4-pound population of trillions of creatures interacts with your body 24 hours a day. They rely on you—who else?—to feed them, while you rely on them to produce metabolites, or by-products, that your body depends on, such as specific fatty acids and vitamins that you cannot manufacture on your own. While microorganisms populating the skin, mouth, and other areas likewise hold implications for health, it's the population in the bowels that holds the greatest consequences for us.

I have found that viewing bowel flora like a backyard garden helps get your arms around these issues. Just as you prepare the soil and plant seeds in springtime and then water and fertilize your garden through the growing season in order to have a rich bounty of juicy cucumbers and tomatoes, you will take a similar approach in cultivating this "garden" called bowel flora. And I want you to take full advantage of this powerful strategy and nurture your "brown thumb."

Fail to nurture this symbiotic relationship or allow external factors to disrupt it and—like other failed relationships involving crying, yelling, and nasty divorce settlements—there will be no happy ending. Unfortunately, just as we have managed to pollute our lakes and rivers, we have also fouled our intestinal tracts for the creatures dwelling there—with serious implications for our health.

One of the ways in which we've fouled our body environment, inside and out, is from an excessive focus on cleanliness. While some forms of cleanliness, such as municipal sewage to avoid dysentery, have been public health successes, others have had unintended adverse consequences. We've gone from a life of hunting animals, sleeping on dirt floors, and bathing whenever the seasonal occasion arose to a life filled with hot running water and toiletries for every surface and orifice, levers that flush away products of human digestion, and hand wipes for every occasion. We reach for hand sanitizers, mouthwash, toothpaste, dental floss, deodorants, and antiperspirants to conceal human body odors. We wash dishes and silverware in dishwashers that don't just clean off food residues, but sterilize. But the day-to-day "dirtiness" of human life was also what kept repopulating our bodies with the organisms needed for health. Witness the body and life of someone who lived before the last few decades, and you would likely be repulsed by the smell, the dirt, the eagerness with which they consumed the organs and meats of the animals they killed, sometimes raw. Yet that is how human life was conducted until modern conveniences like washing machines, supermarkets, and Lysol came along.

Yes, life may have been dirty in our eyes. But the bodies of our primitive ancestors were populated by microorganisms, both internally and externally, different from those that populate us. No matter how much you shampoo your hair, scrub your skin and crevices with soap, or wipe kitchen counters down with disinfectant, your body is still populated by trillions of microorganisms. Modern efforts to sterilize our surroundings have not eliminated microorganisms, but they have *changed* the varieties dwelling in and on our bodies, allowing benign or healthy organisms to be replaced with harmful intruders. Distortions of microorganism populations begin at birth if a child is delivered by C-section, rather than through the vagina, depriving the newborn of essential microbes, as does feeding an infant formula in place of breastfeeding. Throw in the occasional exposure to antibiotics for, say, an earache or urinary tract infection, which temporarily wipes out microorganisms, especially those in your bowels, or the effects of chlorinated and fluoridated drinking water, and modern humans now have an entirely different collection of microorganisms compared to "dirty" primitive people.

I'm not suggesting that you pass up the bathroom and move your bowels in the backyard or reject the use of toothpaste or toilet paper. As exposure to hordes of humans around us has increased (unlike primitive humans who were exposed to only a few dozen other people with limited potential for exposure to disease-causing bacteria), exposure to undesirable organisms, such as staphylococcus from the skin and *E. coli* from the stool, as well as good ones, has increased, too. In fact, a recent London School of Hygiene & Tropical Medicine study found fecal organisms on the hands of 44 percent of people who touched public doorknobs.[1] To a degree, the cleanliness of our age is a necessity arising from the modern populated world, but we've taken it too far.

On top of our modern obsession with cleanliness are countless other factors that alter the human microbes colonizing our bodies: antibiotic residues in meat and nonorganic dairy products, industrial chemicals in food, genetically modified foods with Bt toxin and glyphosate, other herbicides permeating air and water. Just like the grasshoppers and hummingbirds that used to fill backyards and woods but are now nearly gone, so many microorganisms that were supposed to populate our bodies are long gone in modern people, replaced by a collection of newcomers.

Disrupted bowel flora (dysbiosis) is now the rule, rather than the exception. For instance, up to 85 percent of people with the common and "benign" condition irritable bowel syndrome have dysbiosis.[2] Prescription drugs, such as acid-blocking drugs prescribed for gastritis or acid reflux and narcotics (that slow bowel function), alter bowel flora to the point of causing new health problems just from this effect. If you are overweight or have an autoimmune condition, prediabetes, diabetes, constipation, or any number of other common health problems, it is virtually guaranteed that you have dysbiosis sufficient to impact health.

Can we compare the microorganisms of our bodies with people whose bodies have not been corrupted by modern exposures? The Hadza of Tanzania, living in the wild, following the hunter-gatherer life humans practiced for millions of years, never taking antibiotics, unexposed to wheat or grains or soft drinks, allowed the bowel flora from their bowel movements to be analyzed (surely puzzling the simple-living Hadza), which was then compared to the bowel flora of modern Italians. Hadza bowel flora proved strikingly different with, for instance, plentiful spirochetes and *Prevotella*, species that are absent or present in negligible numbers in modern humans.[3] Likewise, bowel flora of the Matsés living along the Javari river in Peru, also isolated from modern life like the Hadza, was compared to bowel flora of Americans from Norman, Oklahoma, revealing that Matsés harbored species entirely unlike modern Oklahomans—but very similar to the Hadza, even though the two groups live on two different continents.[4]

Populations such as the Burkina Faso of northwest Africa and the people of the Tunapuco highlands of Peru who have lifestyles that are intermediate— some hunting and gathering, some agriculture, some trade with modern people for breads and dairy—have bowel flora that is intermediate in composition, in between that of isolated primitive cultures and modern people. Human habits craft the composition of our bowel flora, with bowel flora composition of the Hadza and Matsés likely reflecting Stone Age bowel flora before the mistakes of modern diet entered the picture.

It is clear that modern humans have inadvertently and dramatically changed the composition of their bowel flora. The science surrounding bowel flora is evolving, but it is providing surprising lessons nonetheless. Do we already know enough to make efforts that help us retrace our bacterial legacy and regain some of the potential health benefits of healthy, undisrupted bowel flora? You bet.

It has become clear that just about any disruption of health, such as diabetes or ulcerative colitis, is associated with substantial *further* changes in bowel flora compared to "normal" modern people. It is not clear, however, whether such changes are part of the cause or just a consequence of each process (probably both). Some of the most exciting observations are still in the experimental stage but providing compelling lessons. For instance, when bowel flora of mice with colon cancer is transplanted to normal mice, normal mice recipients develop colon cancer—unhealthy bowel flora causes cancer.[5] The effect of bowel flora on mental and emotional health is proving to be so powerful that researchers now discuss the implications of a gut-brain axis, a two-way line of communication between bowel flora and the brain. (When your 3-year-old son calls his sister a "poop head," he is making an accurate physiological observation.)

Exercising your brown thumb to cultivate a healthy bowel flora garden can yield impressive health benefits, including:

- Reduced symptoms of irritable bowel syndrome
- Reduced childhood infections and infant colic
- Reduced atopic dermatitis (eczema)
- Reduced appetite mediated through appetite hormones such as GLP-1 and ghrelin
- Reduced blood sugar, insulin, and insulin resistance
- Increased absorption of calcium
- Reduced triglycerides and total and LDL cholesterol

- Deeper sleep and reduced daytime anxiety
- Reduced stress via reduction in cortisol and other stress responses
- Reduced blood pressure
- Improved bowel regularity and reduction in factors leading to colorectal cancer
- Higher urinary oxalate levels that lead to calcium oxalate kidney stones[6, 7, 8, 9, 10, 11, 12, 13]

You can appreciate that the microorganisms living in your bowels affect many aspects of health, not just the health of the bowels where they live. These creatures may reside mostly in your colon, but their impact reaches far and wide into body processes. You can also appreciate that nobody in modern health care works to restore healthy bowel flora; instead, countless drugs are prescribed to "correct" many of the phenomena attributable to dysbiosis.

How do you know whether you have dysbiosis? This is like asking "How do I know I've been exposed to industrial chemicals?" or "How do I know whether my teenagers are Snapchatting their friends?" Living in the modern world, it is impossible to *not* be exposed to industrial chemicals through water, air, food, plastics, or hair conditioner, and if you've got a teenager, she is almost certainly among the kids sharing two billion images per day on social media. Likewise, if you breathe, eat, live in a house, take medication, or have ever taken an antibiotic, then you have some degree of dysbiosis. And given the stark differences in bowel flora when comparing modern people to primitive people, one could even argue that *everyone* in the modern world has some degree of dysbiosis.

Unfortunately, methods to formally diagnose dysbiosis are crude. No surprise, gastroenterologists advocate upper endoscopy to obtain a sample of intestinal contents, an effort that misses the majority of cases since only the most severe forms of dysbiosis, labeled small intestinal bacterial over-growth, will be detected this way. The majority of dysbiosis occurs in the colon, 24 feet away from where an upper endoscopy sample is obtained, in the duodenum. There are breath tests that identify altered products of metabolism caused by undesirable bacterial species, though few doctors use them, and there is general disagreement on what constitutes "abnormal."

In truth, the great majority of us do *not* need to undergo such diagnostic efforts. Since virtually all of us begin with various degrees of dysbiosis, why not just follow a simple program that pushes us toward a healthier bowel flora composition? Perhaps we don't have to have poop rich in

U-HAUL, YOUTUBE ... NOW YOU CAN
SEQUENCE YOUR OWN BOWEL FLORA

Control over life and health is being returned to the individual, putting *you* at the center of the effort. The same applies to analyzing the status of your bowel flora.

The company uBiome (ubiome.com) makes a bowel flora assessment easy for just $89. (Don't let the price fool you, though: uBiome uses the same cutting-edge technologies used in the National Institutes of Health Human Microbiome Project.) After a bowel movement, simply take the cotton swab from the test kit provided, swipe it across a piece of toilet paper, insert it into the plastic tube from the kit, and then mail it back for analysis. uBiome technicians extract the bacterial DNA in the sample. In a few weeks, you will be able to review the composition of your bowel flora in exquisite detail.

uBiome is also the perfect example of burgeoning crowdsourced wisdom. After analyzing the composition of your bowel flora in the context of your health issues (or lack of), they add your data (with your permission) anonymously, of course, into a database of hundreds of thousands, soon to be millions, of people who have done likewise. This is already beginning to yield fascinating new lessons.

But there is no need to wait for unfolding crowd wisdom to put at least some of the information to practical use. The uBiome report will help identify patterns in your bowel flora, such as a relative lack of Bacteroidetes and an excess of Firmicutes, a pattern associated with obesity, which you can change over time with efforts such as the Undoctored Wild, Naked, and Unwashed program. In other words, you can monitor the status of your bowel flora on your own and assess whether you are achieving positive changes or not. (uBiome also offers a Gut Time Lapse, which consists of three kits: one to establish a baseline and two follow-up assessments.)

---

spirochetes like the Hadza, but replenishing what are believed to be healthy species does indeed yield health benefits in virtually everyone. This is the Undoctored approach: Accept that we start with a problem that allowed unhealthy conditions to gain hold; correct it using easy, safe, accessible methods; and then watch the wonderful things that happen.

To start your garden of bowel flora, you are going to plant seeds. The two kinds of "seeds" you will use are those found in high-potency probiotics and in lactose-fermented foods.

Probiotics are nothing more than nutritional supplements, usually in capsule form, that contain one or more species of bacteria that have been shown to be beneficial, such as *Lactobacillus rhamnosus, Bifidobacterium lactis, L. gasseri,* and *L. acidophilus.*[14, 15, 16] Given current knowledge, the

Admittedly, most of the information does not yield new insights given current knowledge, as the lessons have not yet been learned. But there are a couple of observations that you can make and begin working on.

● Sample diversity—When comparing the species diversity of your sample with samples from other people, it makes sense to push diversity as high as possible since modern people are plagued by a relative lack of species diversity. The precise goal is uncertain, but I believe that achieving more diversity than 90 percent of other people's samples is a workable goal. Incorporating prebiotic fibers and eating a larger variety of vegetables help accomplish this, as does avoiding disruptive factors on bowel flora (see "No Raccoons in the Garden" on page 258).

● Increase the percentage of Bacteroidetes to exceed the average of the comparison population, and decrease the percentage of Firmicutes (species associated with weight gain) compared to the average.

It's not yet a lot to go on. But I have learned over time that if you pose questions, the answers will come; if you don't ask the questions, the answers will never come. And note that changes in bowel flora composition require months or longer; after an initial assessment, wait at least several months before reassessment.

If this stuff really turns you on, you can participate in crowdsourced microbiome science through projects such as American Gut (americangut.org), which also makes bowel flora testing available. There are also excellent and entertaining discussions on the Human Food Project: Anthropology of Microbes Web site (humanfoodproject.com), including analyses of the Hadza diet, analyses of fiber intake, and founder Jeff D. Leach's description of injecting fresh Hadza poop into his rectum with a turkey baster and then following the changes in his personal microbiome.

best probiotics contain multiple species, preferably at least a dozen, since species diversity has proven, over and over again, to be associated with health. A good probiotic should also contain substantial numbers of organisms (colony-forming units, or CFUs), preferably 50 billion (yes, billion with a *B*) or more in order to exert an effect. They also do not have to be taken beyond the first 6 weeks of the Undoctored program—just as you would not plant seeds in your garden every day of the growing season. So take your high-potency, multispecies probiotic for 6 weeks, and then stop, as this "reseeds" your colon with the species contained. If you obtain early relief from symptoms of, say, bloating or abdominal discomfort with the probiotic but have them recur when you stop, then consider a longer probiotic course (3 to 6 months). Also, people with complex health conditions—especially

CONSTIPATION NATION

I don't want you to strain to understand this, but follow this sequence.

1. Encourage people to consume more wheat and grains that contain glia-din, partially digested to opiates that, like all other opiates, cause consti-pation,[17, 18] and then . . .

2. Encourage people to consume more cellulose fiber to bulk up their stools, and . . .

3. Prescribe stool softeners and laxatives to force bowel movements.

Here's another common scenario.

1. Encourage people to consume more wheat and grains that provoke inflammation and pain (joint, muscle), and then . . .

2. Prescribe nonsteroidal anti-inflammatory drugs (naproxen, ibuprofen, Vioxx, etc.) that alter bowel flora and encourage dysbiosis, thereby ampli-fying inflammation, and then . . .

3. Prescribe narcotics, such as morphine and OxyContin, that cause con-stipation, furthering inflammation via dysbiosis, and then . . .

4. Prescribe prescription drugs like Linzess for constipation.

Constipation is an exceptionally common problem, occupying about half of the counseling time of gastroenterologists. It is a perfect illustration of how conventional dietary advice can build a medical franchise, whether the $500 million-per-year over-the-counter laxative market or the $300-per-month-per-person, $1 billion-per-year sales of Linzess.

Try it, you'll like it: no grains, no drugs provoking dysbiosis, no narcotics causing constipation, no need for over-the-counter or prescription drugs to "treat" stubborn bowels, while easing your way to a healthier life for your bowels free of medical shenanigans.

autoimmune diseases, ulcerative colitis, Crohn's disease, or celiac disease—should consider a longer course of at least a year, as healing and repopula-tion of the intestines with healthy microorganisms requires a longer time period in these instances. And if you need to take antibiotics, resume the probiotic both during and for at least 8 weeks after taking the antibiotic; just don't take the antibiotic and the probiotic at the same time (they should be separated by several hours), or else the antibiotic will kill the organisms in the probiotic. (Studies have demonstrated that antibiotics are actually *safer* when taken with a probiotic, as the feared complication of *Clostridium difficile* overgrowth is reduced.) My top choices for healthy probiotic preparations you can purchase are listed in Appendix D.

Another way to seed healthy species is to include fermented foods in your daily habits, a practice that should extend beyond your 6-week Undoctored program and be continued indefinitely. This is a very simple practice that adds little to no cost to your grocery bill but provides a natural means of further supplementing species such as lactobacillus and leuconostoc. These are microbial species that ferment sugars into lactate, giving vegetables and fruits a tangy sensation and adding health benefits when you consume them. You may even find that you and your family begin to love the unique flavors of, say, spiral-cut fermented beets or caraway seed– and rosemary-infused fermented radishes added to salads. (Fermentation is not the same as pickling; dill pickles and store-bought sauerkraut are *not* probiotic sources and have no beneficial microbial species.)

As wonderful as they are, fermented foods cannot replace a high-potency, multispecies probiotic. The numbers of CFUs provided by fermented foods can reach the billions and add to the benefits of a probiotic, but these foods tend to contain only between one and four different species, which won't give you the species diversity you need. Our "seeds" are therefore a combination of an upfront high-potency, multispecies probiotic with long-term consumption of fermented foods. The basic methods to ferment foods in your kitchen are outlined in Appendix C. I've also included some recipes that incorporate fermented vegetables in Chapter 10.

If probiotics and fermented foods are the seeds for bowel flora, what are the "water" and "fertilizer" that nourish them? These are called *prebiotic fibers*, fibers that you ingest but cannot digest, leaving them for microorganisms in the intestines to consume. Some call prebiotic fibers resistant starch since they are impervious to human digestion and digested by microorganisms. Getting prebiotic fibers is crucial to your health and the success of your diet.

Don't confuse prebiotic fibers with the more commonly recognized cellulose fibers from bran cereals, bran muffins, and whole grains, not too different from wood fiber. Cellulose is not metabolized by you or by bowel flora, thereby providing nothing more than bulk in bowel movements with none of the physiological benefits of prebiotic fibers. If you came to believe that bran products were the answer to health problems, you were once again fooled by the overly simplistic thinking and/or marketing of the food industry, an argument not too different from "you need more sawdust in your

NO RACCOONS IN THE GARDEN

Ever have a backyard garden that you carefully tended, only to have rabbits or raccoons make off with your vegetables and fruits? In other words, just planting seeds and tending the garden may not be enough if there are other disruptive factors at work.

The same applies to the bowel flora garden you are cultivating. There are some simple steps you can take to reduce your exposure to bowel flora–disrupting factors, the "raccoons" in your bowel flora garden. By removing wheat, grains, and processed junk foods, as well as Bt toxin and glyphosate residues that come via genetically modified corn and soy, you have eliminated factors that are known to disrupt bowel flora. But there are additional efforts that you can take to help keep wily varmints out of your garden.

● Filter drinking water to remove chlorine, fluoride, and other contaminants. Drinking water straight from the tap is toxic. If you use tap water to ferment vegetables, the chlorine and fluoride will block fermentation. Likewise, watering houseplants with tap water can make them wither. Yes, municipal water filtration removes most contaminants, but chlorine (or, more recently, chloramine, which is more persistent and resists being boiled off) and fluoride are added after filtration. Chlorine and fluoride are antibacterial, therefore reducing or altering the composition of bowel flora, as well as killing off soil flora when used to water plants.[19] To remove chlorine and fluoride, filter your tap water using a reverse-osmosis process and/or carbon filters. Filtered water is also less likely to contain residues of prescription drugs that are making their way into our water supply. Note that water filtration is a modern necessity for full Undoctored health, but it makes it even more important to obtain magnesium by other means (discussed in Chapter 12), as the good is filtered out with the bad.

● Avoid unnecessary antibiotics. There will be times when antibiotics are unavoidable. But steer clear of them for questionable indications, such as for

diet." Cellulose is not harmful, but it does not provide the outsize benefits of prebiotic fibers. The substantial benefits of fiber come via bowel flora digestion of prebiotic fibers to fatty acids and vitamins, not by having a larger bowel movement from cellulose.

As I've discussed, all the Undoctored strategies are adaptively appropriate (i.e., they are not foreign to the human body and mimic primitive experiences of the sort that helped create modern *Homo sapiens*), and this holds true with prebiotic fibers. The consumption of prebiotic fibers is among the oldest of dietary habits in primate species, dating back to pre-*Homo* species.[24] But the problem is that while primitive humans dug in the dirt with sticks or bone fragments for edible roots and tubers, recognizing which were safe and which a viral illness "just in case" it converts to a bacterial infection. Also, dairy products and meats and poultry can, despite FDA policy, occasionally contain antibiotic residues. Avoid this exposure by choosing organic products whenever possible.

• Minimize or avoid prescription drugs. Acid reflux medications, nonsteroidal anti-inflammatory drugs, and narcotics are among the drugs that alter bowel flora.[20, 21] Severe dysbiosis is not uncommon. There are probably plenty of other prescription drugs that change bowel flora, but this is infrequently explored during the drug development process, so very little data exist. For this and other reasons, the Undoctored program works to help reverse your need for prescription drugs of all sorts, allowing your bowel flora to flourish without disruption.

• Minimize exposure to emulsifying agents. These common processed food ingredients keep components from separating (e.g., keeps peanut butter from separating into oil and peanut protein). But emulsifiers have the potential to disrupt the protective mucosal lining of the intestinal tract, alter the microbial composition of bowel flora, and provoke inflammation, insulin resistance, and colitis.[22] Total avoidance is, however, not practical, as there are natural emulsifiers in otherwise healthy foods, such as eggs (lecithin) and mustard. Therefore, try to minimize your exposure to added or synthetic emulsifiers, such as carboxymethyl cellulose, polysorbate-80, sodium stearoyl lactylate, and carrageenan.

• Avoid aspartame, saccharine, and sucralose. These artificial sweeteners have been shown to modify bowel flora and increase potential for prediabetes, helping explain why sugar-free soda drinkers are no more slender, even heavier, than sugared soda drinkers.[23] Choose natural and benign sweeteners instead, such as monk fruit, erythritol, and stevia.

The efforts we make to avoid such ubiquitous disrupters of bowel flora will be an important ongoing conversation, as new insights are emerging rapidly.

were not, this is tough for modern people to adopt. Not only are wild roots and tubers exceptionally fibrous and tough, but you're busy: You've got soccer practice for the kids, after all, a busy work schedule, and frozen ground part of the year. And imagine what the neighbors would say, seeing you clawing in the dirt and then brushing off roots you pulled out to eat. You won't be invited to the next neighborhood barbecue. So we choose foods containing prebiotic fibers that *re-create* the primitive experience, since perfect replication is impractical.

Here are the foods richest in prebiotic fibers.

GREEN BANANAS AND PLANTAINS—And I mean *green*. Not green-yellow, or a little green at one end, but green. It will be tough to peel and virtually inedible, so slice it lengthwise, shell out the pulp, chop it coarsely, and then use it in one of the prebiotic shake recipes, starting on page 263. You may have to stay alert for when the grocer puts out green bananas, and then either store them in the refrigerator, where they generally stay green for 4 to 5 days, or peel, chop, and store them in a container in the freezer and use as needed.

POTATOES—All potatoes when cooked are high in sugars and low in fiber. But when *raw*, white potatoes in particular are rich in prebiotic fiber—with 10 to 12 grams per one-half medium (3½ inches in diameter) potato—and contain zero sugar. (Sweet potatoes and yams have far less prebiotic fibers. This means that you chance excessive carbohydrate exposure even when they are consumed raw. Eat only small quantities, whether raw or cooked.) Some people actually enjoy eating raw white potatoes like an apple, while others prefer to include them in prebiotic shakes (starting on page 263).

INULIN AND FRUCTOOLIGOSACCHARIDE (FOS) FIBERS—From chicory root, Jerusalem artichoke, and other sources, these fibers can be purchased from health food stores as a purified powder. (Inulin has a longer fiber chain, FOS shorter, but they exert similar or overlapping benefits.) Inulin and FOS are easily added to foods such as the "granola" recipe from Chapter 10 (page 217) or to prebiotic shakes (starting on page 263).

LEGUMES—Kidney beans, black beans, white beans, chickpeas, other starchy beans, and lentils can be rich sources of the galactooligosaccharide, or GOS, form of prebiotic fibers. Hummus (pureed chickpeas) is another convenient source. However, legumes contain the carbohydrate amylopectin C, and while not as digestible as the amylopectin A of grains, it still has the potential to mess with blood sugars. We sidestep this issue while still obtaining a modest 3 to 4 grams of prebiotic fibers by limiting ourselves to small servings—¼ to ½ cup cooked with no more than 15 grams net carbohydrates (total carbohydrates minus fiber). (Use your carb-counting resource to calculate for each form of legume. Don't worry: This gets easy after a few tries.) Several recipes in Chapter 10 also incorporate small quantities of legumes.

Modest quantities of prebiotic fibers (generally around 1 gram per serving) can also be obtained through peas, jicama, turnips and parsnips and other root vegetables, onions, and garlic, as well as apples, oranges, and carrots. Of course, always mind your net-carb counts on these foods.

In summary, try to include prebiotic fiber choices from the following list every day.

GREEN BANANAS AND PLANTAINS: 10.9 grams per 1 medium (7-inch) banana (0 gram net carbs)

RAW WHITE POTATO: 10 to 12 grams per ½ medium (0 gram net carbs) (Avoid any raw potatoes with green skin, as this is a fungus. If encountered, peel off the skin.)

INULIN AND/OR FOS POWDERS: 5 grams per teaspoon (0 gram net carbs)

HUMMUS OR CHICKPEAS: 8 grams per ½ cup (13.5 grams net carbs)

LENTILS: 2.5 grams per ½ cup (11 grams net carbs)

BEANS: 3.8 grams per ½ cup (white beans are the richest with twice this quantity) (12 grams net carbs)

Note: Values for prebiotic content vary depending on the source and the method used to measure.[25, 26, 27]

The average (unhealthy) American obtains between 3 and 8 grams of prebiotic fibers per day, about half from grains. Measurable health benefits begin at a prebiotic fiber intake of around 8 grams per day, while maximum benefits occur at an intake of 20 grams per day. We therefore aim to obtain 20 grams each and every day, including replacing the modest deficit left by grain elimination, to stack the odds in favor of cultivating a successful bowel flora garden. As with eating fermented foods, this practice should be continued for the rest of your life. Most people make a daily shake or smoothie that includes one or more of the foods richest in prebiotic fibers, especially a raw white potato, green unripe banana, or 1 to 2 teaspoons of inulin/FOS. You will find recipes for a few variations starting on page 263.

A word of caution: During the first week of the Undoctored Wild, Naked, and Unwashed style of eating, prebiotic fibers are limited to no more than 10 grams per day (e.g., half a green banana). Exceed this during the first week and you can provoke unpleasant bloating and abdominal distress. So keep intake low the first week, and then increase to 20 grams the second week. In addition to using no more than half a banana or half a white potato in the shake recipes at the start, also omit the optional inulin/FOS powder the first week. You can add it later if your abdominal status seems favorable. If you experience unpleasant symptoms even with the low starting quantity, you probably have a worse-than-usual case of dysbiosis; in this case, a more extended course of probiotics and fermented foods should be followed. Try reintroducing prebiotic fibers after 4 weeks of further probiotic "seeding." If even this causes distress, then it's time to seek help from a healthcare practitioner with expertise in correcting severe dysbiosis (thankfully, an uncommon situation).

Here are a handful of easy recipes for shakes to add prebiotic fibers to your daily routine. A carb count of these shakes will suggest that they are high-carb, but they are not. Nutritional panels do not account for the zero carb count in green bananas or raw potatoes, counting all the prebiotic fibers as carbohydrates or sugars. Rest assured that, provided your bananas are green and your potatoes raw, these shakes do *not* pose any sugar challenges and, over time, *improve* blood sugar levels. These shakes obtain a light sweetness with natural sweeteners, such as stevia or monk fruit, thereby avoiding adding tons of fruit that amp up the carb count. (See Appendix B for a list of safe sweeteners.)

You will need a blender with a strong motor to handle the green banana or raw potato. If your blender stalls, or the end result is excessively lumpy or grainy, then treat yourself to a more powerful blender. (While a Vitamix is the ultimate powerful blender, I used a NutriBullet for all of these shake recipes, and it got the job done easily.)

Chocolate-Mint Prebiotic Shake

Start with cocoa and several variations are possible, such as this chocolate-mint shake. You can make a mocha variation by adding 1 teaspoon of instant coffee or by replacing the cup of milk with ½ cup hot brewed coffee and ½ cup canned coconut milk or heavy cream.

Choose the undutched variety of cocoa for full health benefits.

MAKES 1

> 1 peeled green banana or peeled raw white potato, coarsely chopped
>
> 1 cup unsweetened coconut milk, almond milk, or hemp milk
>
> 2½ tablespoons unsweetened cocoa powder
>
> ½ teaspoon vanilla extract
>
> Sweetener equivalent to 1 tablespoon sugar
>
> 1 teaspoon inulin or FOS powder (optional)

In a blender, combine the banana or potato, milk, cocoa powder, vanilla, sweetener, and inulin or FOS powder (if using). Blend until the banana or potato has been liquefied and mixed well. If the shake is too thick, add water as needed and blend to mix.

Masala Chai Prebiotic Shake

Masala chai tea introduces the heady scent and flavors of cinnamon, cloves, and cardamom. But there's an extra step for this shake: Brew a cup of tea first. The end result is a delightful warm tea drink.

While it may be tempting to use one of the preprepared masala chai teas from the supermarket, they are loaded with huge quantities of sugar, so avoid them. Having to brew your own tea adds a step, but you will know that there are no piles of health-destroying sugars involved.

MAKES 1

> 1 peeled green banana or peeled raw white potato, coarsely chopped
>
> 1 cup (8 ounces) freshly brewed masala chai tea
>
> ½ cup canned coconut milk or heavy cream
>
> Sweetener equivalent to 1 tablespoon sugar
>
> 1 teaspoon inulin or FOS powder (optional)

In a blender, combine the banana or potato, tea, coconut milk or cream, sweetener, and inulin or FOS powder (if using). Blend until the banana or potato has been liquefied and mixed well. If the shake is too thick, add water as needed and blend to mix.

Piña Colada Prebiotic Shake

This tropical combination of pineapple and coconut is a treat. Use unsweetened frozen or, of course, fresh pineapple, instead of canned. I like using frozen pineapple so that I can use just a little bit at a time and save the rest.

MAKES 1

> 1 peeled green banana or peeled raw white potato, coarsely chopped
>
> 1 cup unsweetened coconut milk, almond milk, or hemp milk
>
> ½ cup unsweetened shredded coconut
>
> ¼ cup chopped fresh or frozen pineapple
>
> Sweetener equivalent to 1 tablespoon sugar
>
> 1 teaspoon inulin or FOS powder (optional)

In a blender, combine the banana or potato, milk, coconut, pineapple, sweetener, and inulin or FOS powder (if using). Blend until the banana or potato has been liquefied and mixed well. If the shake is too thick, add water as needed and blend to mix.

Blueberry, Carrot, and Greens Prebiotic Shake

If you are into getting more greens and other nutritious foods through a shake or smoothie, here is one way to combine them with prebiotic fibers.

The spinach is interchangeable with your choice of greens, such as kale or collard greens.

MAKES 1

1 peeled green banana or peeled raw white potato, coarsely chopped

1 cucumber, coarsely sliced

1 cup fresh spinach

1 carrot, coarsely sliced

½ cup fresh or frozen blueberries

1 cup water

Sweetener equivalent to 1 tablespoon sugar

1 teaspoon inulin or FOS powder (optional)

In a blender, combine the banana or potato, cucumber, spinach, carrot, blueberries, water, sweetener, and inulin or FOS powder (if using). Blend until the banana or potato has been liquefied and mixed well. If the shake is too thick, add water as needed and blend to mix.

Key Lime–Avocado Prebiotic Shake

The avocado added to this shake creates a wonderful thick, rich consistency. (The same effect can be obtained in any of the other shake recipes here, as well.) While you can use freshly squeezed key lime juice, the bottled variety also works well.

MAKES 1

> 1 peeled green banana or peeled raw white potato, coarsely chopped
>
> 1 small to medium avocado, pitted
>
> 1 cup unsweetened coconut milk, almond milk, or hemp milk
>
> 2 tablespoons key lime juice
>
> Sweetener equivalent to 1 tablespoon sugar
>
> 1 teaspoon inulin or FOS powder (optional)

In a blender, combine the banana or potato, avocado, milk, lime juice, sweetener, and inulin or FOS powder (if using). Blend until the banana or potato has been liquefied and mixed well. If the shake is too thick, add water as needed and blend to mix.

Eater's Digest: A Work in Progress

As critical as bowel flora is to your health, I'll bet your doctor has never once offered to discuss the importance of this crucial health factor and how to restore it. Doesn't that encapsulate a lot about what is wrong with conventional "health care" and what is right with tackling individual, empowered health without the doctor?

Given the pace of emerging wisdom on bowel flora, we are certain to learn new lessons in coming years. It's ironic that what is accomplished so naturally and unscientifically by primitive people seems so daunting and mysterious to modern people. Should someone create a probiotic preparation that mimics the bowel flora composition enjoyed by the Hadza or Matsés that can be purchased at a health food store? Are there better ways to coddle and encourage healthy bacterial species to extract the greatest benefit from bowel flora? The answers will be emerging over time. And remember: This is not about selling you drugs and medical procedures; this is about putting control over such issues back into *your* hands and bowels, always asking whether a strategy is natural, appropriate for the human condition, and yields genuine benefits.

We've discussed diet and restoration of bowel flora, building on the synergies that are going to emerge when the entirety of the Undoctored program is under way. Now let's address how to correct common health-limiting nutrient deficiencies that when restored, yield even more extravagant benefits.

Chapter Summary:
Your Next Steps to Becoming Undoctored

All of us have bowel flora in our intestinal tracts different from that of our ancestors—changes introduced by prior antibiotics, chlorinated drinking water, and a multitude of other disruptive factors. This has profound implications for health, from blood sugar to emotional health.

View cultivating healthy bowel flora to facilitate health as growing a garden: Probiotics and fermented foods are the "seeds," and prebiotic fibers that nourish microorganisms are the "water" and "fertilizer." While a bit of effort is required, you will be rewarded by health on a level you hadn't thought possible.

CHAPTER 12

Wild, Naked, and Unwashed: Nutritional Supplements to Correct Deficiencies

Scurvy "is caused by the lack of fresh food. It is most common between the ages of six and eighteen months, and its occurrence calls for an immediate change to fresh boiled milk, raw meat juice, and mashed potato, but of course medical advice must be sought."

—D. G. Revell, MD, Rush Medical College, 1906

If you had scurvy and developed bleeding gums, painful open skin sores, incapacitating fatigue, damaged joints, and jaundice, would an intensive jogging program cure it? Would cutting back on fat make it better? Would a program of purging enemas provide relief? How about "fresh boiled milk," as doctors of the early 20th century advised?

I'm trying to drive home the point that if a specific nutritional deficiency exists, such as scurvy from lack of vitamin C, the only way to reverse it, treat it, cure it is—vitamin C. *Nothing* else can take its place. The costliest drugs or high-tech medical procedures can't replace it. You could buy the finest health insurance, take antibiotics for poorly healing skin wounds,

269

undergo MRIs, have your eroded knee or hip joint replaced with a prosthesis by the world's best orthopedic surgeon, but if the real cause is not addressed, then health problems will continue. Scurvy is not among the deficiencies addressed in this chapter, but it serves as a graphic illustration of how pointless medical "treatments" are if a nutritional cause is not pinpointed and corrected.

Despite the outward appearance of plenty in our society, most people have deficiencies of several crucial nutrients. It is therefore critical to identify nutritional deficiencies that develop in modern people and correct them, rather than try to "treat" the consequences of deficiency. This may sound silly until you recognize just how common this situation is in our modern world dominated by the thinking of conventional health care in which, as we've discussed, nutritional supplements cannot treat anything, do not reverse disease, and cannot reduce any symptoms according to the FDA and most doctors, who believe that only drugs can do that. In this chapter, you will learn to recognize the folly of this conventional view. Nutritional supplements can indeed treat health conditions, do indeed reverse disease, and wonderfully reduce or eliminate symptoms—when they are due to deficiency of a specific nutrient and that nutrient is replaced.

We've already addressed one common cause for multiple nutritional deficiencies: grains. I've witnessed, for example, countless women over the years who have undergone repeated blood tests, endoscopies, colonoscopies, and bone marrow biopsies to explain their iron deficiency anemia that fails to respond to iron supplementation, even prescription strength. I've seen women receive blood transfusions when the anemia became severe and life-threatening. The anemia then responds almost immediately to grain elimination, with a rapid increase in blood hemoglobin levels (due to removal of grain phytates that bind iron). Women (oddly, this effect plagues women far more than men) endure years, even decades, of fatigue, feeling chilled all the time, breathlessness, even being unable to carry out everyday tasks because they are too anemic to function. They are trapped by an unexplained disease that stumps doctors, undergoing endoscopy after unnecessary endoscopy, until someone recognizes that it is nothing more than the bagel and cereal for breakfast, the spaghetti or lasagna for dinner, accounting for the entire situation. Once again, if the cause is not identified and addressed, oodles of medical procedures and other useless interventions are aggressively prescribed while health problems pile up.

When the right cause is identified and corrected, the entire situation is transformed. With wheat and grain elimination no longer causing iron deficiency anemia, for instance, fatigue starts to reverse within days, warmth and comfortable breathing return, blood iron and hemoglobin levels climb back to normal—the endoscopies, blood transfusions, iron supplements, all of it entirely unnecessary (although iron supplements can accelerate recovery once grain phytates are out of the picture).

These painful misadventures are not isolated or uncommon, so rare as to make the front page of the newspaper. These are common, everyday issues that plague many people but are "treated" as medical problems. Doesn't it make better sense to always first ask whether any health issue might be due to an easily corrected nutritional deficiency or something wrong with diet, rather than arrive at that conclusion after years of painful symptoms, pointless drugs and medical procedures, and irreversible complications?

So you don't have to needlessly endure these things, this chapter will focus on correcting the common nutritional deficiencies that typically go unrecognized by doctors. You will see that if a nutrient required for a fundamental physiological need is restored, or the blocker of absorption removed, as in the case of wheat and grains, wonderful things happen. Unlike just taking a multivitamin with teensy-weensy quantities of many things, precisely pinpointing deficiencies and correcting them yields outsize, perceptible improvements in health almost immediately. These are the nutrients that fit into the adaptive framework of human life, addressing needs that developed over tens of thousands of generations, with deficiencies developing because of circumstances unique to modern life. Even better, when such deficiencies are corrected following wheat/grain elimination and with cultivation of healthy bowel flora, an extraordinary synergistic effect emerges: *Health improves far more than any one component of the program would explain.*

Conversely, you will not be hearing much about nutritional supplements that do *not* fit into this adaptive framework. There are indeed supplements that provide modest benefits (e.g., rhodiola for low energy or gingko biloba for memory) that fall outside of this adaptive framework, but not the dramatic, life-changing benefits provided by the elements included in the Wild, Naked, and Unwashed nutritional supplement approach that are powerful enough to impact hundreds of health conditions.

In this chapter, you will find strategies that make adaptive sense and provide *big* benefits. Let's run through them one by one.

Living Wild and Naked in the Sun while Gnawing on Liver: Vitamin D

You probably don't want to (or can't) go through your day nearly naked with plenty of body surface exposed, nor do most modern people want to eat liver with any regularity. For those and other reasons, we must address vitamin D, a factor essential for health. It was crucial for primitive humans, so it is crucial for you as a primate dressed in modern clothes. Primitive humans obtained it without conscious effort. But modern life has made it necessary for us to make a conscious effort to re-create this primitive but crucial experience.

Your wild ancestors lived outdoors most of the day, certainly before human populations migrated north and south of the equator. There was no Banana Republic or Ann Taylor, so they made do with anything they could fashion from skins of animals, often leaving much of their bodies exposed to the sun, if they wore anything at all. That was the primary means of obtaining vitamin D, since hairless skin exposed to sunlight activates vitamin D. Unlike modern people squeamish about consuming organs, such as liver, your ancestors relished it, along with bird eggs and fish, all modest additional sources of vitamin D. When deficient, the consequences on health are profound, almost as wide-ranging as the consequences of consuming the seeds of grasses. When replenished, the benefits of vitamin D can be spectacular. Combine the elimination of grains with the restoration of vitamin D, and the combined effects can be life-changing, an especially powerful combination for reversing various forms of inflammation.

A vitamin D deficiency develops when you live far from the equator, wear clothes covering much of the body's surface area, work indoors, gain weight (fat sequesters vitamin D and prevents your body from using it), and grow older, since we lose much of the ability to activate vitamin D in the skin after age 40.[1] Modern life in tropical or subtropical climates, such as Florida or southern California, is therefore no guarantee of having adequate vitamin D levels, as the majority of people even in sunnier climates are deficient.[2] I learned this lesson well in my Wisconsin cardiology practice when retired snowbirds just back from spending the entire winter in Florida, sporting dark leather-brown tans and tiny tan lines, were every bit as deficient as Wisconsinites who weathered the entire winter in Wisconsin.

Bottom line: It is uncommon to *not* be deficient in vitamin D and thereby exposed to all of its consequences: increased inflammation and increased risk for autoimmune diseases, osteopenia/osteoporosis (bone

VITAMIN D DEFICIENCY: DOWNRIGHT DISASTROUS

The consequences of vitamin D deficiency reach far and wide. No organ system is spared from its damaging effects.

Health issues associated with vitamin D deficiency include:

- Greater inflammation (reflected as higher C-reactive protein, interleukins, tumor necrosis factor, matrix metalloproteinase, and other blood markers), resulting in joint pain and arthritis and a greater risk for heart disease, cancer, and dementia
- Higher blood sugar and resistance to insulin, leading to type 2 diabetes
- Autoimmune injury to pancreatic beta cells that produce insulin, leading to type 1 diabetes
- Weight gain
- Greater risk for osteopenia/osteoporosis and fractures
- Periodontal disease
- Higher risk for many cancers, especially breast cancer, prostate cancer, colon cancer, ovarian cancer, and malignant melanoma
- Higher risk for heart attack, heart failure, and overall cardiovascular mortality
- Preeclampsia and eclampsia
- Depression and seasonal affective disorder
- Autoimmune conditions such as multiple sclerosis and rheumatoid arthritis
- Earlier death[3, 4, 5, 6]

The list is extensive and overlaps substantially with health conditions caused by wheat and grain consumption. The combination of wheat and grain consumption with vitamin D deficiency is a potent duo that accounts for an astonishing amount of human illness. Over the years, I've seen thousands of people who were "treated" through conventional medical care—drugs for osteoporosis, anti-inflammatory drugs, drugs and biologics for autoimmune disease—for conditions that reversed completely with the combined strategies of wheat/grain elimination with restoration of vitamin D. It is common for exposure to some component of wheat and grains to *initiate* a condition, and then vitamin D deficiency permits the disease to flourish—what I call a "permissive" effect. For example, people who develop Hashimoto's thyroiditis initiated by the gliadin protein of wheat and related grains are 90 percent likely to have vitamin D deficiency with 25-hydroxy vitamin D levels of 30 ng/mL or less; vitamin D finishes off what wheat and grains started.[7]

Understand the implications of vitamin D deficiency and you are empowered to not allow it to happen. The benefits of vitamin D replacement, on the background of wheat and grain elimination, are profound.

thinning), bone fractures, heart disease, depression, cancer, and dementia—in other words, a wide range of common modern diseases. (See "Vitamin D Deficiency: Downright Disastrous," page 273.) This plays out in some profound ways. For example, children genetically susceptible to type 1 diabetes (an autoimmune disease of the pancreas *initiated* in many, if not most, cases by the gliadin protein of wheat and related proteins of other grains) are more likely to develop the disease when vitamin D deficient, less likely if not deficient (it doesn't cause the disease, but deficiency allows it to emerge).[8] Multiple sclerosis, an autoimmune condition of the nervous system, is more common the farther north and south of the equator you live.[9] Likewise, colon and breast cancers are more common in less sunny regions and with lower blood levels of vitamin D (i.e., vitamin D deficiency permits diseases caused by other factors to emerge).[10]

You can assess vitamin D status by measuring the blood level of 25-hydroxy vitamin D, a simple and inexpensive test that you can even do on your own with a finger-stick.

As with all things Undoctored, we do not aim to achieve an *average* level of any nutrient, yet that is what is typically quoted by laboratories and advised by most doctors. (Imagine the doctor said this out loud: "I help you obtain average health, not ideal health.") What level of vitamin D, measured as 25-hydroxy vitamin D, is *ideal*, however, is open to debate. If we combine observations on diseases permitted by low vitamin D levels with studies that demonstrate reversal of abnormal phenomena with vitamin D supplementation (such as high levels of parathyroid hormone, associated with bone weakening, that drop with increasing vitamin D blood levels), it seems that a 25-hydroxy vitamin D of 60 to 70 ng/mL (or 150 to 180 nmol/L) is the ideal range.[11] Is this level safe? In young people exposed to plentiful sun (e.g., playing on the beach in bathing suits), levels in this range and higher are easily achieved and obviously without toxicity. I interpret that as meaning this vitamin D range is naturally achievable and safe. No toxicity has ever been observed in this range.

The majority of people require vitamin D doses of 4,000 to 8,000 units in oil-based (gelcap) form to achieve the target 25-hydroxy vitamin D value of 60 to 70 ng/mL. Ideally, 25-hydroxy vitamin D should be reassessed every 6 to 12 months to maintain desired levels, as needs can change over time, including *decreased* need 2 to 3 years into your supplementation effort (signaled by an increase in 25-hydroxy vitamin D to unnecessarily high levels; just reduce the dose).

There are some simple rules to follow with vitamin D to increase your likelihood of a successful experience.

- Only choose oil-based gelcaps or liquid drops of vitamin D_3, *never tablets*. Most tablets are erratically absorbed or not absorbed at all, while gelcaps and drops are reliably absorbed.

- Take only vitamin D_3 (cholecalciferol), the human form, *never* vitamin D_2 (ergocalciferol), the nonhuman and, ironically, prescription form. D_2 is not the same, is less effective, does not yield the same benefits, and may even be harmful; there is no reason to take D_2 over D_3.[12, 13] D_3 is widely available in health food stores and big box retailers.

- Ideally, check your 25-hydroxy vitamin D blood level at the start of the program, before starting vitamin D replacement, and then no sooner than 2 to 3 months after supplementation, as it takes that long to rise and plateau (reach "steady state"). Checking too early after starting supplementation yields misleading results. Likewise, if you make a change in dosage, wait at least 2 to 3 months before reassessing your level. The baseline level prior to starting vitamin D can give you a sense of your individual need—the lower the starting level, the higher the dose you are likely to need. (With a starting level of, say, 10 ng/mL—profound deficiency— a higher dosage of 10,000 or 12,000 units can be considered.) Alternatively, just obtain a single 25-hydroxy vitamin D level 3 months or more after starting supplementation to assess whether you have achieved the target level.

- If you enjoy sun exposure for at least some of your vitamin D, do not burn, as this does indeed increase skin cancer risk. (You can also appreciate that conventional advice to severely restrict sun exposure is unnatural, bad advice that increases overall risk for cancer.) Don't be fooled into thinking that sun exposure and a tan are sufficient to restore vitamin D. If you are younger than 40 years old, live in a climate with plenty of sun, and enjoy exposure to sunlight over a large surface area with some frequency, have your 25-hydroxy vitamin D level checked as a means of assessing whether these efforts are sufficient. If you are over age 40, such exposure is typically *insufficient* and oral supplementation is almost always required. Also, consider obtaining at least one midsummer and one midwinter 25-hydroxy vitamin D value to get an idea of whether sun exposure causes an increased level, since there is tremendous individual variation. An occasional person will need to adjust dosage to accommodate the change in season (i.e., lower dose in sunny months, higher dose in cool months).

- People with a history of Crohn's disease, malabsorption, or celiac disease struggle to absorb vitamin D and typically start with more severe degrees of vitamin D deficiency, contributing to their condition worsening. They may not respond to usual doses, particularly in the beginning of a grain-free journey before intestinal healing has had a chance to occur. Higher doses may therefore be required, adjusted by monitoring 25-hydroxy vitamin D blood levels, which is essential. Rarely, absorption is so poor that injectable vitamin D has to be used, at least until intestinal healing has occurred.

- Dark-skinned people require five to ten times more time in the sun to activate vitamin D in the skin than fair-skinned people. (The loss of this activating effect also applies with aging.)

- If you are substantially overweight at the start of your Undoctored program, it is common to require twice as much or more vitamin D to achieve the target level. For people who fall into the obese range with low 25-hydroxy vitamin D levels of, say, 10 to 20 ng/mL, I've seen success starting with 10,000 to 12,000 units per day of D_3 gelcaps, increasing the dose as guided by blood levels several months later and adjusting the dose. As you lose weight on the *Undoctored* process, a reduction in dose is almost always required over time.

Checking blood levels can be a bit of a hassle. I will not be asking you to submit to all sorts of blood testing in the Undoctored approach. But a 25-hydroxy vitamin D blood level is the *one* truly essential measure to obtain beyond routine values like blood glucose.

If your health insurance covers the cost of this blood test (which they nearly always do), then going through your doctor and insisting on a 25-hydroxy vitamin D level will get you the information you need. If your doctor refuses and you don't want to get another doctor, you can do the test on your own. Finger-stick test kits are available from the Vitamin D Council (vitamindcouncil.org/testkit) and ZRT Laboratory (zrtlab.com), as well as direct-to-consumer labs listed in Appendix D.

The benefits of vitamin D restoration are considerable. If children at risk for type 1 diabetes, for example, are given 2,000 units per day, the incidence of type 1 diabetes drops by 88 percent.[14] Women with higher levels of vitamin D reduce their risk for multiple sclerosis by 41 percent and rheumatoid arthritis by 44 percent.[15] Even at a modest dose of 2,000 units per

CALCIUM: THROW IT OUT WITH THE DISHWATER

Calcium supplements have no role in the Undoctored lifestyle. For years, doctors have advised people to supplement calcium to prevent bone thinning and osteoporotic fractures based on the simple reasoning that if something is lacking, taking more of it must be the solution. But clinical trials have repeatedly demonstrated virtually no benefit with calcium supplementation— no slowing of bone thinning, no reduction of osteoporotic fractures. Likewise, people who consume plentiful dairy products containing calcium do not have better bone health. One thing that people who supplement calcium do have is more death from heart disease.[16] It should be a familiar theme by now: Not only has conventional advice *not* worked, it is responsible for *causing* health problems.

Calcium is an ineffective bone health supplement because just taking it orally does not mean it will go where it is needed, just as throwing a pile of bricks in the backyard does not mean that they will eventually form a nice brick patio. It may even end up where you don't want it to go, such as arteries and heart valves, just as the haphazard pile of backyard bricks trips you every time you barbecue.

People deficient in vitamin D start with low blood levels of calcium due to poor intestinal calcium absorption, but they also have elevated levels of parathyroid hormone, PTH, a pituitary hormone that extracts calcium from bones in an effort to compensate for low blood calcium, weakening bones over time. Restore vitamin D, and calcium blood levels increase due to better intestinal calcium absorption and PTH hormone levels drop, a phenomenon associated with better bone health, reduced fractures, and reduced heart attacks.[17] So the solution is not more calcium, but more vitamin D, and calcium naturally follows.

Vitamin D is therefore a powerful control factor over calcium. When replenished, vitamin D increases intestinal absorption of calcium from food, causes calcium to be deposited in bone, and inhibits its deposition in arteries and valves. Calcium is passive; it's the vitamin D that directs its fate. And bear in mind that with the Undoctored lifestyle, we eliminate the plentiful phytates from wheat and grains that block calcium absorption. Combine the calcium absorption–increasing effects of vitamin D, the removal of the calcium absorption–blocking effects of grain phytates, and the drop in PTH, and calcium supplementation is completely unnecessary, as your Undoctored lifestyle restores normal calcium status without the dangers of calcium supplementation.

day, vitamin D is associated with 30 percent reduction in osteoporotic hip fractures.[18] And people with higher vitamin D intakes have 75 percent less risk for Alzheimer's dementia.[19]

Given the power of vitamin D, you'd think that doctors would be experts in managing the vitamin D status of their patients. Ah, but you now know better. It's not a drug, it brings no rich revenue stream, and you can even buy it yourself and finger-stick your own blood levels, so it is essentially off the radar for most physicians. While attitudes among my colleagues are improving, blatant ignorance and imprecision are still rampant. Beyond outright dismissal of its importance, many doctors say things like "you'll be fine with 1,000 units per day" or hand you a prescription for D_2 because of the common assumption that if it comes by prescription, it must be superior. Predictably, drug companies are working vigorously to develop vitamin D analogues that are patent protectable and can be sold at a substantial premium when prescribed by physicians. But we know better: The closer something is to the natural form, the better it is to serve natural physiologic need. Don't let the drug industry do to vitamin D what it did to fish oil. By following the Undoctored approach, you will be far more effective in obtaining the benefits of vitamin D restoration.

Iodine and Thyroid Health: An Old Problem Returns

Those who cannot remember the past are doomed to repeat it—I'm sure you've heard this from your history teacher, if not your dad. That bit of wisdom applies perfectly to iodine.

As I've discussed, up until a century ago, goiters—enlarged thyroid glands protruding from the neck—due to iodine deficiency were exceptionally common. Because the earth's iodine is concentrated in the ocean, people who lived in inland areas suffered the worst, since there is less access to seafood, shellfish, and iodine from crops grown in coastal soil.

Goiters were not just a cosmetic problem. They were also associated with devastating health consequences: impaired growth and learning in children, increased risk for heart attacks and heart failure, weight gain, edema (water retention), and premature death. Pregnant mothers delivered babies that were mentally impaired. Entire inland villages in Europe were sometimes filled with people labeled "cretins," standing barely 4 feet tall, pale, edematous, and mentally impaired—all with visible goiters. In short, goiters were an enormous public health problem.

Conventional health care blamed everything from drinking dirty water to drunkenness. Medical "solutions" were equally bizarre, including burning the thyroid with acid or gunpowder. Since ancient times, people have choked and suffocated as goiters encircled the neck and crushed the trachea and carotid artery and veins. In fact, thyroid surgery is one of the oldest surgeries performed, dating back to ancient Egypt and Greece, a surgery that was lifesaving but resigned the patient to a slow death due to lack of thyroid hormone—hypothyroidism (untreatable in the past due to lack of thyroid hormone replacement).

At various times over the last 2,000 years, sporadic success at reducing goiters was observed by consuming such things as ground seaweed or shellfish and the thyroid glands of animals (which contain iodine). It was finally conclusively demonstrated that goiters were due to lack of iodine, and a systematic public health effort was instituted. In 1924, the FDA, in an effort to provide iodine to illiterate, largely rural Americans, passed a regulation encouraging salt makers to add iodine, followed by nationally broadcasted advice to use salt liberally. Iodine was found to reverse so many health conditions that doctors had a popular saying: "If you don't know where, what, and why, prescribe then K and I" (*K* and *I* referring to potassium iodide as the chemical symbol *KI*).

It worked. Generous use of iodized salt and KI dispensed by pharmacies reversed goiters and other health conditions in millions of people. Up until the early 1960s, children lined up in schools to receive "goiter pills," large doses of iodine. (Ask your grandmother and you will see the glow of recognition: "Yes, I remember. I'd even ask if I could have other kids' pills because they were chocolate!") Iodized salt was hailed as a public health success story on par with municipal water treatment and public sewage.[20]

Those memories have been lost to people in health care, as well as most of the public under age 65. In response to reports that excess salt use in some groups contributed to heart failure and hypertension, the FDA reversed its forgotten stand on iodine and urged Americans to cut back on salt use. Some organizations, such as the Institute of Medicine, advocated that people at high risk cut back to 1,500 milligrams of sodium per day, meaning absolutely no salt added to food (a level that, you may recall, has since been associated with *increased* risk of death from cardiovascular disease), and that everyone else consume no more than 2,300 milligrams per day. You can probably guess what happened next: Yes, goiters have been making a comeback. (I've personally seen many.) But more subtle and widespread, iodine deficiency is a reemerging health problem, with goiters just the tip of the iodine-deficiency iceberg.[21]

I've seen this play out in everyday life countless times. The majority of goiters respond spectacularly to restoration of iodine: The goiter shrinks, and symptoms of hypothyroidism from the lack of iodine needed to

MIMICKING THE NATURAL SITUATION: RESTORING *IDEAL* THYROID STATUS

You've endured a lifetime of misguided dietary advice telling you that wheat and grains are the preferred source of human calories, while most doctors ignored the fact that grains initiate the process of autoimmune thyroid destruction in as many as half the cases of thyroid disease.[22] When initiated by grains (or a handful of other provocateurs), thyroid disease can first show as *hyper*thyroidism (Hashimoto's thyroiditis or Graves' disease), with palpitations, anxiety, weight loss, and other symptoms associated with excessive quantities of thyroid hormone released into the bloodstream due to active thyroid damage. This is typically followed, either naturally or because of medical treatment such as radioactive iodine administration or surgical thyroid gland removal, with lifelong *hypo*thyroidism, or low thyroid hormone status. While Undoctored strategies—especially wheat/grain elimination, vitamin D restoration, and bowel flora cultivation—are wonderfully effective in subduing, even completely "turning off," autoimmune thyroid inflammation (reflected by decreasing levels of antibodies directed against the thyroid, discussed below), these efforts cannot restore thyroid function; once the damage has been done, the thyroid can't really recover lost function, much as an alcoholic who damages his liver cannot undo cirrhosis and liver failure. Most people are left with lifelong hypothyroidism and consequently need thyroid hormone replacement.

This means that, once damaged, people who have had an autoimmune thyroid condition will nearly always need to take thyroid hormones in oral pill form. It is therefore crucial to understand that there are two main thyroid hormones, T_4 and T_3, the *3* and *4* referring to the number of iodine molecules per thyroid hormone molecule (explaining why iodine is necessary for the thyroid to manufacture T_4 and T_3). T_4 by itself doesn't do much, as it is converted to the active T_3 form throughout the body. And it is the conversion of T_4 to T_3 (by the enzyme 5'-deiodinase that removes one iodine) that is crucial to regaining ideal thyroid status.

Problem: Your thyroid can release all the T_4 it wants, or you can be prescribed lots of T_4 as levothyroxine (Synthroid), but we live in a time and place in which many factors block this conversion to active T_3. These blockers include triclosan in hand sanitizers, antibacterial soap, and toothpaste; the common food coloring Red 3 (erythrosine); and polybrominated diphenyl

manufacture thyroid hormones recede. (Uncommonly, an enlarged thyroid can be due to autoimmune thyroid inflammation and will therefore not respond to iodine, or respond with hyperthyroidism, releasing excessive thyroid hormones.) More commonly, however, there is no goiter but there are symptoms of low thyroid hormones, such as inappropriately cold hands and feet, low energy, and weight gain or inability to lose weight no matter how ethers, a flame retardant found in clothes and bedding.[23] Unfortunately, while we can indeed avoid such products for future exposure, no one has yet worked out a way to remove these blockers from the body from prior exposure (since some persist in the body for years) to allow unrestricted T_4-to-T_3 conversion, so we are left with having to address T_3 status through replacement of T_3.

A common situation arises when someone is prescribed a dose of T_4 as levothyroxine but T_3 status is not addressed: Symptoms improve but do not reverse fully, so the person continues to feel inappropriately cold and fatigued and fails to lose weight. The solution is to assess and correct T_3 status. The easiest solution for the majority of people is to replace levothyroxine with preparations that contain both T_4 and T_3, such as Armour Thyroid, Nature-Throid, Thyrolar, and others—widely available and inexpensive.

As you now know, doctors do not always incorporate new information, especially information originating from outside their immediate specialty. This is a problem, since much of the awareness about blockers of T_4-to-T_3 conversion have come from the world of toxicology, and toxicologists do not often talk to practicing physicians and vice versa. Also, much physician "education" is provided by drug salespeople, who advised doctors for many years that non-generic, expensive T_4 preparations were superior to low-cost T_4+T_3 preparations. Physicians were also advised that the T_4+T_3 combination products were sloppily controlled or impure, although this is untrue, even prompting FDA cease-and-desist actions against the drug manufacturers to make them stop these deceptive sales claims. Nonetheless, over 90 percent of physicians bought the sales pitch and prescribe T_4-only preparations.

So most people prescribed thyroid hormone take only T_4, with the majority (about 80 percent) suffering persistent hypothyroid symptoms. The key is to identify a healthcare practitioner, typically someone in functional or integrative medicine, who will assess, then correct, your T_3 status and relieve you of uncorrected hypothyroidism. The effects can be subtle to dramatic. Another way to identify a willing and informed practitioner: Contact a compounding pharmacy in your area (pharmacies that fill prescriptions for custom-made medications) and ask what healthcare practitioners prescribe compounded thyroid preparations. This usually identifies practitioners who go the extra mile in managing thyroid issues.

Bottom line: Challenge your doctor if you are prescribed T_4 alone. More than likely, you will have to identify a new practitioner to get this situation corrected.

serious the effort, symptoms your doctor tries to pointlessly "treat" with antidepressants, diuretics, and other drugs.

The solution: iodine, obviously. I say "obviously" because it is shocking that, even in the 21st century, thyroid removal surgery—the crude solution dating back thousands of years—is still advised, when the real, safest, simplest solution in the vast majority of cases is a few pennies' worth of iodine.

However, as you now know, health care often has nothing to do with health, but plenty to do with maximizing revenues from sickness, even "sickness" that is readily, safely, and inexpensively reversed.

That said, iodine is one of the handful of nutritional supplements included in the Undoctored Wild, Naked, and Unwashed approach that can pack a powerful punch by correcting a common deficiency, yet another component of the combined synergistic Undoctored strategies.

Here are some of the benefits of iodine restoration.

- Restoring iodine reverses 20 to 30 percent of cases of hypothyroidism; people likely to respond begin with a goiter and/or have a characteristic pattern on thyroid testing (see the "Eisenhower, *The Andy Griffith Show*, and Thyroid Testing" section on page 284), with a TSH (thyroid-stimulating hormone) slightly above ideal (1.5 mIU/L) and free T_4 thyroid hormone at the low end or slightly below the reference range quoted by the laboratory. Because some people correct thyroid status just by obtaining the iodine they need, it is best to allow 2 to 3 months to pass while supplementing iodine before committing to repeat thyroid testing and thyroid hormone replacement pills containing T_3 and T_4.
- Iodine protects the thyroid and other organs against halogenated industrial compounds, meaning chemicals containing fluorine, chlorine, and bromine, toxic compounds that are everywhere, from drinking water to swimming pools to herbicide residues on nonorganic vegetables to bread. Iodine is also a halogen and thereby partially blocks the toxic effects of other halogens.
- Iodine blocks the thyroid-blocking activity of cruciferous vegetables (I cringe when people declare, "I avoid all cruciferous vegetables—such as broccoli, kale, cauliflower, horseradish, collard greens, radishes, turnips, and cabbage—because they block the thyroid"). Cruciferous vegetables are nutritious, including amping up cancer-protecting properties via chemical detoxification pathways in the liver. Eliminating them is foolhardy and unnecessary—if iodine intake is adequate. Hypothyroidism from eating foods like broccoli and kale is virtually unheard of, though it can occur with consumption of millet (a grain).[24]
- Iodine protects against or can reverse fibrocystic breast disease. Fibrocystic breast disease, believed to be a precursor to some forms of breast cancer, occurs to greater degrees in women with iodine deficiency and can be reversed in many women with iodine restoration.[25]
- Iodine may be protective for oral health, as the salivary glands also concentrate iodine for secretion into saliva. While I've discussed how we

want to obtain some "dirty" microbes, salivary iodine may limit our exposure to excessive quantities in some situations.[26]

If you start your Undoctored program with iodine deficiency, the benefits of iodine restoration can be spectacular. If you are not deficient at the start, iodine is still worth supplementing because it provides a protective effect against many industrial chemicals and will prevent future deficiency.

This question arises commonly among people who have had their thyroid glands removed: Is there still a need for iodine? While iodine is critical for thyroid health, you can see that it is also important outside of the thyroid, especially for breast and oral health.

What is the dose of iodine required? Once again, we aim for the ideal intake, not an adequate or average intake. The Recommended Dietary Allowance, RDA, for iodine in adults is 150 micrograms per day, the quantity set many years ago as the intake required to not have a goiter. But just not having a goiter, you may appreciate, is probably not the same as the ideal intake, especially when factoring in nonthyroid benefits such as breast health. Even judged by the lax RDA measure, many Americans are deficient, with 28 percent markedly deficient in a recent national survey.[27] Examination of worldwide iodine intake patterns reveals some extreme variation. The Japanese, for instance, commonly have average intakes of 3,300 micrograms per day. Unfortunately, there are no detailed explorations to establish an ideal intake, but I have advised 500 to 1,000 micrograms per day for many years and have witnessed assured iodine replacement that includes reversal of hypothyroidism and many cases of fibrocystic breast disease, with not a single instance of iodine toxicity.

While you could obtain iodine by consuming the thyroid glands of animals, most instead opt for easier and more palatable potassium iodide drops or kelp tablets (dried seaweed tablets). Typical potassium iodide drops contain 100 to 150 micrograms per drop. I do not advise using a preparation called Lugol's iodine solution, a highly concentrated form of potassium iodide sold in some health food stores and pharmacies that, with even a minor miscalculation, can yield iodine toxicity in a few months. (I've seen this happen in a number of people.) The two forms I advocate, the low-potency drops or kelp tablets, have never yielded toxicity when used properly, are widely available, and are inexpensive, not costing more than a few dollars for a several-month supply.

One caution: If you have an autoimmune thyroid condition, such as Hashimoto's thyroiditis or Graves' disease, wheat/grain elimination and vitamin D supplementation should be pursued for at least several months while tracking the decline in thyroid antibodies that signal receding autoimmune inflammation before supplementing iodine. If and when the antibody values fall back to normal, that is the time to consider adding iodine. Add it too early, while autoimmune inflammation is active, and you can reactivate autoimmune inflammation. When inflammation subsides, I've had success adding iodine starting with very small doses of potassium iodide drops of 50 micrograms per day, increasing by 50 micrograms per day increments every 4 weeks until the target dose (e.g., 500 micrograms per day) is achieved, backing off if inflammation is triggered.

Eisenhower, *The Andy Griffith Show,* and Thyroid Testing

Get your thyroid tested at a conventional doctor's office, and you'd swear that President Eisenhower still held office and new episodes of *The Andy Griffith Show* with Andy, Aunt Bee, and Barney were airing on the black-and-white TV—that is how far out of touch many doctors are about thyroid health in an age of rapid information exchange and enlightenment.

Testing for thyroid status by most doctors means a single value, a TSH level. It also means adhering to outdated standards of what levels should be regarded as "normal." Greater levels of hypothyroidism (i.e., low thyroid hormone status) are signaled by higher levels of TSH. In other words, someone with a TSH level of 8 mIU/L has a lower thyroid hormone status, or more severe hypothyroidism, than someone with a TSH value of 2.5 mIU/L. Doctors continue to advise people that TSH values of 4.5 or 5.5 mIU/L are normal, ignoring the newest evidence over the past decade revealing that ideal—not average, not acceptable—thyroid status is 0.2 to 1.5 mIU/L.[28] It is therefore an exceptionally common situation for someone to have a TSH of 3.5 mIU/L accompanied by symptoms of cold hands and feet, unexplained fatigue, and inability to lose weight, as well as high cholesterol, high blood pressure, and thinning hair, and have a doctor advise that everything is fine—that it's all in that person's head. No, it's in the doctor's failure to factor in the newest information, the flood of data that fly in the face of old practices.

Another issue: A TSH value alone is insufficient to understand everything you need to know about thyroid status. How about levels of free (i.e., unbound to proteins, only the free and active) T_4 and free T_3? Those are important, too. How about levels of antibodies trying to damage the thyroid, such as thyroglobulin and thyroid peroxidase antibodies? These values can be important because they identify whether an autoimmune destructive process is at work and whether, if autoimmune inflammation is present, thyroid status should be expected to change, sometimes wildly, over time. Antibody levels also give you something to track to assess whether efforts such as grain elimination and vitamin D supplementation are causing antibody levels to drop as autoimmune inflammation subsides.

There is also the issue of reverse T_3, a T_3 hormone lookalike (mirror image) that blocks the action of the real T_3 and creates symptoms of hypothyroidism even when all other values appear normal. It is not entirely clear why some people develop this situation, though it appears to be more common in the presence of adrenal gland dysfunction and prolonged emotional or physical stress.[29]

A full thyroid assessment includes:

- TSH—aiming for an ideal range of 0.2 to 1.5 mIU/L.
- Free T_3 and free T_4—aiming for an ideal range in the upper half of the "reference range" provided by the lab. (Note that weight loss and acute illness can transiently drop T_3 levels that rebound over time and do not require replacement.)
- Thyroid antibodies—with levels above the reference range suggesting increasing levels of thyroid inflammation damaging the thyroid.
- Reverse T_3—with levels above the reference range suggesting increasing levels of blocked T_3 status. Reverse T_3 status can change over time, shifting your need for T_3 replacement. This can be especially true with Undoctored program benefits such as weight loss, reversal of inflammation, and cultivation of healthy bowel flora.

There's another level of complexity to factor in: We live in the age of endocrine disruption. We are increasingly exposed to industrial chemicals such as bisphenol A (BPA), phthalates in shampoos and conditioners, vinyl chloride from plastics, pesticides, herbicides, polychlorinated biphenyls (PCBs), perfluorooctanoic acid from Teflon, and many, many others that are proving to be potent disrupters of the endocrine system.[30] Although the thyroid gland is responsible for producing thyroid hormones, it's the hypothalamus and pituitary gland in the brain that control the thyroid. Every step of the way—hypothalamic control over pituitary function and pituitary control over thyroid function, for example—is susceptible to endocrine-disrupting chemicals. Bottom line: The simple rules doctors, including endocrinologists, follow to identify thyroid dysfunction no longer apply. In short, many doctors fail to recognize a thyroid problem even if it bit them.

The most common mistake is following the advice of a doctor who declares, "Your TSH of 3.8 mIU/L is in the normal range. You're fine." You can now appreciate how inadequate that assessment can be. Once again, the solution is to find a healthcare practitioner who empowers you and does a more comprehensive job of evaluating, then correcting, the increasingly common problem of thyroid dysfunction. On rare occasions, you may not be able to find such a person in your area, in which case there are ways to take back control over your thyroid status on your own, discussed below.

Going Commando on Thyroid

What if, despite your best efforts, you encounter nothing but resistance, ignorance, or indifference in your quest for ideal thyroid health? Every doctor you consult scoffs, laughs, or hustles you out of the office with advice to leave it alone or just shut up and take your levothyroxine.

Well, while it is not an ideal situation, this may be the time to become fully Undoctored and go commando on your thyroid—do it without the doctor.

If you find yourself in such a situation, here are some basic rules to follow.

- Read and reread this section on thyroid health so that you are fully aware of issues such as the importance of free T_3, the ideal range for TSH, and the effect of reverse T_3.
- Get the full panel of thyroid testing (see "Eisenhower, *The Andy Griffith Show*, and Thyroid Testing" on page 284) on your own. You can get tested through one of the direct-to-consumer labs listed in Appendix D or perform the testing in your kitchen or living room using finger-stick test kits provided by ZRT Laboratory (zrtlab.com).
- Use the do-it-yourself-at-home thyroid assessment strategy of checking a first-upon-arising oral temperature with a digital thermometer. Any temperatures consistently below 97.3°F suggest hypothyroidism; the farther below this value you get, the more likely hypothyroidism is present and the more severe it generally is. This method can also be used to track the adequacy of thyroid hormone replacement, with consistent oral temperatures of 97.3°F representing adequate replacement. (Consistently higher temperatures can suggest hyperthyroidism.)
- If thyroid hormone replacement is necessary, you can obtain thyroid hormones without a prescription from several overseas sites. I've ordered

Nature-Throid from the UK, for instance, without a prescription. The price is a bit higher than in the United States, but it circumvents all the costs that doctors add. Doses generally start at 1 grain (60 to 65 milligrams) in the morning on an empty stomach, with nothing to eat afterward for a minimum of 30 to 60 minutes (very important). Doses can be increased by one-half grain (30 to 32.5 milligrams) every 3 to 4 weeks as you monitor thyroid values and/or oral temperature.

- Monitor thyroid values—especially TSH, free T_3, free T_4—and first-upon-arising oral temperatures to assess progress. With any increase or decrease in thyroid dose, wait 3 to 4 weeks before any reassessment, as the T_4 component requires this amount of time to exert full effect.

And use the online communities that I and others have established to obtain feedback when you need it. In addition to the Undoctored site (undoctoredhealth.com), Stop the Thyroid Madness (stopthethyroidmadness.com) is an excellent resource. Pose a question, and receive oodles of useful responses.

Restoring iodine and attaining ideal thyroid status are vital components to remaining Undoctored. Failure to do either results in effects such as the inability to lose weight or flagrant weight gain, low energy and excessive need for sleep, higher total and LDL cholesterol, higher triglycerides, higher blood pressure, thinner hair, dry skin, increased risk for heart attack and cardiovascular death, and increased risk for heart failure—health issues that, of course, provide plenty of opportunities for conventional health care to intervene while never addressing the original cause.

The importance of thyroid health and much of the medical community's failure to address all the issues surrounding it are emblematic of the problems in modern health care. If diagnosing hypothyroidism and replacing T_4 and T_3 was a $10,000-per-patient effort, thyroid issues would be managed meticulously. But it is a low-cost, low revenue–return activity, despite how ubiquitous thyroid dysfunction is, and thus miserably neglected in medical circles.

As you now know, this does not mean that you have to sacrifice your thyroid health. It is a perfect area for you to seize control over, Undoctored.

Your Choice: Brain Stew or Fish Oil Capsules

If you tried to mimic some primitive human behaviors, you'd find them not just inconvenient but also abhorrent.

Obviously, primitive people did not obtain the two primary omega-3 fatty acids, eicosapentaenoic acid (EPA) and docosahexaenoic acid (DHA), from fish oil capsules. Nor did they come from plants, nuts, or seeds that contain no EPA and DHA (they contain only linolenic acid). There are only two concentrated sources of EPA and DHA available to us: seafood and the brains of animals—yes, the brains of animals. After all, DHA in particular is the most plentiful fatty acid in the human brain, just as it is in the brains of elk, gazelle, wild boar, and other creatures humans have consumed. Humans can obtain omega-3 fatty acids from consuming fish and shellfish, but not all primitive human populations were coastal or had the ability to fish. But we did kill land animals without cringing at the thought of consuming the liver or heart, and we certainly did not throw away the brain. If I have a hard time persuading modern people to add back a little braunschweiger (liver sausage), it's going to be practically impossible to convince them that a healthy slice of calf or pig brain is worth including with dinner now and then. Like with prebiotic fibers and vitamin D, you will re-create a primitive, but essential, experience using strategies more palatable to modern tastes. (There is also the recent issue of prion diseases, such as mad cow disease in cattle fed the brains and body parts of other cows, a man-made problem that makes human consumption of the brains of cows hazardous due to the perverted things humans have done to them.)

We brain-free folk are, for all practical purposes, left with consuming fish rich in omega-3 fatty acids. But there's a problem here, too: Increasing industrialization of the earth (especially coal burning) has caused fish to accumulate mercury and other contaminants, particularly species that consume other fish and thereby concentrate contaminants, a process called biomagnification. As a result, consuming fish high on the ocean's food chain (tilefish, king mackerel, shark, swordfish, ahi tuna) can cause accumulation of heavy metals and other chemicals in creatures who consume them, such as us. (Problems with mercury bioaccumulation are also emerging in people who consume plentiful merganser duck and other waterfowl that consume fish in large quantities.) Once again, it would be wonderful if we could mimic the behavior of a primitive human and just eat plenty of fish, but in today's world, that virtually guarantees mercury toxicity.[31] Our practical compromise is to eat fish no more than two or three times per week, preferably not those listed as the worst at biomagnification, while taking up the slack in omega-3 intake with fish oil, since the process of fish oil purification removes nearly all mercury and other contaminants.[32] (Cod liver oil is the exception, with unacceptable levels of contaminants, especially PCBs.)

There are plenty of good reasons to supplement omega-3 fatty acids.

Omega-3s are essential, not optional, fatty acids, with a very clear deficiency syndrome when they are lacking (impaired mental performance, depression, impaired childhood development, dry skin, dermatitis, and neuropathies). Many clinical studies demonstrate that higher intakes and blood levels of EPA and DHA yield reductions in sudden cardiac death, heart attack, heart rhythm disorders, autoimmune inflammatory conditions such as rheumatoid arthritis and lupus, and a variety of cancers, as well as improved brain development in children.[33, 34, 35, 36] (Recent controversy over the magnitude of benefit has arisen given that early studies demonstrated a dramatic reduction in cardiovascular events, while more recent studies demonstrate lesser or no benefits; this has been attributed to a blunting of benefit due to the ubiquitous prescription of statin drugs in study participants.[37]) Potential benefits apply only to the EPA and DHA of fish oil, not to the linolenic acid of meats, flaxseed, chia seeds, and walnuts. While linolenic acid is biochemically an omega-3 fatty acid and is, for other reasons, a healthy fatty acid, it does not yield the same benefits provided by EPA and DHA; only EPA and DHA can do that, just as only vitamin C can correct vitamin C deficiency.

You can observe the effects of EPA and DHA on triglyceride levels, typically reduced by 30 percent.[38] Among the other benefits of EPA and DHA are:

- Modest reduction in blood pressure (around 5 mmHg reduction in systolic pressure and 3 mmHg reduction in diastolic pressure)
- Modest reduction in risk for stroke
- Modest reduction in symptoms of rheumatoid arthritis
- Modest reduction in some measures of ulcerative colitis
- Modest reduction in measures of depression[39, 40, 41, 42, 43]

Although the reduction in triglycerides is substantial, most of the other benefits are relatively modest when EPA and DHA alone are used as treatment. However, the real power of EPA and DHA does not become evident until they are added to the other Undoctored strategies, reflecting the extraordinary synergy of this program. Triglycerides, for example, starting at a high level of 500 mg/dL can be reduced with 3,600 milligrams of EPA and DHA to around 300 mg/dL. But if combined with wheat/grain/sugar elimination, vitamin D restoration, iodine/thyroid normalization, and bowel flora cultivation, a final level of 45 mg/dL would be typical—complete reversal to healthy levels due to the breathtaking synergies built into the Undoctored menu of strategies. Likewise, reduction in blood pressure with

EPA and DHA alone is small, but when combined with all the other Undoctored strategies, the effects can be profound, typically sufficient to be able to stop several blood pressure drugs. Living Undoctored does not mean following only one of the strategies, but following the program *in its entirety*.

Fish oil supplements and seafood are the only reliable source of EPA and DHA. Krill oil, while interesting for its astaxanthin content (a carotenoid, similar to beta-carotene), provides only a trivial quantity of EPA and DHA and, unless you take huge quantities, cannot achieve the protective blood levels of EPA and DHA we need. (Those misleading marketing claims of "40 times more potent than fish oil" refer to the antioxidant potential of the astaxanthin, not to the omega-3 fatty acid content.) Krill oil is often marketed as containing a more highly absorbed phospholipid form of omega-3s, which is true, but the quantity contained in krill is so small that an entire bottle would have to be taken every day to yield a sufficient quantity of EPA and DHA.

I recommend an EPA + DHA intake of 3,000 to 3,600 milligrams per day (the dose of omega-3 fatty acids within fish oil, not the fish oil itself), divided in two (e.g., before breakfast, before dinner). This is the quantity that yields a level of omega-3 fatty acids in the bloodstream of 10 percent or more (i.e., 10 percent or more of all fatty acids in red blood cells are composed of EPA and DHA). (You can obtain your RBC omega-3 fatty acid level with a finger-stick blood test you perform at home; test kits are available from OmegaQuant at omegaquant.com. Wait several months after initiating supplementation before checking a level.) At this level, health benefits are maximized, especially protection from cardiovascular disease and dementia and reduction of body-wide inflammation.

The best fish oils are the liquid triglyceride form, as the triglyceride form is better absorbed (particularly up to threefold improved absorption of the DHA) and re-creates the natural form of omega-3s in fish. (See Appendix D for a listing of brands.) Properly processed liquid fish oil is nonfishy in odor but must be stored in the refrigerator tightly sealed. Most fish oil in capsule form is the ethyl ester form, the form that results when the triglyceride form is treated with alcohol. You can still do just fine with the capsule form, though absorption will simply not be as favorable as with the triglyceride form. Whether liquid or capsule, look for higher-potency preparations, as this makes obtaining our target level easier. For example, a fish oil capsule that contains 750 milligrams EPA and DHA means that four or five capsules per day will be needed to achieve our goal, while a capsule that contains 300 milligrams EPA and DHA means 10 to 12 capsules per day will be needed. Most liquid fish oil contains 1,500 milligrams or more of EPA and DHA per teaspoon.

JULIE IS UNDOCTORED

St. Louis, Missouri

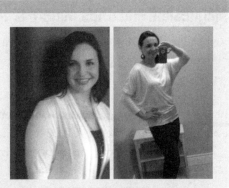

I am a registered nurse and mother of four. I have struggled with my weight since I was a child. I have tried every single diet imaginable.

I was diagnosed with polycystic ovary syndrome. After my third baby, I was experiencing fatigue, joint pain, constant hunger and cravings, acid reflux, hormonal acne, and terrible depression and anxiety. I was only 31.

As a nurse, I did what I thought I was supposed to do, which was to join Weight Watchers. I obsessed over points and went to bed hungry every day. Not only that, but my joint pain was getting worse. How was I going to take care of my kids if this was the way I was destined to feel the rest of my life? I felt hopeless.

My mother has rheumatoid arthritis, and her physician gave her a copy of the book *Wheat Belly* and told her to read it. Although she wasn't too convinced that this was the way she should change her life, she gave the book to me, and it was like I had finally found the missing piece of the puzzle. As a nurse, I understood what insulin was and how it worked, but I had no idea that my hormones were causing all of my trouble and that what I was eating was controlling my hormones. "Healthy whole grains" and sugar were putting me on a blood sugar roller coaster.

I made immediate changes to our diet as a family. I use probiotics and magnesium daily, take D_3, and use a raw prenatal with omega 3s and iodine. I lost 15 pounds in 2 weeks, and my skin cleared up. After a month, my joint pain was gone and I continued to lose weight, ultimately losing 45 pounds. My acid reflux is completely gone, and I have more energy most days than I know what to do with. My anxiety and depression are completely controlled as long as I don't stray from eating this way. I'm never hungry and eat delicious food every day. When I wanted to have one more child, I got pregnant without medications. I had no acid reflux during my pregnancy unless I overindulged in sugar, and I didn't have high blood pressure with my last pregnancy even though I was much older. I have been able to lose all of the baby weight again effortlessly, and now that I am almost 36, I can't believe that I am in so much better shape mentally and physically than I was in my twenties.

Your information completely changed my life, and I know that my four daughters will not have to struggle the way that I did. Thank you, thank you, thank you!

Magnesium and Other Minerals: Think Positive

Remember those darned phytates in wheat and other grains that bind magnesium and other positively charged minerals in the intestinal tract, preventing absorption and causing you to pass them into the toilet? It means that for years minerals were prevented from being absorbed whenever any phytate-consuming grain was in the vicinity, blocking the absorption of even mineral supplements. Advice to include grains in every meal and snack predictably caused deficiencies of positively charged minerals, especially magnesium, calcium, iron, and zinc.

Magnesium is at the top of the list of minerals that have been depleted. Have a breakfast of cereal with fruit, and nearly all the magnesium from breakfast is lost in the toilet due to phytates. Have a lunch of turkey breast on whole wheat bread with lettuce and tomatoes—and, once again, nearly all the magnesium from this meal was bound and passed. Popular acid-blocking drugs (PPIs) like Prilosec, Prevacid, Nexium, and others also block magnesium absorption.[44] Those with diabetes and prediabetes typically have the most severe magnesium deficiencies, as they lose magnesium through their urine.[45] Combine the magnesium absorption–blocking effect of grain phytates and PPIs with the removal of magnesium from drinking water via water filtration, both municipal and home, as well as the reduced magnesium content of modern crops,[46] and magnesium deficiency is now the rule. We therefore start the Undoctored process with profound, body-wide magnesium deficiency.

This has real health implications. Because magnesium participates in many essential body processes, depletion is disruptive. Among the effects of magnesium deficiency:

- Higher systolic and diastolic blood pressure. Ironically, the number-one preferred starting treatment for high blood pressure among primary care physicians is thiazide diuretics, such as hydrochlorothiazide and chlorthalidone, which cause increased urinary loss of magnesium (and potassium) and have thereby been associated with increased sudden cardiac death.

- Higher or erratic blood sugar, since magnesium is required for the body's enzymes to process blood sugar. Accordingly, each 100-milligram increase in daily magnesium intake decreases risk for diabetes by 15 percent.

- Muscle cramps, particularly in the calves and fingers, since magnesium modulates muscle tone.

- Heart rhythm disorders, especially premature atrial and ventricular con-
  tractions, atrial fibrillation, even life-threatening rhythms such as ventricular tachycardia and torsade des pointes.
- Higher risk for sudden cardiac death and heart attack. People with lower
  magnesium levels have double the risk of people with higher magnesium
  levels.
- Osteopenia and osteoporosis. Since over half of body magnesium is contained in bones and provides a "cross-bridging" function for structural
  bone proteins, lack of magnesium can have devastating long-term implications for bone health.
- Constipation. Ever notice that many laxatives are nothing more than
  forms of magnesium, such as milk of magnesia (magnesium hydroxide)?
- Migraine headaches, with magnesium injections providing relief in some
  instances.[47, 48, 49, 50]

The power of magnesium to even be lifesaving in acute deficiencies is
evident in hospitals, where it is administered intravenously to subdue
life-threatening heart rhythms and does so immediately and dramatically.
But we, of course, do not want to allow such acute, life-threatening deficiencies to develop.

As with other Undoctored strategies, restoration of magnesium
reaches across numerous health issues because it addresses an intrinsic,
fundamental human need, thereby providing outsize, sometimes
life-changing, benefits. Because most of us don't want to drink from a
nearby stream or river flowing over rocks and minerals or forage for wild
foods, we are left with nutritional supplementation. When done properly,
magnesium supplementation can be powerful. When done improperly
(which is what most people who supplement magnesium are guilty of), you
may be obtaining only the benefit of a laxative without restoration of this
essential mineral.

The trick with restoration of magnesium is to choose the form that is
best absorbed. Forms that are not well absorbed exert an osmotic effect in
the intestine (i.e., they draw water into the intestine and yield loose stools
and diarrhea). Loose stools can cause even greater magnesium loss, meaning
that the wrong magnesium supplement can *worsen* magnesium deficiency.
Choose the following forms for their greater absorptive potential.

- Magnesium malate, in tablet or capsule form (malic acid is a common
  component of fruit).

- Magnesium bicarbonate. This is the most highly absorbed form, but it is available only as a liquid that you make yourself (see Appendix C).
- Magnesium glycinate. While not absorbed as well as malate, it is a reasonable choice.
- Magnesium citrate. This is the preferred form if you desire a modest laxative effect or if you have a history of calcium oxalate stones (as both magnesium and citric acid inhibit formation of kidney stones).

I do not recommend magnesium oxide; although it is the most inexpensive and most common form, very little of it is absorbed and the laxative effect is quite prominent.

You want to obtain between 400 and 500 milligrams per day of magnesium, often called elemental magnesium (the weight of magnesium only, without the weight of the acid, such as malate). Confusingly, some supplement manufacturers will list the weight of the total capsule or tablet. For example, one 1,250-milligram tablet of magnesium malate provides 150 milligrams of elemental magnesium—the 1,250 milligrams is immaterial; you are only interested in the quantity of elemental magnesium. If you find a brand that only lists the total weight, skip it and find one that lists elemental magnesium.

Although the health benefits of restoring magnesium aren't as dramatic as that of vitamin D restoration or wheat/grain elimination, it can still yield some perceptible and measurable benefits, including reduction in systolic/diastolic blood pressure, relief from muscle cramps, reduction in heart rhythm disorders, less erratic blood sugars, more regular bowel movements, and fewer or less severe migraine headaches. Magnesium is also a crucial component of any effort to restore bone health, such as reversing osteopenia/osteoporosis, and to prevent or even reduce kidney stones (calcium oxalate). Because magnesium deficiency is the rule in modern people, since you cannot obtain sufficient quantities through modern foods or water, and because the health implications of deficiency are so great, everyone needs to restore magnesium. (The only exception is people with kidney disease who abnormally retain magnesium.) And as with all other Undoctored efforts, the real power of restoring magnesium shows itself when combined with the synergies of all the other Undoctored program components.

What about the other minerals blocked by prior grain phytate exposure and other factors? Deficiencies of calcium, iron, and zinc can be prominent at the start of your Undoctored program but, for most, do not require a specific replenishing effort, as removal of grain phytates, coupled with healing of the gastrointestinal tract, automatically corrects deficiencies of these three minerals without supplementation. Calcium status, for example, is corrected by removing all grains (which cause urinary calcium loss), restoring vitamin D, and correcting dysbiosis (which increases intestinal calcium absorption), making further efforts unnecessary. However, there can be exceptions in which some additional effort may be required.

IRON—Some people, females more than males, can begin with iron deficiency anemia (worsened by menstrual cycle loss). This is identified by a low hemoglobin level (below the reference range) coupled with a low MCV (mean corpuscular volume) value (describing red blood cell size) and low ferritin level (a storage form of iron). Common symptoms include low energy, feeling inappropriately cold, dizziness, breathlessness worsened with exercise, and pale skin and fingernail beds.

After wheat/grain elimination, eating foods rich in the organic heme form of iron—such as beef, liver, pork, poultry, fish, and shellfish—restores iron. Supplemental iron intake is only necessary if low levels of the iron storage protein, ferritin, or iron deficiency anemia are present. In these situations, several months of supplemental intake, either over-the-counter or prescribed, can accelerate correction, including more rapid relief from symptoms such as fatigue. The richest sources of nonheme iron are spinach, chard, kale, molasses, pumpkin seeds, lima beans, and kidney beans.

Unlike the RDA for iodine and some other nutrients, the RDA for iron is reliable. It is 8 milligrams per day for adult males, 8 milligrams for females not experiencing menstrual cycles, 18 milligrams for menstruating females, and 27 milligrams for pregnant females. (All quantities refer to elemental iron—the weight of the iron alone.) Note that growing teenagers require 50 to 100 percent more iron than nonmenstruating adults. Vegans and vegetarians require up to 200 percent higher intakes of nonheme iron sources, since they avoid heme iron sources.

Look for iron supplements in the ferrous form: ferrous fumarate, ferrous sulfate, and ferrous gluconate, of which the fumarate is best absorbed (33 percent absorption) and gluconate the least (12 percent).[51] Avoid ferric forms, which are poorly absorbed. Because of limited absorption, even of the ferrous forms, typical dosing regimens of prescription forms of iron provide 50 to 60 milligrams of elemental iron per day, divided in two or three doses to maximize absorption, generally taken for only 1 to 2 months. (Doses this high should only be taken with regular hemoglobin and ferritin assessments to avoid iron overload.) Heme iron forms are also available that provide advantages in absorption and reduced gastrointestinal upset.

Here are some other unique situations surrounding iron.

- People with celiac disease and Crohn's disease may require iron supplementation for longer than usual to compensate for the reduced absorptive function.

- Mild iron deficiency, especially mild degrees represented by low levels of ferritin, is common in competitive athletes, such as swimmers, runners, and tennis players. Serious athletes should therefore consider an assessment of iron status. Female and vegetarian athletes, in particular, should consider a low-dose supplement to correct any abnormalities and/or prevent deficiency.

- People with hypochlorhydria, or low stomach acid, which can result from years of grain consumption, may require prolonged iron supplementation to correct iron deficiency.

ZINC—Zinc absorption from meats and organs likewise improves dramatically with grain removal, since the same phytates that impair iron absorption also impair zinc absorption. Zinc deficiency is common and accounts for a variety of symptoms, from skin rashes to distortions of taste to unexplained diarrhea. Zinc deficiency shows itself as impaired growth and development in grain-dependent children, increased susceptibility to infection, poor wound healing, gastrointestinal distress, impaired learning, and other chronic health problems. Grain-consuming vegans and vegetarians begin with the most severe zinc deficiencies since nearly all zinc sources are in animal products.[52]

Adults need 15 milligrams of zinc per day to permit all zinc-dependent immune, neurological, reparative, and other functions to proceed normally, especially important in the first few grain-free months as gastrointestinal health recovers and bowel flora is restored. The RDA for zinc for adults is 11 milligrams per day for males, 8 milligrams for females, 11 milligrams for pregnant females, and 12 milligrams for lactating females. Unfortunately, lab testing for zinc is not very helpful, as blood levels underestimate tissue levels. Nonetheless, if a blood level is obtained and is below or at the lower end of the quoted reference range, zinc deficiency is very likely.

Much of daily zinc needs can be obtained through food, especially animal products. For example, 6 ounces of beef chuck roast provides 6 milligrams of zinc; 2 slices of pork loin provides 5.8 milligrams; 4 ounces of chicken breast provides 1 milligram; and 3 ounces of Alaskan king crab provides 6.5 milligrams. Lesser quantities are obtainable from vegetables, nuts, and cheese and other dairy products, generally less than 1 milligram per serving.

While not at the top of the list in the Undoctored program, it is worth adding an inexpensive daily zinc supplement if you avoid meats or consume them infrequently; if you have struggled in the past with immune issues (especially rheumatoid arthritis), skin rashes, distorted taste, or unexplained loose stools; or if you have an inflammatory intestinal condition, such as Crohn's disease, ulcerative colitis, or celiac disease.[53] In these cases, zinc supplements—such as zinc gluconate, zinc sulfate, and zinc acetate—can enhance dietary intake. As with magnesium and iron, look for the quantity of elemental zinc in the preparation, not total weight. Because zinc supplements are indeed meant to supplement dietary intake, a modest additional intake of 10 to 15 milligrams per day is reasonable.

Vegans and vegetarians—due to the absence of zinc-rich animal products, along with common reliance on legumes that, like grains, contain phytates that block zinc absorption—typically need higher supplemental intakes, such as 15 to 25 milligrams per day, but it is wise to not exceed 35 to 40 milligrams total (dietary and supplemental intakes) per day. People who have inflammatory bowel diseases, such as ulcerative colitis or Crohn's disease, have other malabsorptive conditions, or take thiazide diuretics (hydrochlorothiazide, chlorthalidone, metolazone) can begin their grain-free journey with a severe zinc deficiency; supplementation with higher levels, similar to doses taken by vegetarians, can be helpful. As intestinal healing proceeds, a reduction in dosage will be required.

Unique Nutrient Situations

I've discussed the nutrient deficiencies that apply to everyone that need to be corrected at the start of your Undoctored journey. But there are also occasional nutrient deficiencies of vitamin B_{12} and folate in some people that you should be aware of.

VITAMIN B_{12}—The absorption of this nutrient requires the participation of two components: the so-called intrinsic factor, a protein produced by the parietal cells of the stomach, to bind the B_{12} and a healthy distal ileum (just before the colon) to absorb it. Disruption of either will impair vitamin B_{12} status. Wheat germ agglutinin from wheat, rye, barley, and rice blocks the intrinsic factor, while gliadin from wheat and related grains provokes antibodies against the intrinsic factor and stomach parietal cells. People with Crohn's disease are especially vulnerable, since an inflamed distal ileum may require months to years to recover the ability to absorb B_{12}. Should vitamin B_{12} deficiency be present, it is suggested by symptoms such as impaired mental performance, deteriorating nervous system function, low energy, an enlarged liver, a cherry-red tongue, and macrocytic anemia (anemia with an abnormally high MCV).

Vitamin B_{12} deficiency is identified by measurement of cobalamin or holotranscobalamin on a blood test, as well as increased levels of methylmalonic acid, which can suggest milder degrees of deficiency. Look to achieve cobalamin and holotranscobalamin levels in the upper half of the reference range, as levels in the lower half can still be associated with persistent neuropathy, impaired balance, and memory.[54]

You may recall that removing grains, restoring vitamin D, and cultivating healthy bowel flora help reverse autoimmune inflammation but that some organs, such as the thyroid or the beta cells of the pancreas, are poor at recovering; once autoimmune damage has been done, there is low likelihood of recovery of organ function. The same can be true for autoimmune damage to the stomach's parietal cells that produce the intrinsic factor required for vitamin B_{12} absorption: You can remove the original cause of their damage, but the parietal cells may not recover. This is signaled by a long-term dependence on vitamin B_{12} supplementation, with levels dropping if supplementation ceases. For the great majority, oral (or sublingual—beneath the tongue—if poor absorption is suspected) supplementation with higher doses in the 500 to 1,000 micrograms per day range get the job done; rarely are injectable forms required.[55] Because vitamin B_{12} is most plentiful in animal products—such as meat, liver, and eggs—vegans and vegetarians should consider lifelong B_{12} supplementation. The best form of B_{12} is methylcobalamin, rather than the more common cyanocobalamin, as the methylform is better absorbed and sidesteps the question of potential cyanide toxicity with the cyano- form.[56]

FOLATE—Folate supplementation is mostly an issue for pregnant mothers, as well as for people with celiac disease and inflammatory bowel diseases.

Adopting a grain-free diet based on real, whole foods—compared to a folate-depleted diet of chips, pizza, and other junk food—improves intake of folate without supplementation. However, because the consequences of folate deficiency in pregnant mothers are so profound, such as spina bifida in the newborn baby, and because the grains we reject are supplemented with folic acid (a synthetic form of folate), folate supplementation during pregnancy is still a good idea as added insurance against this lifelong birth defect. Likewise, people with inflammatory bowel diseases should consider long-term supplementation.

The RDA for folate is 400 micrograms per day for adult men and women, 600 micrograms per day for pregnant females, and 500 micrograms per day for lactating females. Conventional advice for females contemplating pregnancy is to start taking 400 micrograms per day of folic acid at least 1 month before becoming pregnant.

Rich food sources of natural folate include beef liver (430 micrograms in 6 ounces), spinach (262 micrograms per cup cooked), asparagus (178 micrograms in eight spears), Brussels sprouts (156 micrograms per cup cooked), romaine lettuce (64 micrograms per cup), and eggs (66 micrograms in three eggs).[57] In general, green vegetables (*folium* is Latin for leaf), nuts, seeds, meats, fish, legumes, and eggs all contribute to a healthy total folate intake.

If you are interested in documenting your folate status, insist on measuring the quantity of folate in red blood cells (an RBC folate), a superior measure compared to the blood (serum or plasma) levels of folate.[58]

Even though government agencies advise pregnant mothers to supplement 400 micrograms of synthetic folic acid per day, advice that has indeed reduced the incidence of congenital spinal deformities, studies suggest that intake of folic acid (not folate) of 800 micrograms or more per day increases risk for colon cancer.[59, 60]

Regardless of the situation, if you choose to supplement folate in some form, it is preferable to supplement with the 5-methylfolate form, rather than folic acid, as the 5-methylfolate form does not result in abnormally high levels of unmetabolized folic acid in the bloodstream associated with cancer risk, and it is better metabolized by the substantial proportion of the population that struggles to metabolize folate (via MTHFR genetic variants).[61] The 5-methylfolate form has also been shown to be more effective in the treatment of depression, with several clinical trials demonstrating dramatic responses with or without conventional antidepressant therapy.[62] Anyone, including pregnant mothers, concerned about folate intake on a grain-free lifestyle can do fine by supplementing 400 micrograms per day in the methylfolate form—enough to address deficient intake from diet but not enough to invite questions about cancer.

Just one caution: Anyone choosing to supplement folate in some form should consider making sure that vitamin B_{12} status is favorable, as adding folate supplements in the presence of vitamin B_{12} deficiency, particularly when the characteristic anemia is present, can have nervous system consequences.

Just What Is So Special about the Undoctored Strategies?

Nutritional supplement articles and ads try to convince you that St. John's wort, black cohosh, ashwagandha, saw palmetto, theanine, gamma-aminobutyric acid, ginseng, turmeric, berberine, raspberry ketones, green coffee bean extract, garcinia cambogia, and some foul concoction that tastes like an elixir of something-the-cat-dragged-in are all essential to your future health and that without them you will be unhealthy, tired, irretrievably depressed, and overweight—if only you could pick and choose the right ones. There are hundreds of such supplements, some of which do indeed provide modest benefits, many of which do not. Surely, if such things provided the magnitude of benefits they claim, just taking, say, 30 different nutritional supplements would put you back on course to high energy, weight loss, and ideal health. Of course, they do not. But hidden in that pile is a handful of answers that holds enormous potential.

If you've gotten this far into the Undoctored discussion, I suspect that you are interested in more than just fitting into a dress one or two sizes smaller or being able to stop a prescription drug or two. I expect that you want huge; rule-shattering; life-changing; family, friend, and coworker head-turning benefits, changes that allow you to stop lists of prescription medications and walk or ride a bicycle without joint pain or stiffness, while full of energy, free of rashes and gastrointestinal struggles, looking sexy and 10 or 20 years younger than you are. Such ambitious changes won't come by taking ginseng or turmeric. They come by understanding that a common collection of nutritional blunders and deficiencies apply to most people, given the circumstances of modern life and the disinformation campaign that accompanies it. These deficiencies reflect unmet fundamental, intrinsic human needs and thereby yield enormous benefits when corrected.

There's also something special about the specific combination of strategies included in the Undoctored program: While each strategy on its own provides benefits, it is the combined effect of all the strategies that yields a larger, synergistic effect. For example, elimination of wheat/grain phytates, restoration of vitamin D, and cultivation of bowel flora all contribute to normalizing calcium status. Elimination of wheat/grain amylopectin A, correction of vitamin D and magnesium deficiencies, and cultivation of bowel flora all contribute to reducing high blood sugars and reversing type 2 diabetes as much as possible. Neglect just one Undoctored strategy and the whole will suffer. In short, you need to do them *all*.

You asked for a 1973 Buick LeSabre with no more than 150,000 miles on it, and I give you a 2017 shiny new Ferrari ready to blow the doors off anyone who tries to pass you. Follow this Undoctored path, and you will likewise be blown away by what you can accomplish long after you told your doctor that his waiting room, prescription pad, misguided agenda, and indifference were no longer an impediment to your health success.

Next, let's discuss some of the odds and ends in your Undoctored lifestyle, a handful of additional strategies that provide other outsize benefits.

Chapter Summary:
Your Next Steps to Becoming Undoctored

The Undoctored nutritional supplement program restores nutrients that address intrinsic human needs. Here are the most important ones.

- Vitamin D provides far-reaching and magnificent benefits when restored. We aim for a 25-hydroxy vitamin D blood level of 60 to 70 ng/mL, typically achieved with 4,000 to 8,000 units per day of vitamin D_3 in gelcap form. Delay measuring blood levels for at least 2 to 3 months after initiating or changing dosage to allow the full effect to develop.

- Calcium is *not* part of the Undoctored process as it does *not* yield bone health and poses increased risk for cardiovascular disease.

- Iodine is an essential trace mineral that is increasingly deficient in modern populations. We aim to obtain 500 to 1,000 micrograms of iodine per day from kelp tablets or iodine drops.

- Fish oil and seafood are the only reliable sources for the omega-3 fatty acids EPA and DHA, as the ideal daily intake of 3,000 to 3,600 milligrams EPA and DHA is only achievable by this route (and not with linolenic acid–containing foods, such as chia or flax, or krill oil).

- Magnesium is the most commonly depleted mineral from prior grain consumption—with restoration yielding substantial benefits.

(continued)

We aim for a daily magnesium intake of 400 to 500 milligrams of elemental magnesium.

- Zinc, iron, vitamin B_{12}, and folate can be deficient in some people, so awareness of how to identify and correct these deficiencies can be important in some situations.

While each strategy on its own yields advantages, it's the synergistic power of the combination added to the unique nutritional program that gives this Undoctored approach such unexpected and powerful benefits.

A Final Health Hodgepodge: Sleep, Exercise, Toxin Avoidance, and Breaking Weight Plateaus

Healing is a matter of time, but it is sometimes also a matter of opportunity.

—Hippocrates

Here is a hodgepodge of issues that, while not as crucial as the issues discussed earlier, can still play big roles in health, particularly if you want to stack the odds in favor of not calling on the doctor. First, I dispel some common misconceptions about sleep and tackle why sleep management is really part of something much bigger and fundamental to health: restoration of the natural circadian rhythm. I then put exercise in proper perspective, dispel common misconceptions, and explain how and why it can facilitate success on your Undoctored journey. Toxic exposures are, in our modern world, ubiquitous and unavoidable, but we can take some basic measures to minimize exposures and their impact on endocrine health and cancer risk. Lastly, because of factors such as prior thyroid damage from grain consumption and toxic exposures, many people will encounter frustrating weight plateaus despite the power of the Undoctored program to promote weight loss. I therefore review a handful of additional factors to consider to get back on course and achieve the weight loss you desire.

One of the reasons why the Undoctored process can be accomplished by non-health-professionals is because we now have tools to not just *detect* a health issue but also *track* it. This is a critical innovation, because if we can track something, we have the potential to improve it: Track and reduce blood pressure, track and reduce blood sugar. Some of the ideas discussed in this chapter provide those opportunities, which can be both fun and hugely empowering.

Sleep Tight

In conventional health care, poor sleep is a reason to prescribe sleeping pills or to perform a sleep study to diagnose sleep apnea. But there are a number of avenues to explore to improve individual sleep and take full advantage of the metabolic, emotional, cognitive, and other health benefits of adequate, undisrupted sleep, as our modern age seems to conspire to do everything possible to upset this balance.

You already know that poor or abbreviated sleep makes you feel lousy and impairs daytime performance. It also amplifies appetite, particularly for snacks, making poor sleep a weight gain factor all by itself. People who chronically lack sleep can easily gain 10, 20, or 30 pounds over the course of a year just from this effect.[1] Poor sleep can even contribute to risk for dementia (with greater brain plaque deposition from sleep deprivation) and increase mortality.[2] For example, people who habitually sleep less than 6 hours per night (except the occasional person who functions perfectly well on such quantities) experience increased likelihood of earlier death, particularly cardiovascular death.[3] Sleep can literally be, at least over an extended time period, a life or death matter.

All life on earth follows the natural rhythm of the planet, and you are no exception. Sleep is really just one aspect of the broader and fascinating issue of circadian rhythm (i.e., biological rhythms that humans have developed to acclimate to the 24-hour day-night cycle of life on this planet). Not only are you active during the day and sleeping at night (or at least supposed to), but multiple body processes also follow a similar rhythmic pattern, including hormones, the nervous system, white blood cells, the immune system, blood pressure, blood sugar, and even some species of bowel flora.

RESTORING CIRCADIAN RHYTHMS IN LIGHT OF THE TECHNOLOGICAL AGE

A number of new devices/technologies—or their avoidance—can help get you back on track with your circadian rhythm.

If possible, it is helpful to avoid electronic screens for at least 1 hour before bedtime. The screens of modern smartphones, tablets, computers, and TVs are dominated by light in the blue wavelength, which can "reset" human circadian rhythm, causing your brain to act as if it were bright daylight even late at night while you're reviewing e-mails or shopping online, stimulating alertness and cognitive activity (e.g., not being able to "turn off" thinking about life stresses) and suppressing melatonin release.[4] Reading on a tablet an hour before sleep reduces melatonin release by half and reduces alertness upon awakening, effects not provoked, of course, by reading an old-fashioned book made of paper.[5]

If you must use screens prior to bedtime, you can purchase yellow-tinted glasses that block the blue wavelength or have your prescription eyeglasses yellow-tinted (though this last solution is problematic in that it blocks blue light during the day when you desire it; consider having two pairs of glasses: one for the day, one for the night, if you think night screen exposure is an issue for you).

A simple, no-cost solution: Download the f.lux application for your computer (justgetflux.com), which automatically adjusts the blue wavelength of your computer screen according to time of day, reducing it as evening approaches. Search your app store for similar software solutions for your smartphone or tablet.

In addition to numerous computer programs and apps that provide soothing music, nature sounds, white noise, and auditory signals intended to lull brain waves into patterns to allow sleep, there are tools that can reset circadian rhythms, such as Re-Timer (re-timer.com). These are useful if you struggle to sleep, travel across time zones, work nighttime or revolving shifts, or have seasonal affective disorder.

Some wearable devices that track heart rate, such as the Jawbone UP, can also provide feedback on the quality of sleep (generally by monitoring body movement). The Withings Aura device (withings.com) is devoted strictly to monitoring sleep phases. There are, of course, smartphone apps that also monitor sleep, such as Sleep Cycle (sleepcycle.com). You may find such devices useful if, for example, you struggle with low daytime energy and sleepiness. Assessing your sleep quality can suggest whether there could be a problem with sleep patterns underlying your energy struggle. These devices can also awaken you at an appropriate time at the end, rather than middle or deeper phases, of a sleep period (sleep occurs in approximately 90-minute cycles throughout the night), a practice that increases daytime alertness.

These strategies are just the tip of the iceberg in the evolving science of circadian rhythms, with new devices and strategies emerging rapidly.

Disruptions of the 24-hour circadian rhythm are proving to be common in modern humans as we are exposed to indoor artificial light at all hours of the night and day, computer screens, TVs, phones, intermittent sleep deprivation, shift work, jet lag, caffeine, excessive alcohol, etc. It is becoming clear that circadian disruption has implications that go beyond the effects of sleep deprivation alone, potentially disturbing endocrine, nervous system, cardiovascular, and immune system health, adding to risk for conditions as disparate as irritable bowel syndrome, depression, and various cancers.[6]

Melatonin is the modulator of circadian rhythm in the body. It is released by the brain at night and lowers body temperature, slows brain waves, brings on sleep, and increases the time spent in deeper phases (REM) of sleep, thereby increasing the restorative power of sleep.[7] Any factor that interferes with melatonin release will impair sleep and have other health implications. Exposure to indoor lights after sunset is a major factor, for example. Unfortunately, avoidance of artificial light is impractical for most people. The simple commonsense Undoctored approach is not to have you sit in dark rooms after dinner. Rather, it is to avoid disruption of melatonin release and, as a result, encourage sufficient quantities of deep restorative sleep both naturally and via restoration of melatonin. (See "Restoring Circadian Rhythms in Light of the Technological Age," page 305.)

I'm sure that you don't need me to give you obvious advice to improve sleep, such as avoid caffeine after noontime, don't exercise at night, block all light into your bedroom during sleeping hours, and keep your bedroom comfortably cool. Beyond such "sleep hygiene" efforts, consider supplemental melatonin.

Consistent with the Undoctored philosophy of only employing strategies that are part of normal human physiology and thereby serve an intrinsic need, melatonin falls into that category as the prime regulator of human circadian rhythm secreted by the brain's pineal gland. Melatonin levels, as well as tryptophan levels that trigger melatonin release (see below), are lower in some health conditions, such as irritable bowel syndrome, and are responsible for disrupted sleep, an effect that reverses over time on the Undoctored program.[8] Melatonin should be the first nutritional supplement choice for restoring sleep patterns.

Melatonin is not a sleeping pill, as it does not share the characteristics of prescription sleeping pills: It does not adversely modify sleep patterns, it does not become habit-forming, and there is no withdrawal process when stopped. It simply "resets" your circadian clock to make your brain and body receptive to sleep. Numerous other benefits have been identified, including 70 percent reduction in tension headaches, 50 percent reduction in migraine headaches, reduction in chronic pain, and reduction in symptoms of irritable bowel syndrome and other gastrointestinal effects of stress. Melatonin has also been shown to improve prediabetic measures, such as reduction in triglycerides, reduction in blood pressure during sleep (reducing an important risk factor for cardiovascular disease called nondipping, in which blood pressure fails to drop during sleep, like it normally should), and modest reduction in waist size. Accumulating data also suggest advantages in preventing, even treating, breast, prostate, and ovarian cancers.[9, 10, 11, 12] Because insufficient or disrupted sleep contributes to weight gain, you'd expect that improved sleep via melatonin supplementation would result in weight loss, and it does, though the effect is modest, about 5 pounds over 4 months.[13] No sleeping pill can accomplish the range of positive health effects achieved by this potent hormone of circadian rhythms.

Melatonin, available at health food stores and drugstores, is easy to use. Start with a small dose (e.g., 0.5 milligram) about 1 hour prior to bedtime, and increase the dose with every use until you achieve the desired effect. Doses can range as high as 12 milligrams per day or more. If you manage to fall asleep but struggle to stay asleep, consider either a higher dose and/or converting to a time-release preparation. If you experience a "hangover" effect that persists upon awakening, take your dose earlier in the evening. The younger you are, the earlier you should take your melatonin dose. Adolescents, for instance, who wish to fall asleep at 10:00 p.m. may need to take it as early as 7:00 p.m., while people over 60 years old generally do fine by taking it 30 minutes before the desired sleep time.

You can add to the melatonin effect by supplementing tryptophan, an amino acid that also triggers melatonin release from the brain and increases serotonin levels, making it useful for improving mood over time, as well.[14] Tryptophan can be taken alone or, even better, with melatonin. Doses start at 500 milligrams at bedtime and range up to 3,000 milligrams; as with melatonin, start with a low dose, and then increase it with each nighttime use until you achieve the quality and duration of sleep (and mood) you desire.

Given the substantial health benefits of melatonin, should *everyone* take measures to increase it, regardless of whether sleep/circadian issues are present? This is not yet clear. But even if you don't struggle with sleep issues, melatonin supplementation should be considered for any form of endocrine disruption—such as thyroid disease, adrenal dysfunction, or infertility—given that this regulator of circadian rhythm modulates numerous hormonal levels.[15] It should also be considered as you age, as over age 50 or so, circadian hormonal rhythms are blunted, leading to dysfunction of several hormonal systems, such as reductions in testosterone and growth hormone, partially restored by melatonin supplementation.[16]

How much sleep is enough? First of all, sleep occurs in "packages" lasting 90 minutes (with some individual variation). This means that total sleep duration should occur in multiples of 90 minutes (e.g., 7½ hours). You can appreciate that advice to sleep 8 hours, for instance, would cause you to be awakened by your alarm midcycle, leaving you with reduced daytime alertness and energy. This is where one of the new devices that detect your sleep stage can be helpful, as they awaken you when you have emerged from the deepest sleep phases. Alternatively, you can set your alarm for a period of time that represents some multiple of 90 minutes. You probably already have a good idea of what your ideal total sleep time should be. A good rule of thumb would be the amount of time you sleep when on vacation, after having caught up on lost sleep—it might be 7½ hours, it might be 9 hours, or you might simply be among the lucky few who can get away with 6 hours or less unimpaired by daytime sleepiness. Any amount of sleep that leaves you with daytime sleepiness should make you suspicious that your ideal sleep time is longer than you think it is.

And stay alert to this issue. As with bowel flora, the power of circadian health is only beginning to be appreciated and has the potential to provide important and individually empowering strategies for those of us living the Undoctored life.

Exercise: Hop, Skip, Jump—With a Smile

Conventional dietary and health "wisdom" advise us to increase exercise as a means of compensating for continued consumption of sugary sodas and grains. (Some authorities advocate as much as 90 minutes of exercise per day to combat a poor diet—no kidding.) In other words, follow the advice of agencies such as the Academy of Eat Anything You Want, and you will need to exercise more to not become obese and diabetic. Clearly, I've got some myths to dispel.

Let me first add that you should not regard this as an attempt at providing a comprehensive, everything-you-need-to-know guide to exercise, since there are oodles of resources to help you get started on this, from a local personal trainer to Zumba and CrossFit classes. This is simply an effort to equip you with some important insights that increase your odds of success in applying exercise effectively to your Undoctored lifestyle. As in other areas of the Undoctored message, I dash false gods while uncovering some hidden gems of insight that can make substantial differences in your health success.

Exercise Is Ineffective for Weight Control

If you live a sedentary lifestyle or engage in minimal physical activity, then beginning a moderately vigorous program will yield weight loss. But that is not the situation for the majority of us, many of whom exercise to moderate or higher levels with some regularity yet fail to experience any weight loss— this is exceptionally common.[17] The human body quickly adjusts to consistent exertion, and weight loss does not result. Extreme exercise, like running a marathon, can also yield weight loss (at least initially), but I am referring to much more common levels of effort that most people engage in, such as using an elliptical machine for an hour or running 3 miles several times per week. It would be highly unusual for such efforts to cause weight loss. Diet remains the primary effort to control weight, not exercise. Don't frustrate yourself by using exercise as a weight-loss tool—it just does not work for the majority of us. And *never* persuade yourself that you don't have to mind your diet because you engage in serious exercise—this is absolutely false. Diet trumps exercise, hands down, and you can readily overpower the benefits of exercise by choosing unwise foods.

Exercise Is a Useful Health Tool

Despite the ineffectiveness of regular exercise for achieving weight loss, daily physical activity is an important component of an overall effort to maintain or regain health. The health risks of poor physical fitness may even be greater than that of obesity.[18] Physical activity and exercise are therefore a part of your Undoctored effort.

Exercise is effective in achieving many health benefits, including reducing blood sugar; reducing insulin resistance; reducing blood pressure; improving mood and reducing depression; reducing anxiety; reducing risk for diabetes, heart disease, and heart attacks by 30 to 50 percent; and reducing risk for osteoporosis and fractures, cancer, and dementia.[19] Because exercise causes you to sweat, it can also be an important means of removing heavy metals, such as cadmium and mercury, from your body (discussed below). Being physically fit is part of your ability to be resilient, to adjust and adapt to stressful emotional and physical situations. Exercise has even been found to encourage neural plasticity (i.e., the brain's ability to change, even expand in volume), which helps maintain vigor later in life and reduce the potential for dementia; the hippocampus of the brain, in particular, a major center for memory formation and balance, has been shown to enlarge modestly with exercise, a major advantage in reversing the potential for dementia.[20] Exercise can also modestly reverse endocrine disruption of the hypothalamic-pituitary-adrenal system and dysfunction of the autonomic nervous system, both involving excessive cortisol release (the stress hormone). It can also improve immune system response; reduce inflammation and inflammatory mediators/markers, such as C-reactive protein; and even contribute to healthier and more diverse bowel flora.[21] In other words, a sedentary life impairs health in numerous ways, and regular physical activity and exercise improve health in far more ways than weight management.

But how much exercise is required to obtain full benefit? The majority of health benefits are obtained by engaging in a moderate level of physical activity, like walking at a moderately brisk rate for 30 minutes five times per week.[22, 23, 24] The additional incremental benefit from upping moderate levels of exercise to high levels is measurable, but small. In other words, jogging 5 miles provides more benefit than walking 3 miles—but only by a little.

One thing is becoming clear: Adding brief bursts of high-intensity exercise (e.g., 20 to 60 seconds of all-out bike pedaling, sprinting, rapid walking, etc.) several times during the course of an otherwise casual exercise effort can reproduce many of the metabolic health benefits of prolonged exercise, but without the wear-and-tear strain of, say, jogging 5 miles.[25] Incorporating such bursts is also incredibly time-saving, yielding the benefits of an hour-long bike ride in 20 minutes, for example.

Here are some essential features of any form of physical activity or exercise you choose.

- Include some form of strength training or moderate-to-heavy physical work (digging in the garden, rock climbing, etc.). Strength training increases muscle mass that, in turn, builds bone density, contributes to weight management and normalization of insulin resistance, helps stabilize hormonal status, and prevents falls later in life. This does not mean hanging around with bodybuilders at the gym for hours; rather, it means engaging in just 15 minutes of strength training once or twice per week, for example.[26] You will find that the Undoctored lifestyle of banishing all grains also curiously helps preserve or increase muscle mass and strength, though the explanation for this is unclear. (It might be due to the higher testosterone levels that occur very commonly in both males and females, compounded further by loss of visceral fat).

- Include motions that involve axial impact, such as jumping rope, doing high-impact aerobics, hiking, jogging, stairclimbing, playing tennis or volleyball, or any other activity that involves jumping, hopping, or skipping. Such activities introduce stress to the long axis (top-to-bottom) of the spine, hips, and legs, which encourages bone growth and helps prevent osteoporosis, with sometimes dramatic effects.[27] Benefits begin with efforts as simple as jumping 10 to 20 times twice per day for several weeks, with even greater benefits with more prolonged, repetitive efforts.[28]

- Consider new forms of activity. Don't just walk or run; add tai chi, yoga, square dancing, swing dancing, Wii Fit, rock-wall climbing, walking briskly on a sandy beach, taking classes in self-defense or martial arts, biking to work or school, and walking new and scenic trails.

- Reduce sitting time (computer work, desk work, TV watching, etc.). Because prolonged sitting uninterrupted by physical activity has been associated with increased risk for diabetes, heart disease, lower-back pain and other musculoskeletal complaints, and death, taking intermittent brief standing or walking breaks to break up sitting periods is a good idea.[29] This risk is not reduced by exercise outside of sedentary periods. Some people have adopted standing desks and treadmill or stationary bicycle desks as another way to decrease sitting time while working.

- Choose activities you enjoy. I've seen too many people think that exercise must be tedious torture, then give up. It is far better to choose activities that make you spring out of the bed in the morning and say, "Wow, today is Wednesday, the day I _____." It might be walking with a friend, it could be ballroom dance lessons, it could be yoga class, or it could be building the new stone wall around your flower garden.

But too much of a good thing can also be bad. As more people come to believe that exercise is the key to everything in health (it is not) and/or seek the "high" of extreme exercise, more pathological bone fractures (especially hip); long-term wear-and-tear injuries; heart rhythm disorders, such as atrial fibrillation and atrial flutter (fivefold increased likelihood); and even sudden cardiac death are being observed. This does not happen with moderate or even high levels of exercise, but with what most of us would regard as extreme exercise: running marathons or ultramarathons with some regularity, repeatedly biking 100+ miles at high intensity, etc. Two-thirds of people running the Boston Marathon, for instance, release heart muscle proteins (cardiac enzymes) that approximate the level experienced during heart attacks, signifying heart muscle damage with each 26-mile effort.[30] Some people who engage in extreme levels of exercise, for instance, develop enlarged right ventricles of the heart that make the heart electrically unstable, a situation that encourages ventricular fibrillation and sudden cardiac death, identified at autopsy.[31, 32] This is due to the extreme blood-volume stress placed on the normally low-stress right ventricle of the heart, which provokes fibrous tissue that should not be there to be deposited (a process cardiologists call remodeling). Exercise is wonderful, but not extreme exercise. It should be a health advantage, not a cause for disease and death.

You may already know that your smartphone is an exercise-quantifying device that can count steps or track miles walked. Wearable devices—such as the Fitbit, Apple Watch, and numerous other devices all the way down to a $20 digital pedometer—can also help quantify activity. Smartphones and some devices—such as those from Fitbit, Garmin, and Jawbone—allow you to upload your data to a smartphone app or computer to track it over time, allowing you to correlate the data to other measures, such as blood pressure or blood sugar. (Most of these devices will also provide insights into sleep patterns if worn to bed.) If you enjoy using such devices to track steps taken, aim for a minimum of 5,000 steps (2.5 miles) per day from your walking, more from daily life activities, with at least some of that time spent at a walk rate of 60 steps-per-minute or 1 step-per-second or more.[33] Even Spotify has a running app that pairs music with the pace of your stride. In addition to the steps/miles walked counter on your smartphone, there are apps such as MyFitnessPal, a popular app that tracks calories consumed and burned. Despite the proliferation of apps and devices that purport to help you lose weight by counting calories burned, remain aware that exercise (as well as calorie counting) is not an effective means of controlling or losing weight, so use the calorie-burn measurement as nothing more than a tool for feedback, a fun tool to track your activities. (This is an area in which tracking is more gimmick than real advantage.) Serious athletes, of course, may find additional uses for such devices, such as tracking running or biking times or distances, that fall outside of our general health concerns.

Exercise and be physically active while throwing in a bit of strength training. It can be unregimented, or it can be quantified and tracked, if you are into such things. But don't go overboard. And, above all, enjoy it.

Minimize Toxic Exposures

Because industrial chemicals are so ubiquitous in the modern world, particularly in North America, avoiding them altogether is no longer possible. Our air, water, soil, food, cosmetics, toiletries, and other commercial products all contribute to cumulative exposures. The best we can manage at present is to *minimize* exposure.

Think polychlorinated biphenyls, PCBs, for example, that were used in hundreds of industrial processes and products, banned in the United States in 1979, restricted use in Europe enforced in 1985, after it became clear that they were potent endocrine disrupters (especially thyroid), neurotoxins, and carcinogens. Despite the ban, PCBs persist at high levels in the environment over 30 years later since there are few natural means to degrade them to harmless breakdown products.[34] Dioxins are another carcinogenic, immune and endocrine systems disrupter, banned after being widely used in numerous industrial processes. Despite the ban, their unusual environmental persistence, as well as their persistence in the human body upon exposure measured in decades, means that, without exception, everyone has measurable dioxin levels in their bodies. Continued exposure comes through ingesting water and food and even using modeling clay, many years after dioxins are no longer used by industry.[35]

The issue of toxic exposure is the worst in the United States because of the business-friendly federal policy provided by the woefully outdated Toxic Substances Control Act that allows chemicals to be introduced for commercial and consumer applications without having to prove safety; safety is only questioned if adverse effects are encountered after the substance is used. Hundreds of new pesticides, herbicides, plasticizing agents, paint additives, etc., are therefore added to the environment every year with no assurances of public safety. Nor are Canadians or Europeans spared these effects, even when these toxins are banned within individual countries, as environmental toxins are spread via air, clouds, and oceans and even found in the polar ice caps. It is a worldwide problem with implications you can see even in your own backyard (I haven't seen a grasshopper, hummingbird, firefly, or butterfly in years, despite seeing such creatures everywhere just 30 or 40 years ago).

The dangers of chemical exposures can be passed down through generations with, for example, exposure to parabens in toiletries or BPA (bisphenol A) from canned foods, conveyed to children or even grandchildren via epigenetic effects (i.e., changes in the proteins regulating gene expression), a concerning new insight.[36] It means that your exposure, for example, to the parabens in shampoo yield effects in your children and grandchildren even if they are personally unexposed, another example of unintended consequences of releasing chemicals without understanding the implications.

Obviously, these issues range far beyond what you and I are trying to accomplish in this individualized Undoctored experience. As you may already appreciate, toxic exposures are simply not addressed in conventional healthcare interactions, predictably, because there are no drugs, procedures, or other revenue-generating activities applicable, so the entire issue is ignored. And, as you are already aware, just because something is overlooked by your doctor doesn't mean that it is not important for health. We cannot personally clear the environment of banned chemicals, or even of chemicals in active use today, such as the glyphosate being sprayed on your neighbor's lawn to kill dandelions or the triclosan in antibacterial hand soaps and hand sanitizers. But we can choose to avoid ongoing exposures in our homes.

Here are some steps you can take to reduce your exposure to industrial compounds and other health disrupters.

Supplement Iodine

I've already discussed iodine at length. But know that iodine can also be part of your protection from industrial chemicals. Many environmental poisons are halogens (compounds containing bromine, chlorine, and fluorine), whose effects are partially blocked by iodine. It does not make you impervious, but it provides some measure of protection.

Filter Your Water

Even though most (not all) municipalities and cities do a good job of filtering water, most add back chlorine (or the longer-acting chloramine) or fluoride, both—as you now know—halogenated compounds. As discussed earlier, chlorine and fluoride are antibacterial in water and on kitchen counters but also in your gastrointestinal tract, where we want microbes to thrive. Filtering your water with a reverse osmosis or charcoal filter system, or both, is a good practice to remove these halogenated compounds. It is also added assurance against water contaminated with atrazine, perchlorates, polybrominated diphenyl ethers, arsenic, and lead from home plumbing.

Grow Your Own or Buy Organic

There is no longer any question: Consuming organic foods provides greater quantities of nutrients, especially antioxidants and polyphenols (which provide much of the health benefits of vegetables and fruits); lower levels of the toxic metal cadmium; and dramatically reduced quantities of herbicides, pesticides, and antibiotic-resistant bacteria.[37] Critics argue that while that all may be true, the difference in health is small to nonexistent. I believe, however, that they fail to consider that choosing organic foods reduces *overall* exposure to industrial chemicals on the background of daily, ubiquitous exposure, that some of the chemicals encountered *accumulate* in the human body, and that organic farming is a more environmentally friendly and sustainable method than conventional farming.

The effects of choosing organic foods can be measured. A recent study, for example, found that people choosing organic produce had lower urine levels of the common herbicide glyphosate and that healthy people had lower glyphosate levels than people with a variety of chronic diseases.[38]

Minimize Use of Products with BPA

Bisphenol A, or BPA, is widely used in consumer products, especially the resin lining of cans (canned foods) and plastic bottles made of polycarbonate. It is even in plastic baby bottles. The FDA and its European counterpart, the European Food Safety Authority, declared BPA safe based on two studies conducted by manufacturers, discounting hundreds of independent, noncommercial studies demonstrating otherwise. Noncommercial studies have demonstrated that BPA is an endocrine disrupter and has been associated with increased risk for diabetes, congestive heart failure, infertility, disruption of the hypothalamic-pituitary system, and prostate and breast cancers.[39] For these reasons, despite the industry-friendly bias of official agencies, we should minimize use of canned foods (unless designated BPA-free) and plastic bottles with recycling code #7.

Seek Out Safe Toiletries and Cosmetics

Shampoos, hair conditioners, hand/body creams, lipsticks, lip balms, and other toiletries and cosmetics are landmines of industrial chemicals, the vast majority of which have never undergone human safety testing and are often not even listed on the label. The most obnoxious culprits are parabens (endocrine disruption and breast cancer) and phthalates (endocrine disruption and cancer), so look for products without such problem ingredients.[40, 41] Burt's Bees, Beautycounter, MyChelle, Jouvé, and Natural Organics are among the manufacturers who have consistently obtained favorable ratings from the Environmental Working Group (see below).

Avoid Products with "Fragrance"

The term *fragrance* provides a loophole for industry to conceal hundreds of chemicals in perfumes, colognes, deodorants, cosmetics, and toiletries, since the FDA does not require manufacturers to disclose what is contained within fragrances. As a result, we cannot tell what is contained in fragrances, nor will the manufacturer divulge that information to consumers. Sidestep this issue by avoiding cosmetics and toiletries that list "fragrance." You can safely continue using colognes and perfumes by spraying them on clothing (testing an inconspicuous area for staining first) but not directly on skin or on clothing surfaces in direct contact with skin.

We've only just scratched the surface of this huge topic. For further information on the safety or dangers of consumer products, the Environmental Working Group (EWG)—a nonprofit, nonpartisan consumer advocacy organization based in Washington, DC—maintains a database of commercial products along with a detailed rating system on the safety of each product. The group assigns an "EWG Verified" designation to personal care products, making it easier to shop without having to consult long lists of chemicals for the no-no's. EWG has a smartphone app that can also make shopping for safe products easier.

Detoxify

In addition to avoiding exposure to chemicals, we can also try to extract what is already in our bodies. Unfortunately, this is an area in which fairy tales and empty promises abound, an area in which the science is also skimpy.

One advantage may be found in enthusiastic consumption of cruciferous vegetables, such as Brussels sprouts, cabbage, broccoli, kale, and cauliflower, as they contain a class of natural compounds called glucosinolates that amplify the activity of liver enzymes that accelerate detoxification reactions, causing chemicals to be harmlessly excreted into the stool and then out of the body.[42] This may account for the reduction in a variety of cancers in people who consume plenty of crucifers.

Recent studies have also uncovered the potential role of Nrf2, which controls dozens of human genes involved in detoxification; Nrf2 activators are found in many of the Undoctored strategies, including the omega-3 fatty acids EPA and DHA; vegetables, especially cruciferous vegetables, and fruit; sulfur compounds from allium vegetables, such as garlic, shallots, chives, and onions; and carotenoids from yellow and green vegetables.[43]

Metals such as arsenic, cadmium, lead, and mercury are known carcinogens and increase cardiovascular risk. Sweating is proving to be an important detoxification mechanism for such heavy metals, whether achieved via exposure to hot ambient temperatures, exercise, or use of a sauna. Levels of arsenic, cadmium, lead, and mercury in sweat exceed that of the blood or urine, suggesting that sweating has the potential to concentrate such metals, released from the body the more you sweat.[44]

Loose regulations, lax or nonexistent enforcement, failure to incorporate new scientific findings—I don't think we should wait for legislation and enforcement to catch up, hoping that regulatory agencies will come to our rescue. In the meantime, you and I can take personal action to protect ourselves and our families from the onslaught of industrial compounds. Growing our own vegetables, choosing the simplest cosmetics and toiletries without toxic ingredients, and incorporating simple detoxification strategies are our way of taking back individual control as part of an Undoctored effort.

Breaking Weight Plateaus

This may seem a bit out of place back here in our little collection of Undoctored program strategies. But this is such a common question that I thought it would be helpful to tackle specifically.

First of all, all the strategies articulated in the Undoctored program achieve substantial, often dramatic, reductions in body weight and in measurements because they eliminate numerous weight-increasing effects, such as the gliadin-derived opiates from wheat/grain that stimulate appetite, high blood sugars from the amylopectin A of grains, the weight loss–impairing/inflammatory effects of dysbiosis, and iodine deficiency. Correcting these issues alone is a huge weight-loss advantage. Each and every strategy in the Undoctored program plays a role, and each strategy interacts and alters the effects of other strategies—leaving out just one Undoctored strategy can impair not just weight-loss success but also health success. Losing 15 to 18 pounds in body weight and 4, 5, or 6 inches off the waist are common during the first month—but not for everyone. But it is important to not misread failure to lose weight as failure of the program or personal failure; it is most commonly due to the presence of *one or more factors that are blocking your weight-loss success*. It is therefore crucial that you identify these factors and take steps to correct them, which nearly always yields weight-loss success.

Here are some of the factors that can block your weight-loss success.

- **PRESCRIPTION AND OVER-THE-COUNTER DRUGS.** These include beta-blockers (metoprolol, nadolol, carvedilol, bisoprolol, propranolol), all antihistamines (diphenhydramine or Benadryl, fexofenadine or Allegra, cetirizine or Zyrtec, cyproheptadine or Periactin, and others), antidepressant drugs (amitriptyline or Elavil, nortriptyline or Pamelor, doxepin or Sinequan, paroxetine or Paxil, and trazodone or Desyrel, and others), anti-inflammatory drugs (naproxen, ibuprofen, Vioxx, prednisone), Lyrica for fibromyalgia and pain, valproic acid (Depakote) for seizures, Actos and Avandia for prediabetes and diabetes, and injectable insulin (in all forms, responsible for not just failed weight loss but also astounding quantities of weight gain). All these common drugs can prevent weight loss regardless of how serious your efforts to adhere to this lifestyle are, no matter how meticulous your food choices or your exercise efforts are. If you take one or more of these drugs, a serious conversation with the prescriber is in order, as some drugs cannot just be stopped but need to be tapered down. Insist on replacing with agent(s) that do not block weight loss. The need for many, if not most, of these drugs also reverses with the Undoctored lifestyle, making them unnecessary.
- **FAILURE TO INCREASE FATS AND OILS.** Even today, after the science has conclusively demonstrated that there is no health or weight advantage to cutting fat, we are still bombarded with the message to cut fat (and thereby cut calories and heart disease risk—absolute nonsense). So I shall stress this once again: Do not restrict fat, and never eat low- or nonfat foods of any sort. Buy fatty cuts of meat, and don't trim off the fat. Use more lard, tallow, organic butter, or coconut oil in your cooking, and use more extra-virgin olive oil in your salads.
- **DAIRY.** No, it's not the calories, or the fat; it's the properties of the whey protein of dairy, yes, the protein that so many people regard as healthy

for exercise, muscle growth, etc. Whey protein has the peculiar capacity to increase insulin levels dramatically in about 20 percent of people, an effect that can completely shut down any hope of weight loss. The only way to test this question is to eliminate dairy completely for a 4-week period; if you lose, say, 8 or 9 pounds, then you are among those with an exceptional sensitivity to this whey protein effect. If nothing happens, then dairy products are not the culprit, and you can add them back (with all the caveats discussed earlier, such as choosing organic, full-fat, etc.).

- **IODINE DEFICIENCY AND HYPOTHYROIDISM.** I shouldn't really have to mention this here because I included an extensive discussion on iodine deficiency and hypothyroidism in Chapter 12. But I list it again because it is shocking how many people are frustrated with low energy, abnormal lab tests, feeling generally awful, low mood, and continual weight gain but still fail to have a thyroid assessment or are wrongly advised by their doctors that their thyroid status is normal. Or they simply believe that iodine is not really necessary. Never accept doctors' pronouncements such as "Your thyroid is fine" or "You don't have a thyroid problem, so forget about it." Iodine deficiency is increasingly common, thyroid dysfunction likewise. You can share your thyroid values on thyroid forums, Undoctored discussions (undoctoredhealth.com), and others to obtain virtually immediate and insightful feedback that will, more often than not, make your doctor look like an unskilled factory worker trying to perform rocket science.

- **EXCEEDING THE NET-CARB LIMIT OF 15 GRAMS PER MEAL.** This is a very common tripping point. The key is to endure the modest hassle of counting your net carbs (you will be shocked at how often foods you thought were safe were actually booby-trapping your weight-loss program). Invest the modest effort and, for a surprisingly large number of people, the answer will be found in the Mexican refried beans you love or the gluten-free or low-carb pasta you thought was safe.

- **ELEVATED BLOOD SUGAR LEVELS.** Added confidence in blood sugar/insulin management is obtained by checking blood sugars immediately prior to a meal and then 30 to 60 minutes after starting the meal, aiming for no change. In other words, if your blood sugar premeal is 100 mg/dL, it should be no higher than 100 mg/dL 30 to 60 minutes later when the blood sugar peak occurs. If blood sugar rises to, say, 140 mg/dL, you ate something that not only raised blood sugar to unhealthy levels but also turned off any hope of weight loss for at least the next 24 hours. Should you identify such a blood sugar effect, review the meal and reduce or eliminate the food responsible, which will be some form of carbohydrate.

- **INADEQUATE SLEEP.** I'm guilty once again of reiterating something I've discussed elsewhere. But because people too often dismiss sleep as an inconvenience or sacrifice sleep due to time pressures, it is all too often an impediment to weight loss, as well as to overall health. Recognize that inadequate sleep quality or quantity has potent metabolic consequences, such as increased cortisol levels, increased appetite for snacking on junk, and other metabolic distortions that impair health and weight loss. You cannot neglect sleep and hope to succeed by compensating in other ways—period.

- **EXTREME STRESS/ADRENAL DYSFUNCTION.** I lump these two weight loss–blockers together because they are typically one and the same: Anything that causes extreme and longstanding stress—financial struggles, unrewarding work stress, a bad relationship, caring for an impaired child or parent—provokes excess cortisol release from the adrenal gland. Cortisol is a steroid hormone, therefore making stress not too different from taking the anti-inflammatory drug prednisone, typically associated with extravagant weight gain. Unfortunately, being freed of stress and/or reversing adrenal/cortisol dysfunction can be among the toughest of issues to resolve. Typical symptoms include morning energy followed by a dramatic drop-off in the afternoon and evening, or low daytime energy with an inappropriate nighttime surge that prevents sleep. Quantify and characterize your individual pattern of cortisol release with a four-sample salivary cortisol test kit from services such as ZRT Laboratory (zrtlab .com), or, of course, identify a functional medicine or integrative health practitioner with an interest in adrenal health.

- **DYSBIOSIS.** I've discussed the steps required to start the journey back to healthy bowel flora: a high-potency, multispecies probiotic at the start, fermented foods, and prebiotic fibers to nourish bowel flora. Unfortunately, some people are so far down the path of having unhealthy bowel flora that even these commonsense and mostly effective efforts are inadequate. This situation can be suggested by an adverse response to prebiotic fibers, such as excessive bloating and diarrhea. Start by following the discussions provided in Chapter 11 on how to deal with mild degrees of dysbiosis by simply delaying the introduction of prebiotic fibers for several weeks while continuing a probiotic. Should this fail to yield relief from a weight plateau and/or from abdominal symptoms, then this is one of those occasional situations in which a doctored solution may be required, involving a formal analysis of bowel flora followed by correction.

- **SEVERE INSULIN RESISTANCE.** An occasional person does everything right, but it may not be enough due to marked inability to respond to insulin, which blocks weight loss (i.e., persistent high blood levels of insulin prevent the mobilization of fat for disposal). While all the Undoctored strategies help reverse this situation, you can push it further by achieving ketosis, a natural physiologic state in which you eliminate virtually all dietary carbohydrates, forcing your body to draw from fat for energy. The key is to cut net-carb intake to 10 grams or less per meal (below the usual cutoff of 15 net grams) and load up on fat—not protein, as it will block ketosis. And for a serious effort, monitor blood ketones using Abbott's Precision Xtra device for testing finger-stick ketone levels (which is preferable to the less reliable urinary ketone checks); you will need both the device and ketone test strips. While the device is relatively inexpensive (around $25), the test strips are pricey, running around $4 per test strip (available via online retailers such as Amazon). Finger-stick ketone levels, checked only occasionally, should be maintained in the 1 to 3 mmol/L range. Maintaining a ketotic state over several weeks can break weight plateaus for many. (Those with type 1 diabetes should not use this strategy, as they can develop dangerous levels of ketones, which does not occur in people without this form of diabetes.)

Recognize that excess weight and obesity are virtually unknown in cultures that follow primitive diets and lifestyles. You, too, can return to that state, sporting a BMI of less than 25 and having to endure jealous criticisms from neighbors and friends that "you're too skinny," though you would indeed look pretty darned good if you donned a loincloth. If the Undoctored lifestyle is followed as written, and weight loss eludes you, then it is time to pinpoint the reason(s) why you cannot retrace steps back to ideal health and weight—not be discouraged or just give up.

And don't blame the *wrong* factors and waste time and effort in directions that are unlikely to yield success, such as cutting calories or portion sizes, cutting fat, or increasing exercise.

Chapter Summary:
Your Next Steps to Becoming Undoctored

Healthy sleep is an unavoidable requirement to maintain health and reverse established health conditions, though it is among the first health habit sacrificed in modern life. Melatonin is the key to sleep, as it is the prime regulator of circadian rhythms, restored via efforts such as reducing exposure to evening light and electronic devices and supplementation.

Exercise is a generally ineffective means of losing weight, but it is an important component of your effort to maintain or regain health because it reduces insulin resistance, improves bone density, and reduces the heavy metal burden in the body through sweat. The key is not to achieve extremes, however, but to introduce variety and enjoy the process.

Part of maintaining a long-term life of Undoctored health is to reduce toxic exposures, especially from drinking water, toiletries, cosmetics, and food. While complete avoidance is impossible, you can take several commonsense steps to reduce exposure. You can also incorporate more cruciferous vegetables and recognize that sweating, especially via exercise and use of saunas, is an important accelerator of detoxification.

Should you encounter a weight plateau, don't be discouraged. Instead, recognize that there are almost always identifiable, correctable reasons for it, such as sensitivity to dairy, use of certain prescription drugs, or other factors. And know that identifying and correcting the one or more factors nearly always yields weight-loss success and thereby improved health.

CHAPTER 14

Breathe, Drink Water, and Be Undoctored

You can't be that kid standing at the top of the water slide overthinking it. You have to go down the chute.

—Tina Fey, *Bossypants*

You're in my office of neutral wallpaper and beige carpeting, month-old magazines on the table. You sit in a thread-worn chair and wait an hour or two, an indifferent staff behind glass partitions accustomed to dealing with impatient patients. I finally see you and I sit, dressed in my white coat, barely uttering a word while pecking away at my laptop. I make an attempt at a pleasantry or two and then pull a prescription pad out and proceed to write you a few prescriptions. What do you do now?

You . . . run!

I hope you passed this test, as I was only trying to see if you've been paying attention. If you've stuck with the conversations in *Undoctored* this far, then you should know that genuine insights into health—not health care—don't happen this way. Crack up your car, and there will be an ambulance to transport you to the hospital. Develop a high fever and confusion a week after you return from Costa Rica, and a family member will need to dial 911. But you now recognize that the majority of healthcare interactions are not quite so urgent or dramatic. Most healthcare issues are slow, chronic, and long term—and constitute the bulk of issues in health. There is no need to inject the urgency of life-threatening medical situations into everyday issues of health, even though the modus operandi of medical care is to use such scare tactics, all part of the effort to make you kowtow at its altar.

You have personal control—extraordinary control—over much of what is labeled "health care," thereby rejecting what are largely efforts cleverly repackaged to generate revenue and control for healthcare insiders. Just as the wily mechanic at the local garage knows that the unsuspecting woman bringing in her Jetta because it's making a funny noise can be convinced that a major overhaul is needed, healthcare insiders know they have the power to persuade you that no simple dietary change, nutritional supplement, or blood test can accomplish what an MRI, CT scan, endoscopy, laparoscopic surgery, or organ transplant can. But I hope you now understand that if you correct the handful of factors that allow numerous health conditions to develop in the first place, those conditions will reverse in the majority of people. It can indeed be as simple as that.

I regret that I can only cover so much in just one book. But know that if you do nothing else but engage in the handful of strategies discussed in the Undoctored Wild, Naked, and Unwashed program, this alone will yield health benefits that most of the people around you, unaware of these basic principles, will never achieve, as they continue to struggle needlessly with weight, multiple health problems, and feeling awful, despite the solutions being so simple. Take Ms. Fey's advice and don't overthink things: Every Undoctored strategy is as natural as breathing or drinking water, a restoration of the way things should have been all along. There is no advantage in hesitation, just go ahead and jump. Following these strategies in their entirety—and I stress in their *entirety*, not one, not some, but all—restores a level of health that you may find shocking. It's what I call the 2 + 2 = 11 effect: The total is greater than the sum of the parts, magnificently greater. Add fish oil by itself, for instance, and a few good things happen, such as reduced triglycerides and blood pressure. Just take iodine, and you might feel warmer, your hair may grow thicker, and your breast cysts may recede. Just eliminate wheat and grains from your diet and you will lose plenty of belly fat, drop blood sugar, and reverse most of the symptoms of Crohn's disease and ulcerative colitis. But incorporate *all* the strategies of the program and even bigger, more astounding things happen because there are synergies shared among each and every strategy in the program, powerful interactions that yield health on a scale you thought was impossible or lost. Neglect just one strategy and you will obtain far less.

Some effects will be perceived, such as increased energy, relief from skin rashes and acid reflux, and reversed inflammation, while others will not be perceived but can be measured, such as reduced blood sugar, reduced blood pressure, reduced triglycerides, reduced intestinal permeability, and reduced glycation that would have led to arthritis and dementia. But it all adds up to a marvelous transformation in health, weight, and appearance that will have friends and family in awe, begging to know what you did to look so good.

And we engage in this journey as a community with global reach, experiencing results that we can share, track, and compare with other people's results. We all share in this quest to discover health outside of the medical system. We are as close as having a virtual town square to rub elbows over coffee and discuss issues, receive feedback, learn new lessons, and hear about new ideas, facilitated by all the new technological tools coming our way. Never before have we had access to so much information, interactive and tracking potential; never before have we had hopes of finding so many answers to health problems so quickly, so easily.

Putting It All Together

Because we've covered a lot of territory on this journey to beat a path away from the doctor's office and the healthcare system, here's a summary of the essential strategies of the Undoctored program.

FOLLOW THE UNDOCTORED PROGRAM—in its entirety, not just one, two, or a few strategies, but the entire program, in order to take advantage of the powerful synergies among all its components—and achieve extraordinary and glowing health.

FOLLOW THE DIET YOUR BODY IS ADAPTED TO. We revert to eating foods our bodies have adapted to consuming, rejecting those that are destructive recent additions, regardless of what misinformed government agencies, dietitians, or doctors tell us. Specifically, we reject all grains and sugars and do not limit healthy fats or oils, choosing real, whole foods as often as possible, returning to a choice of foods we followed for over 99 percent of human time on this planet. Because of the widespread presence of insulin resistance/diabetes/prediabetes, we also manage carbohydrates by restricting ourselves to no more than 15 grams net carbs per meal. Further health success emerges from the loss of inflammatory visceral fat. You get thinner because you become healthier.

CULTIVATE BOWEL FLORA. Everyone begins with varying degrees of disrupted bowel flora (dysbiosis). We restore healthy bowel flora by viewing it as a garden: We start with a high-potency, multispecies pro-biotic and fermented foods as the "seeds" and then add daily prebiotic fibers as the "water" and "fertilizer" that nourish the seeds, aiming for an eventual daily intake of 20 grams prebiotic fiber per day, the level that yields maximum benefit. This contributes to both intestinal and body-wide health.

RESTORE VITAMIN D. Take a daily dose of vitamin D in oil-based gelcap form to achieve a 25-hydroxy vitamin D level of 60 to 70 ng/mL, typically achieved by adults with doses in the 4,000 to 8,000 units per day range. Vitamin D restoration exerts beneficial effects on virtually every organ system in the body, especially the immune system and skeletal health. Calcium is not part of the Undoctored program, as it adds risk without benefit and intestinal calcium absorption is natu-rally increased by Undoctored strategies.

RESTORE IODINE AND REGAIN IDEAL THYROID HEALTH. Iodine is an essential trace mineral obtainable through iodine drops or kelp tablets; a daily intake of 500 to 1,000 micrograms per day is likely ideal. We also aim for ideal thyroid function, as the thyroid is the most commonly disrupted endocrine gland in modern life and an increasing number of people are experiencing health disruption from thyroid dysfunction.

RESTORE OMEGA-3 FATTY ACIDS. EPA and DHA are essential fatty acids that are increasingly deficient in modern people, easily restored and an important component of the complete Undoctored collection of strategies. We aim for a daily intake of 3,000 to 3,600 milligrams of EPA and DHA, the dose that yields maximum benefit on cardiovas-cular, metabolic, and neurological health and exerts maximum syn-ergy with other Undoctored strategies.

RESTORE MAGNESIUM. Magnesium is the mineral most likely to be made deficient by prior dietary habits. We restore magnesium by taking magnesium bicarbonate (that we make ourselves as Magnesium Water, page 351), magnesium malate, or magnesium glycinate. Magnesium citrate is the preferred form if you desire a modest laxative effect and/or have calcium oxalate kidney stones (see Appendix A). We aim for an elemental magnesium intake of 400 to 500 milligrams per day to restore magnesium tissue levels to the ideal. Iron, zinc, vitamin B_{12}, and folate are other nutrients that need to be considered individually.

Listed like this, it may not seem like much, but an astonishing amount of health-restoring power is built into this simple collection, a simple and synergistic prescription to get you started.

It Doesn't End with the Undoctored Experience

You will see that an impressive range of health conditions recede with the Undoctored experience. It is not uncommon to reverse several health conditions and be able to stop numerous medications following these strategies because we regain overall health by reversing shared factors that underlie related conditions. It is common, for example, to reverse the entire "package" of hypertension, high triglycerides, high cholesterol values, enlarged male breasts or female infertility, disrupted sleep, fatigue, depression, and breathlessness along with type 2 diabetes—because all these conditions share overlapping causes reversed with the Undoctored approach. (No drugs, by the way, achieve the same range of benefits because they target only one mechanism underlying a disease, not the physiological foundation that permitted a collection of diseases to develop in the first place, explaining why people end up being prescribed not one but many drugs.) It also means that drugs prescribed to "treat" hypertension, high triglycerides, hormonal disruption, poor sleep, depression, and diabetes can also be reduced or eliminated, amounting to lists of drugs being stopped.

Even today, I continue to learn new lessons about health conditions that improve or disappear with this approach. For example, despite seeing thousands of people face-to-face over the years reverse conditions as widely disparate as rheumatoid arthritis and acid reflux, I did not observe reversal of conditions such as plantar fasciitis or endometriosis until this lifestyle was followed by hundreds of thousands, then millions, of people. The expanded experience—a crowdsourced phenomenon—provided numerous examples of relief from the debilitating foot pain of plantar fasciitis and the chronic abdominal/pelvic pain of endometriosis. Anecdotal experiences, of course, do not provide any indication of what percentage of people can expect relief (that will come in the future), but there is *no downside* to this lifestyle. Unlike drugs or procedures (such as repeated exploratory laparotomies—open abdominal procedures—for endometriosis), you obtain broad health benefits even if you do not experience relief from, say, the abdominal/pelvic pain of endometriosis. The fact that many females with endometriosis will experience partial or total relief also raises many new questions about our understanding of such diseases, questions that may lead, in the future, to better insights and better answers.

There are, however, going to be exceptions to the Undoctored process, conditions that do not fully respond. Perhaps you're feeling better after having lost 27 pounds, with less pain, swelling, etc., down from three prescription drugs to one, but you'd like to go the full mile and regain total health with *no* medications. Or you have a condition that doesn't respond at all to the core Undoctored strategies. This includes conditions such as calcium oxalate kidney stones, osteoporosis/osteopenia, and coronary disease (the condition that launched Undoctored principles in the first place). These conditions require *one or more additional steps* that fall outside of the core collection of strategies included in the Undoctored Wild, Naked, and Unwashed program. I've included a number of protocols for various conditions in Appendix A, additional strategies worth strongly considering that hold potential for additional improvement. New protocols for other conditions will be added over time to undoctoredhealth.com.

I also find that failure to respond to the Undoctored strategies can even serve as a therapeutic test, meaning the combined Undoctored strategies are so effective that, in the minority of people who fail to respond, it suggests that there is indeed a medical problem present, like a genetically determined predisposition or an anatomical anomaly, factors that cannot be corrected with even the healthiest approach. Should you be among the minority who do not respond after a genuine effort, consider returning to the healthcare system to pinpoint the cause and solution. But hopefully you do so with greater overall health and an appreciation for what the system can and cannot do for you.

There are, undoubtedly, going to be lessons learned along the way, and new protocols added, but that is the nature of our effort: learn, apply, get feedback, learn, apply, get feedback. The protocols as written represent the best information, the most effective and safe strategies, that have been shown, for example, to prevent or to reduce calcium oxalate kidney stones but are rarely ever conveyed by doctors to people who suffer from this (painful) condition. The Undoctored methods used are always natural, accessible, and safe; nothing is lost in the process of trying and learning.

I hope that I have also succeeded in stirring up your curiosity, a desire to learn more about your health and recognize how much you are capable of accomplishing. As new direct-to-consumer technologies are released at breathtaking speed, you might find that a better, sleeker, more elegant, less costly effort is just around the corner. These will be among the online discussions I shall be cultivating in the future, as well. Imagine, for instance, that the new software to track parkinsonism, once available to the broad public, leads to generating fortuitous observations from the "crowd" that slow, even stop or reverse, progression of the condition that you can track on your own, solutions that may have nothing to do with drugs or procedures. Such revelations are going to come flooding our way in coming years, as more and more people embrace the world of self-empowered health.

Empowering Innovation on a Personal Level

Conventional health care in some form is here to stay, of course, as there will always be, at least, a need for catastrophic care for injury and infection. But we are going to cut health care down to size, our David to their Goliath, taking back control over many, more likely most, chronic conditions that are mismanaged by a system whose interests are different from ours. Cataclysmic disruption of health care is on the horizon.

Kodak was, in its heyday, a $16 billion-per-year, 140,000-employee success story, listed on the New York Stock Exchange for over 70 years, providing "Kodak moments" for millions of people, that nearly disappeared with the emergence of disruptive digital technologies. Blockbuster rentable DVDs can be added to a list that includes eight-track tapes, floppy disks, and IBM Selectrics, just another remnant of technologies long past. Would you trade any of these old technologies with your view-immediately-upon-demand cable, satellite dish, iTunes, cloud memory, or laptop?

Empowering innovation (i.e., advances that change the ground rules, slash costs, and improve results) has the potential to end careers and shut down entire industries, as well as provide life-altering benefits. In other words, innovation can involve pain and loss, as it surely did with Kodak's downsizing and near shutdown, but it can then lead to a better life for many. (Digital photography itself may not have led to a better life, but data digitization has transformed our lives in so many other ways.) Empowering innovation is disruptive to the status quo, but something better is left in its place.

Health care is, probably more than any other industry, ripe for disruption. It is dominated by complacent insiders who provide a product that is unsatisfactory on so many levels and who follow rules of pricing that have no basis in reality and cripple family finances and the national economy. Industries are not disrupted by insiders, but by outsiders, people who introduce an entirely new way to provide *better services at a fraction of the cost*. Even though you are a healthcare consumer, you are also the consummate industry outsider. You can be among those who disrupt the healthcare industry by choosing to acquire health on your own while obtaining massively superior results, and while also helping to cut back this huge and unsustainable wealth transfer. Multiply your contribution by millions of people, all displaying health, slenderness, and freedom from health problems mismanaged by the medical system, and we can get a sense for what the future of health—not health care, but *real* health—holds.

Our health innovations, as with all other disruptive innovations, will undoubtedly fuel the birth of new industries. For example, imagine a health-care insurer who comes to recognize (as we collect and tabulate results on a large scale) that people following the Undoctored lifestyle don't require medications, rarely have hypertension or heart disease, don't have acid reflux or migraine headaches, don't go to emergency rooms or hospitals very often, and incur dramatically lower healthcare costs. Healthcare insurers will understand that such people can be insured for far less than the average person, and as a result, the cost of health insurance will plummet and new companies will appear in the business of insuring only those of us engaging in such a health-powering lifestyle. Other innovative changes will ripple over time across other aspects of conventional health care.

Ironically, industry insiders are often among the last to recognize that their industry is being disrupted. Kodak continued to focus on conventional photographic equipment and film, even scrapping a prototype digital camera for fear it would disrupt existing business—until people on the outside did it for them. Likewise, doctors will poke fun at any notion of people or crowds of people tackling issues on health, drug companies will continue to advertise their products to an increasingly indifferent public, while hospitals won't even see us coming as this movement takes root and grows.

So don't expect pats on the back from doctors, or nods of understanding from nurses or hospital executives, and don't expect a disclaimer at the end of TV drug commercials saying, "This may not apply to people managing their own health." Instead, expect criticism and skepticism, outright accusations of foolhardy and childish behavior—all while you feel and look better than *all* of them.

Undoctored and unbounded. Nothing undecided or unexplorable here. It's *all* open to our unrelenting, unrestrained, Undoctored efforts. And in the not too distant future, you will know you have finally arrived in this world of the Undoctored when you find yourself sitting in the doctor's office for whatever reason—an insurance physical, a splinter in your finger—and the doctor does a double take and asks, "Just what is it you're doing to look so terrific?"

Acknowledgments

I regard this book as a bold experiment that charts new territory in how we think about health and health care. I'll be honest: Getting here was not without its contentious discussions, differences of opinion, and a fair share of emotion and loud voices.

At its core, the *Undoctored* premise is upsetting and unsettling, as it requires us to question not just the practices of modern health care, but its honesty and motivations. I view this as a sort of group psychotherapy: Diving deep into this thing we've collectively created called health care exposes some less-than-admirable impulses—greed, selfishness, the need for control—that play far larger roles than most are willing to admit, an Oedipal-like examination that can yield nightmares and a regretful recounting of prior healthcare interactions that likely yielded unsatisfactory outcomes. But this is part of the therapeutic catharsis that leads to something better. Thankfully, I've had the assistance and input of many people over the years that I've considered the issues summed up in this book.

My agent, Rick Broadhead, despite being an exceptionally polite and considerate sort of guy, has been fearless in urging me to get this book to publication. Having been my agent through the *Wheat Belly* adventure, Rick proved every bit as supportive for this new chapter called *Undoctored*. I actually proposed an early version of *Undoctored* at least 8 or 9 years ago that got pushed aside because of the momentum that the *Wheat Belly* message enjoyed. But Rick never forgot about this provocative idea and encouraged me all along.

I need to compliment the people at my publisher, Rodale, as it takes courage and chutzpah to support a book as contrary as *Undoctored*. My editors, Marisa Vigilante and Jennifer Levesque, understood the message I was trying to convey and stood behind it every step of the way. The rest of the Rodale staff has likewise helped me convey what is a contentious and controversial message. To all of you a big thank-you.

I owe my public television producer, Niki Vittel, who has seen me through some pretty dramatic highs and lows over the past several years, a special thanks for her feedback on how I delivered this message. Niki's eye for detail, her devotion to delivering a message clearly, and her knack for storytelling, lessons honed during her many years working with the late and wonderful Dr. Wayne Dyer, helped make *Undoctored* a better book.

My New York publicist, Gretchen Crary, has been fearless in helping me promote these ideas. She has also proven to be an insightful and tough critic and sounding board for ideas. She brings her many years in television journalism to the table in weighing arguments, never mincing words but providing important feedback.

My friend from the frigid north, Paul MacInnis of Halifax, Nova Scotia, provided support and feedback throughout the process, even spending a week with me while preparing practically every meal, putting his talents as a former professional chef to work. Paul has proven a spiritual and intellectual sounding board for the *Undoctored* ideas, and I found his observations priceless.

I have thanked my good friend in Milwaukee, Chris Kliesmet, many times in previous books, but his deep tolerance for contentious discourse over coffee or wine has helped me refine many of the *Undoctored* ideas. More than anyone else, Chris has helped me evolve these concepts, throwing in his unique notions of the "empowered patient." I may disagree (loudly) with his politics, but on these issues we find solid common ground.

I owe my social media team, Mary Agnes Antonopoulos, Johanna Spinoza, Lynn Douglas, and Tommy Antonopoulos a big thank-you for the many hours they have devoted (and continue to devote) to help spread the message I am trying to propagate. Best of all, in addition to being supremely smart and capable, they "get" it: They grasp the enormity of the issues being considered and have made these campaigns their own.

I also owe a debt of gratitude to the many people who, through Wheat Belly social media and now Undoctored sites, have helped develop and refine these ideas. This is not a journey or a book conceived in isolation; it is a group effort that draws from the varied knowledge and experience of thousands and thousands of devoted participants. Know that your views and opinions count and that they will continue to help chart a course of answers to health questions that are logical, accessible, effective, and help keep you free of this thing we should rarely need called health care.

Appendix A

Undoctored Protocols:
Additional Steps to Take in Specific Health Situations

The Undoctored Protocols target specific health situations that are not fully addressed by the basic Wild, Naked, and Unwashed program. I wish I could tell you that every disease known to man is addressed by the basic program, but that is simply not true. Numerous health conditions are indeed addressed, among them the most common and most debilitating long term (such as type 2 diabetes, autoimmune diseases, and hypertension), but there are going to be exceptions.

I tackle some of the more common exceptions here by providing Undoctored Protocols of additional strategies that you add to the basic Undoctored program for further benefits. Note that these protocols do not stand on their own; they are designed to be added onto the basic Undoctored strategies. Failure to follow the basic Undoctored strategies while only following the items in each protocol is a recipe for failure: That is how powerful the basic program can be.

In the future, through undoctoredhealth.com, I shall be asking you to provide some demographic data (age, sex, basic health information, etc.— voluntarily and anonymously, of course) so that I can track the combined group results of each protocol and then, over time, report the findings. You take nothing on faith here, as the long-term results will be conveyed so that you know what the community has or has not experienced. In time, I will also be adding new protocols for other conditions, such as gout and gallstones, not covered by these first protocols.

Calcium Oxalate Kidney Stones

People who have had the painful experience of passing a kidney stone remember well what this feels like, a pain described as worse than childbirth. Over 7 years, 50 percent who have had an episode will have a recurrence, with a greater proportion experiencing a recurrence over a longer period. The majority of kidney stones are made from calcium oxalate.

UNDOCTORED PROTOCOL

HYDRATE. Think of kidney stones like the rock candy you made as a kid: You dissolve as much sugar as possible in boiling water and then allow the solution to cool, causing sugar to crystallize on a piece of string. A similar process causes the formation of calcium oxalate kidney stones: If urine is allowed to become saturated with calcium and oxalate, calcium oxalate crystals form and, over time, become "stones" that can block urine if lodged in the ureters (leading to the bladder). These stones can lead to blood in the urine as well as excruciating pain. A key strategy is to keep urine diluted to prevent calcium and oxalate from crystallizing, achieved by hydrating well.

Gauging individual hydration, however, is imprecise. Rules such as "drink half your weight in water per day," unfortunately, do not factor in level of physical effort, time of year/ambient temperature, clothing, variation in sweating, or individual urine concentrating ability, so they are potentially misleading. One crude method is to look at urine color and hydrate to keep it from becoming amber, maintaining a light-yellow tint at all times. Another way is to test your urine with dipsticks (widely available in pharmacies), never allowing urine-specific gravity to exceed 1.010. Several manufacturers are developing portable devices that measure sodium concentration of sweat, an indirect gauge of hydration status. Stay tuned for online Undoctored discussions about these devices as they become available.

REBUILD BOWEL FLORA. Supplement with a high-potency, multi-species probiotic, as in Chapter 11; be certain that your preparation contains at least one, preferably several, of the following species: *Bifidobacterium infantis, B. lactis, B. breve, B. longum, Lactobacillus paracasei, L. acidophilus, L. plantarum,* or *L. gasseri.* These species reduce urine levels of oxalate dramatically, leaving less oxalate to form crystals. Garden of Life RAW products and Renew Life Ultimate Flora Extra Care are two excellent choices with several of these species in each. Though not yet on the market, there will likely be probiotics that include *Oxalobacter formigenes,* an enthusiastic consumer of oxalate, further reducing urinary oxalate levels. It is not yet clear how long a probiotic must be taken for full benefit, or on what schedule (e.g., 4 weeks every 6 months?), particularly when combined with a prebiotic fiber program, like the one in *Undoctored.* For full assurance of benefit, taking the probiotic chronically or on a repetitive schedule ensures continual reseeding of bowel flora; I shall update everyone as new data emerge.

TAKE MAGNESIUM CITRATE as your magnesium supplement. Ideally, 400 milligrams three times per day. Both magnesium and citrate (citric acid) block the formation of calcium oxalate crystals, making magnesium citrate a convenient means of obtaining both.

TAKE VITAMIN B$_6$. Taken as the most active form, pyridoxal 5'-phosphate (rather than the less-well-metabolized pyridoxine), vitamin B$_6$, at 50 milligrams per day, also blocks calcium and oxalate from forming crystals in the urine in some people.

REFERENCES

Abratt, V. R., and S. J. Reid. "Oxalate-Degrading Bacteria of the Human Gut as Probiotics in the Management of Kidney Stone Disease." *Advances in Applied Microbiology* 72 (2010): 63–87.

Oppici, E., S. Fargue, E. S. Reid, et al. "Pyridoxamine and Pyridoxal Are More Effective Than Pyridoxine in Rescuing Folding-Defective Variants of Human Alanine:Glyoxylate Aminotransferase Causing Primary Hyperoxaluria Type I." *Human Molecular Genetics* 24, no. 19 (October 2015): 5500–5511.

Reddy, S. V., A. B. Shaik, and S. Bokkisam. "Effect of Potassium Magnesium Citrate and Vitamin B-6 Prophylaxis for Recurrent and Multiple Calcium Oxalate and Phosphate Urolithiasis." *Korean Journal of Urology* 55, no. 6 (June 2014): 411–16.

Constipation

It's uncommon, but some people can continue to struggle with constipation even after all the bowel health–restoring strategies of the Undoctored approach, including iodine/thyroid normalization, magnesium supplementation, and bowel flora cultivation. There are a few modest efforts that you can add if you still struggle with constipation.

UNDOCTORED PROTOCOL

HYDRATE. The same hydration strategies discussed in the section on calcium oxalate stones apply to preventing or reversing constipation.

TAKE MAGNESIUM. Here is where choosing a less efficiently absorbed form of magnesium may be preferable. Such forms cause an osmotic effect, pulling water into the intestines, a benign process compared to irritative laxatives like phenolphthalein or senna that exert low-grade damage over time and are even associated with cancer risk. Taking 400 milligrams of magnesium citrate two or three times per day is a good place to start. If nothing happens after 24 hours, one or more doses of 800 to 1,200 milligrams will usually do the trick; then back down to the 400-milligram dose two or three times per day.

TAKE ADDITIONAL FIBER. Only a rare person needs to add fiber beyond the prebiotic fibers that we supplement to cultivate bowel flora in the Wild, Naked, and Unwashed program. If you are among those who do better with supplemental fiber for "bulk," ground golden flaxseed, chia seed, and psyllium seed (e.g., 1 tablespoon added to foods) are benign forms. Just be sure to hydrate even *more* to prevent a stool-hardening effect.

Coronary Disease

Every component of the Undoctored Wild, Naked, and Unwashed program plays a role in reducing risk for coronary heart disease. The nutritional program reduces or eliminates small LDL particles, raises HDL cholesterol, reduces triglycerides, and reduces postprandial (after-meal) lipoproteins. Omega-3 fatty acids from fish oil also reduce triglycerides, raise HDL, help reduce small LDL particles, reduce postprandial lipoproteins, and normalize blood clotting. Iodine/thyroid normalization helps maintain normal thyroid status and avoids/corrects the common hypothyroid situation that magnifies heart disease risk. Magnesium reduces blood pressure and the likelihood of abnormal heart rhythms. Vitamin D reduces blood pressure, insulin, parathyroid hormone, and inflammation and exerts a multitude of other positive health effects that add up to reduced cardiovascular risk. Cultivation of healthy bowel flora reduces LDL values, reduces triglycerides and blood sugar, and further improves all other measures that add to coronary risk. Put them all together, and they add up to a huge advantage in preventing, even reversing, coronary disease. These strategies can stand alone for the majority of people to reduce or eliminate risk for coronary disease. However, given the complexity of the causes for this condition, there are several additional strategies that should be considered for people at high risk, such as those with family members with heart disease before age 65.

UNDOCTORED PROTOCOL

CONSIDER A CT HEART SCAN. This safe, low-cost (typically around $200), low-radiation test yields a coronary calcium score; zero signifies no coronary atherosclerotic plaque and thereby virtually zero risk for heart attack for the next 5 years, while increasing scores signify increasing quantities of plaque and increasing risk for heart attack. No score, no matter how high, mandates any heart procedure if there are no symptoms of heart disease (e.g., chest discomfort, excessive breathlessness with exercise), but it provides you with a tracking tool. The only test that might be considered is a stress test in some form for higher scores, particularly scores of 500 and greater. Also, beware of the closely related test, CT coronary angiography, which is rarely necessary and exposes you needlessly to extremes of radiation (but yields lots more revenues for the testing center). If you have a zero score, terrific. Your risk for heart disease is virtually zero for the next 5 years, and simply carrying on the core Undoctored strategies will help keep it that way. If your score is above zero, it will serve as a starting place for future comparison when in, say, 1 or 2 years you undergo a repeat scan. Without any Undoctored efforts, you can expect the score to increase at the horrifying rate of 25 to 30 percent per year; with the Undoctored efforts, minimal increase or even a decrease in score is typically achieved.

I cannot stress how important 100 percent adherence to the Undoctored nutritional program is, as this is the most common reason for continuing excessive increases in heart scan scores (e.g., a once-per-week "indulgence" in some grain or sugary product that provokes formation of small LDL particles that last for 5 to 7 days with each indulgence).

GET AN ADVANCED LIPOPROTEIN ANALYSIS. This test should be run instead of the crude, imprecise cholesterol ("lipid") panel. We aim to have no more than 20 percent of all LDL particles in the small category. There are a number of laboratories that run these tests (see Appendix D). Your healthcare provider can obtain the order forms from the company's customer service department, or you can obtain the test yourself from the company and have the blood sample drawn on your own from one of the labs listed. Interpretation is the key: Feel free to share your results with the Undoctored community for useful feedback. Most commonly, an excess of small LDL particles persists that requires you to "tighten" your dietary approach of wheat, grain, and sugar elimination.

HAVE LIPOPROTEIN(A) ASSESSED. This measure can be obtained with your advanced lipoprotein analysis. If you carry this genetic factor, I have found that an increase in omega-3 fatty acids (EPA + DHA) to 6,000 milligrams per day (divided into two doses) magnifies protection from this factor. Also, strive to achieve ideal free T_3 thyroid hormone and TSH levels (as discussed in Chapter 12). This approach may or may not reduce lipoprotein(a) levels, but it has been associated with reduced progression of coronary disease.

OBTAIN BLOOD SUGAR MEASURES. Fasting glucose and hemoglobin A1c (HbA1c) should be tracked and brought into the ideal range of fasting glucose no higher than 90 mg/dL and HbA1c of 5 percent or less. (See the protocol for diabetes on page 340 for strategies.)

REFERENCES

Diffenderfer, M. R., and E. J. Schaefer. "The Composition and Metabolism of Large and Small LDL." *Current Opinion in Lipidology* 25, no. 3 (June 2014): 221–26.

Pauletto, P., M. Puato, M. G. Caroli, et al. "Blood Pressure and Atherogenic Lipoprotein Profiles of Fish-Diet and Vegetarian Villagers in Tanzania: The Lugalawa Study." *Lancet* 348, no. 9030 (September 21, 1996): 784–88.

Siri-Tarino, P. W., Q. Sun, F. B. Hu, and R. M. Krauss. "Saturated Fat, Carbohydrate, and Cardiovascular Disease." *American Journal of Clinical Nutrition* 91, no. 3 (March 2010): 502–9.

The Emerging Risk Factors Collaboration. "Glycated Hemoglobin Measurement and Prediction of Cardiovascular Disease." *JAMA* 311, no. 12 (March 26, 2014): 1225–33.

Cholesterol—Total and LDL

This is an area in which I will be guilty of oversimplification. But even over-simplified, it will vastly outstrip your doctor's focus on total cholesterol, LDL cholesterol, and statin drugs. Unfortunately, most doctors have fallen for the marketing disguised as statin drug "research," paid for by the drug industry. Statin drugs do indeed provide a very small benefit—but with substantial health (and financial) costs.

The Undoctored Wild, Naked, and Unwashed strategies address these issues quite aggressively. For example, wheat/grain elimination reduces tri-glycerides dramatically, often by several hundred points (in mg/dL); raises HDL cholesterol over time; and reduces or eliminates one of the most powerful causes of heart disease—small LDL particles. Omega-3 fatty acids from fish oil reduce triglycerides, removing the distorting effect of excessive triglycerides on other lipoproteins and reducing heart disease risk. Cultivation of bowel flora likewise reduces triglycerides and improves insulin response, along with reducing cholesterol values (via increased growth of bacterial species that yield bile salt hydrolase enzymes that prevent intestinal cholesterol reabsorption). In other words, the basic Undoctored strategies improve the values on the standard cholesterol panel dramatically. Some people, however, are left with higher total and LDL cholesterol values, so it is important to understand several issues surrounding these two values.

Total cholesterol is virtually worthless, as it includes HDL cholesterol. If HDL goes up (as it nearly always does on the Undoctored program) by 40 mg/dL (which is great), total cholesterol will also go up by 40 mg/dL, but many doctors try to "treat" this rise with statin drugs, which makes no sense whatsoever. There is no useful information in total cholesterol, so this outdated value should be ignored.

LDL cholesterol is usually not even measured; rather, it is calculated from the other three values (total cholesterol, HDL, triglycerides). The calculation is outdated (over 50 years old), based on crude and inaccurate assumptions, and unreliable. It also ignores variation in LDL particles—size, duration of persistence in the bloodstream, potential for oxidation (since oxidized LDL particles are especially bad), etc. For these reasons, I call LDL cholesterol "fictitious LDL," since it is wildly unreliable. On this lifestyle in which we sharply curtail carbohydrates (which modifies lipoprotein composition), it becomes even more unreliable, essentially invalidating the calculation.

We therefore turn to superior methods to quantify LDL particles and measure their size. (See Appendix D for a listing of lab services.) Small LDL particles—by far the worst (they persist much longer, are more prone to oxidation, and are more adherent to artery walls to form atherosclerotic plaque)—are triggered by consumption of carbohydrates; large LDL particles—more benign—are caused by fats. Among lipoprotein testing methods, I believe that the NMR method is the best choice for accuracy and provides the most information. A typical NMR lipoprotein test result in someone with heart disease risk would be: total LDL particles 1,800 nmol/L (the units signify number of particles per volume) and small LDL particles 900 nmol/L—meaning that 50 percent of all LDL particles are the undesirable, heart disease–causing small variety caused by grain and sugar consumption, reduced with their elimination. Other methods, though distant second choices, are to measure apoprotein B (apo B)—since each LDL particle contains one apo B molecule, which therefore serves as a virtual count of LDL particles—or direct LDL measurement. However, both apo B and measured LDL provide no indication of size and therefore do not suggest a dietary solution to correct the excess of small LDL particles.

The goal is to minimize small LDL particles (no higher than 20 percent of the total), while the goal for total LDL particles is not yet worked out, as it is not clear whether large LDL particles even contribute to heart disease risk and at what level. Stay tuned to Undoctored conversations for clarification of this issue.

REFERENCES

Diffenderfer, M. R., and E. J. Schaefer. "The Composition and Metabolism of Large and Small LDL." *Current Opinion in Lipidology* 25, no. 3 (June 2014): 221–26.

Meeusen, J. W., C. L. Snozek, N. A. Baumann, A. S. Jaffe, and A. K. Saenger. "Reliability of Calculated Low-Density Lipoprotein Cholesterol." *American Journal of Cardiology* 116, no. 4 (August 15, 2015): 538–40.

Diabetes, Type 2/Prediabetes

As with the other protocols listed here, each and every strategy in the Undoctored Wild, Naked, and Unwashed program makes an important contribution to reducing blood sugar and resistance to insulin, thereby reducing or reversing type 2 diabetes and prediabetes. Leaving out any component will compromise your results. Cultivation of bowel flora is especially crucial as this helps restore your body's responsiveness to insulin. Also, factor in time: If you are on, for example, injectable insulin and three oral drugs and have 100 pounds of excess weight to lose, reversal of diabetes can take at least several months, with results blunted by the process of weight loss that can keep blood sugars high (due to the flood of fatty acids that is part of the natural process of weight loss). Once weight plateaus, you will observe that blood sugars plummet. So time and patience are part of the process.

However, there are some additional strategies that can add to your success in minimizing or fully reversing type 2 diabetes and prediabetes. Please note that if you have type 1 diabetes or the latent autoimmune diabetes in adults (LADA) form (uncommon, in about 5 percent of people labeled type 2), then the following strategies do *not* apply, as you risk diabetic ketoacidosis, a dangerous situation, due to your pancreas's inability to produce insulin. This is one of the situations in which you have to ask your doctor whether the LADA form is present.

Uncommonly, people who follow the protocol but are still left with high fasting and/or after-meal blood sugars may be among the minority who have damaged their pancreatic beta cells that produce insulin and cannot reverse diabetes, only minimize it, no matter how serious the effort. In this situation, oral medications to reduce blood sugar can indeed be helpful.

UNDOCTORED PROTOCOL

OBTAIN BLOOD SUGAR MEASURES. Fasting glucose and hemoglobin A1c (HbA1c) should be tracked and brought into the ideal range: fasting glucose no higher than 90 mg/dL and HbA1c of 5 percent or less. Ideally, you track glucose values yourself with use of a glucose meter and test strips. You can obtain both from your doctor (who can typically provide them at no cost), or you can purchase them at pharmacies and department stores. OneTouch Ultra, Accu-Chek, Bayer's Contour, FreeStyle, and the Walmart device (the most affordable) have all worked well with consistently reliable results.

FOLLOW THE NO-CHANGE RULE. In addition to closely adhering to the Undoctored strategy of no more than 15 grams net carbs per meal, following blood sugars around meals can be a great advantage. Using finger-stick blood sugars, obtain an immediate premeal blood sugar and a 30- to 60-minute after-meal (i.e., after the start of eating) blood sugar and aim for no change. If blood sugar prior to the meal is, for example, 110 mg/dL, the 30- to 60-minute blood sugar should be no higher than 110 mg/dL. If it is higher, say, 140 mg/dL, examine the contents of the meal and reduce or eliminate the food (that contains a carbohydrate) responsible, and then retest the next time you eat that food or meal to ensure no change.

ACHIEVE KETOSIS. This strategy is for those who do everything right, including using the No-Change Rule, yet continue to encounter high fasting blood sugars and/or cannot keep after-meal blood sugars from rising, even with removal of all carbs. Ketosis is the natural and safe physiologic state (in people who do not have type 1 diabetes or LADA) obtained when no carbohydrates are in the diet and ketones are formed from the mobilization of fat. Ketosis is achieved by keeping net carbs even lower, generally no higher than 10 grams per meal, loading up further on *fats* (not proteins, as this will reverse ketosis). You can track blood levels of ketones using Abbott's Precision Xtra blood sugar device that also allows finger-stick ketones to be assessed, though test strips specifically for ketones will be required (cost about $4 per strip). Maximum benefit is obtained by maintaining ketones in the 1 to 3 mmol/L range, measured at random times throughout the day (only on occasion, given the expense). Provided you concurrently continue efforts at cultivating bowel flora with prebiotic fibers, you can maintain ketosis for as long as you like.

ENGAGE IN INTERMITTENT FASTING. Not eating for variable periods (e.g., 15 to 18 hours or longer) can help restore insulin resistance and thereby accelerate recovery from type 2 diabetes. There are many variations. One easy way is to have a healthy breakfast, skip lunch and dinner, and then resume eating the next morning. Or eat breakfast and lunch, skip dinner, and delay breakfast the next morning or wait until lunch before resuming food. The key is to hydrate well during the brief fast. If you are taking prescription beta blockers, clonidine, or diabetes medications, a reduction in dose is often necessary during the fasting period that will have to be managed with the help of your doctor (though the lack of need of the drugs during the fasting period almost always suggests that the drugs will not be necessary as you proceed through the program). It is absolutely crucial that you do not permit any hypoglycemia (low blood sugars) to develop if you are taking insulin or diabetes drugs, especially glyburide, glipizide, and glimepiride. For example, most people need to cut insulin dose by 50 percent during any fasting period.

Intermittent fasting should not be undertaken until you have completed the entire 6-week Undoctored process. The longer the fasting period, the more fatty acids are released from fat stores, and the more blood sugar will be temporarily disrupted and go higher, but this is a transient effect that reverses when you resume eating.

REFERENCES

Halberg, N., M. Henriksen, N. Soderhamn, et al. "Effect of Intermittent Fasting and Refeeding on Insulin Action in Healthy Men." *Journal of Applied Physiology* 99, no. 6 (December 2005): 2128–36.

Fatty Liver/Nonalcoholic Fatty Liver Disease

Provided these efforts are undertaken relatively early before cirrhosis sets in (which is irreversible), fatty liver is magnificently reversed with the Undoctored strategies, particularly with eliminating wheat/grains, limiting carbohydrates, taking omega-3 fatty acids from fish oil, and cultivating bowel flora. It is uncommon for liver function blood tests (AST, ALT) to *not* return to normal within several weeks of these strategies. If you have a lot of excess weight to lose and/or severe resistance to insulin from type 2 diabetes, then it may take longer than usual; once again, consistent effort and patience pay off.

UNDOCTORED PROTOCOL

AVOID ALCOHOL COMPLETELY. Alcohol is obviously a liver toxin, as well as a brake on weight loss and reversal of insulin resistance. Complete avoidance can therefore stack the odds further in your favor.

ENGAGE IN INTERMITTENT FASTING. See the discussion in the diabetes section above. The same process of intermittent fasting that helps reverse type 2 diabetes can be used to reverse fatty liver.

REFERENCES

Halberg, N., M. Henriksen, N. Soderhamn, et al. "Effect of Intermittent Fasting and Refeeding on Insulin Action in Healthy Men." *Journal of Applied Physiology* 99, no. 6 (December 2005): 2128–36.

Neuschwander-Tetri, B. A. "Carbohydrate Intake and Nonalcoholic Fatty Liver Disease." *Current Opinion in Clinical Nutrition and Metabolic Care* 16, no. 4 (July 2013): 446–52.

Osteopenia/Osteoporosis

The diet, vitamin D, and magnesium protocols in the core Undoctored program provide the bulk of bone health benefits through a variety of mechanisms, including increased intestinal calcium absorption, reduced urinary calcium loss, and reduced levels of the parathyroid hormone that weakens bones. We also reject calcium supplements, as the effects of vitamin D and the increased intestinal calcium absorption that develops after eliminating calcium-binding phytates from grains make them unnecessary, even dangerous. There are two additional strategies to consider.

UNDOCTORED PROTOCOL

GET VITAMIN K_2 AND K_1. Vitamin K_2 is obtained via fermented foods, such as cheeses and natto (Japanese fermented soybean), as well as in lesser quantities in animal products. An uncertain quantity of vitamin K_1 from green vegetables is also converted by some species of bowel flora to K_2 in the human intestine. I therefore suspect that the apparent need/benefit from K_2 supplementation in rebuilding bone density (and reducing cardiovascular risk) may be yet another expression of modern dysbiosis. Because K_2 supplementation is benign, it is a reasonable strategy to adopt to stack the odds in favor of rebuilding bone or preventing osteopenia/osteoporosis, especially since the precise way to encourage bacterial conversion of K_1 to K_2 has not been worked out.

Vitamin K_2 has been demonstrated to increase bone density and reduce fractures. (In Japan, K_2 is prescribed as a drug to treat osteoporosis.) The long-acting MK-7 form, rather than the short-acting MK-4 form, is the most effective at a dose of 180 to 200 micrograms per day, such as contained in the Life Extension Super K preparation.

Getting 4 to 5 servings every day of green vegetables that provide plenty of vitamin K_1 as well as other health benefits is also helpful. Vitamin K_1 supplementation, as opposed to getting it from green vegetables, does not appear to hold the same bone density–increasing potential, and consuming plenty of green vegetables seems to be a more effective means of obtaining bone health, as well as other health benefits.

Note that people taking the blood thinner warfarin (Coumadin) will need to work with their healthcare providers, as both K_1 and K_2 supplementation will counteract the effect of the drug, an effect that can pose dangers if supplementation is not done properly (e.g., low doses of K vitamins, either K_1 or K_2, taken in consistent amounts every day to avoid excessive fluctuations of the INR value). Another option would be to convert to a blood thinner that does not interact with the K vitamins.

DO AXIAL-IMPACT EXERCISES. Exercise that involves impact to the spine ("axial" impact), like jumping rope, jogging, stairclimbing, hopping in place, and dancing, but not swimming or biking (though healthy for other reasons), has dramatic effects on increasing bone density. Jumping in place 10 to 20 times, for instance, once or twice per day achieves measurable increases in bone density.

REFERENCES

Cheung, A. M., L. Tile, Y. Lee, et al. "Vitamin K Supplementation in Postmenopausal Women with Osteopenia (ECKO trial): A Randomized Controlled Trial." *PLoS Medicine* 5, no. 10 (October 14, 2008): e196.

Greenway, K. G., J. W. Walkley, and P. A. Rich. "Impact Exercise and Bone Density in Premenopausal Women with Below Average Bone Density for Age." *European Journal of Applied Physiology* 115, no. 11 (November 2015): 2457–69.

Huang, Z. B., S. L. Wan, Y. J. Lu, L. Ning, C. Liu, and S. W. Fan. "Does Vitamin K_2 Play a Role in the Prevention and Treatment of Osteoporosis for Postmenopausal Women: A Meta-Analysis of Randomized Controlled Trials." *Osteoporosis International* 26, no. 3 (March 2015): 1175–86.

Iwamoto, J. "Vitamin K_2 Therapy for Postmenopausal Osteoporosis." *Nutrients* 6, no. 5 (May 16, 2014): 1971–80.

Knapen, M. H., N. E. Drummen, E. Smit, C. Vermeer, and E. Theuwissen. "Three-Year Low-Dose Menaquinone-7 Supplementation Helps Decrease Bone Loss in Healthy Postmenopausal Women." *Osteoporosis International* 24, no. 9 (September 2013): 2499–507.

Appendix B

Hidden Sources of Grains and Safe Sweeteners

Watch Out for Hidden Sources of Wheat and Grains

You need to be careful when you shop, as grains, especially wheat and corn, can be found in an incredible variety of forms in processed foods—hidden as additives, thickeners, coatings, or cheap "bulk." So it is important to recognize these aliases to remain safely grain-free. Of course, the best way to avoid hidden sources of grains is to eat whole foods that don't require labels in the first place, such as vegetables, eggs, and meats. But on those occasions when you need something with a label, such as premixed salad dressing or mayonnaise, it's important to be aware of such hidden landmines, listed below. Also note that many medications and nutritional supplements contain wheat or corn.

People with extreme gluten sensitivities, an allergy to a grain component, or increased sensitivity to various grain components that can develop the longer a grain-free diet is maintained, all need to be aware of the potential for cross-contamination (i.e., grain contamination from utensils, cooking surfaces, airborne particles, or liquids). If a food is labeled "gluten-free," then it should have been prepared in a facility where cross-contamination should *not* have occurred. Potential for cross-contamination is greatest in restaurants, since few have the ability to avoid it. However, increasing numbers of restaurants are taking on the challenge as the market for gluten-free grows. (Yes, we have to play the gluten-free game in restaurants, as they will not understand if you say "grain-free.") This means reserving a section of the kitchen with utensils and work surfaces segregated from the rest of the kitchen. (Unless airflow is managed, airborne contamination remains a potential source of exposure, though much reduced in likelihood.)

For foods sold in stores to qualify as "gluten-free," the FDA requires that the product must contain no more than 20 parts per million (ppm) gluten and be produced in a gluten-free facility to prevent cross-contamination. When in doubt, contact the customer service department for the product to inquire whether a gluten-free facility was used. More and more manufacturers are starting to specify whether products are gluten-free or not gluten-free on their products or their Web sites.

Here are the not-so-obvious foods and ingredients that are really wheat. A question mark (?) following an item means it is either variable or uncertain (given manufacturers' reluctance or inability to specify the source).

Hidden Wheat

Baguette

Beignet

Bran

Brioche

Bulgur

Burrito

Caramel coloring (?)

Caramel flavoring (?)

Couscous

Crepe

Croutons

Dextri-Maltose

Durum

Einkorn

Emmer

Emulsifiers

Farina

Farro

Focaccia

Fu (gluten in Asian foods)

Gnocchi

Graham flour

Gravy

Hydrolyzed vegetable protein

Hydrolyzed wheat starch

Kamut

Maltodextrin

Modified food starch (?)

Orzo

Panko (a bread crumb mixture used in Japanese cooking)

Ramen

Roux (wheat-based sauce or thickener)

Rusk

Rye

Seitan (nearly pure gluten used in place of meat)

Semolina

Soba (mostly buckwheat but usually also includes wheat)

Spelt

Stabilizers

Strudel

Tabbouleh

Tart

Textured vegetable protein (?)

Triticale

Triticum

Udon

Vital wheat gluten

Wheat bran

Wheat germ

Wraps

Hidden Corn

While some corn-containing foods, like corn on the cob, cornmeal, high-fructose corn syrup, and popcorn, are obvious, there are also hidden sources.

And there are hundreds of common food ingredients derived from corn, such as dextrose, dextrin, maltodextrin, high-fructose corn syrup, fructose, maltitol, polydextrose, ethanol, caramel coloring, and artificial flavorings, that will not be identified on the label as being corn-sourced. However, the process to generate these products from corn reduces zein protein content to negligible levels, so they are generally not a problem for grain exposure for the majority (though these ingredients, especially sugars like fructose, pose problems of their own).

Because of the many ways that corn-derived ingredients can make their way into processed foods, the best policy for the ultrasensitive is to avoid processed foods as much as possible.

Grits

Hominy

Hydrolyzed corn protein

Hydrolyzed corn starch

Maize

Mixed vegetable oil/vegetable oil

Modified food starch

Polenta

Zea mays

Safe Sweeteners

If you are going to need something sweetened, stick with the safest sweeteners, not ones that rot your teeth, raise blood sugar, mess with bowel flora, or cause weight gain. This eliminates aspartame, acesulfame, saccharine, and sucralose, as well as sucrose or table sugar, agave, coconut sugar, cane sugar, and other forms of sugar.

Among the top picks for safe sweeteners is stevia, a natural sweetener from the stevia plant. Unfortunately, some people experience an undesirable metallic aftertaste with stevia. Combining sweeteners can therefore be a useful strategy. Combine stevia with monk fruit and/or erythritol, for example, and less stevia will be required and the aftertaste will be reduced or eliminated.

Here are some safe sweetener choices.

Stevia

Stevia is the natural sweetener from the stevia plant. Purchase only pure liquid stevia, pure powdered stevia, or powdered stevia with inulin; avoid stevia with maltodextrin, since maltodextrin is a form of sugar.

Monk Fruit

Also known as lo han guo, monk fruit is gaining popularity in the benign sweetener world. Monk fruit has a clean, sweet taste without the aftertaste perceived with stevia. It may be tough to find, but it is becoming increasingly available.

Erythritol

Erythritol is a natural sweetener found in fruit. Although it is only about 70 percent as sweet as sugar, combined with the increasing sensitivity to sweetness that develops after eliminating grains, you can use erythritol, spoonful for spoonful, just as you would sugar. It is especially useful combined with stevia and/or monk fruit.

Xylitol

Xylitol, another natural sweetener found in small quantities in fruit, is the most sugarlike of the sweetener choices, and it is useful for obtaining glazing and streusel effects for baking. Use xylitol in limited quantities, however, as it has a modest capacity to raise blood sugar. And dog owners should know that xylitol is toxic to dogs.

Inulin

Inulin is a fiber with a light sweetness that is best used in combination with other sweeteners. It also acts as a prebiotic fiber that can, unlike other prebiotic fibers, be resistant to heating and not degrade to sugars. (Other prebiotic fibers degrade to sugars when heated during cooking.)

Sweetener Combinations

TRUVÍA—Available widely in supermarkets, Truvía is a combination of Rebiana, an isolate from stevia with less bitterness, and erythritol. Though the erythritol is sourced from corn, which we try to avoid, the corn protein residues are negligible.

SWERVE—A combination of erythritol and inulin, this sweetener is available in granular and confectioners' sugar consistencies.

VIRTUE—This unique combination of monk fruit and erythritol from Wheat-Free Market Foods (wheatfreemarket.com) has four times the sweetness of sugar, teaspoon for teaspoon, allowing a little to go a long way. It is currently available through the company's Web site and in selected health food or specialty stores.

LAKANTO—A combination of erythritol and monk fruit blended to make it replaceable with sucrose 1:1, Lakanto is available through the company's Web site (lakanto.com) and in some stores.

Appendix C

Additional Recipes: Magnesium Water and Fermenting Vegetables

Magnesium Water

The most highly absorbable form of magnesium is magnesium bicarbonate. Because of an unusual tendency to absorb water in dry form (e.g., tablet or powder), no supplement manufacturer sells it. But you can make it in your own kitchen quite easily using readily available ingredients. Use Magnesium Water *in place of magnesium supplements*—i.e., don't take both—to avoid long-term magnesium overload.

A 4-ounce (1/2-cup) serving of Magnesium Water provides 90 milligrams of elemental magnesium; 4 ounces twice per day adds 180 milligrams of elemental magnesium to your daily intake. You can drink up to 16 ounces per day (8 ounces, or 1 cup, twice per day), which provides a total of 360 milligrams of magnesium per day, especially useful during the first few weeks of your Undoctored experience to rapidly restore magnesium.

Because of better absorption, Magnesium Water yields faster relief from muscle cramps and migraine headaches, even abnormal heart rhythms. Such benefits are also more likely to occur with the 360-milligram-per-day total dose.

Note that the milk of magnesia used in the recipe must be unflavored, as flavoring will block the reaction creating the magnesium bicarbonate. Label your bottle of Magnesium Water to prevent unsuspecting people from drinking it (which can result in diarrhea). Magnesium Water does not need to be refrigerated if consumed within 1 week. Because the reaction involves carbonic acid (from carbonated seltzer) and magnesium oxide (milk of magnesia), the end result is magnesium bicarbonate and water, with little to no carbonation remaining.

Add several drops of your choice of natural extract, such as orange, lemon, coconut, or berry if desired for flavor. If some sweetness is desired, add a few drops of the flavored stevias available in place of the extract or add your choice of sweetener, such as several drops of liquid stevia or monk fruit, to the mixture. I used 20 drops of berry-flavored SweetLeaf Sweet Drops, which yielded a light sweetness, subtle enough to allow sipping over ice without being overly sweet. And be sure to choose a carbonated seltzer without sugar or high-fructose corn syrup. (This is why we avoid tonic water.)

YIELD: 2 LITERS

2-liter bottle of seltzer (not tonic water)
3 tablespoons unflavored milk of magnesia
Naturally flavored extracts and/or sweetener

Uncap the seltzer and pour off a few tablespoons. Shake the (unflavored) milk of magnesia, and pour out 3 tablespoons. (Most brands come with a handy little measuring cup that works perfectly.) Pour the milk of magnesia into the seltzer slowly, followed by the extract and sweetener.

Cap the bottle securely, and shake until all the sediment has dissolved. Let the mixture sit for 15 minutes and allow to clarify. If any sediment remains, shake again. Drink as instructed above.

Fermenting Vegetables

Fermenting vegetables is a low- or no-cost way to supplement your efforts to cultivate healthy bowel flora. The process is really called anaerobic lactic acid fermentation, a process that allows microorganisms ordinarily present on produce to proliferate when no oxygen is available, yielding lactic acid that provides a familiar "zing" to fermented vegetables.

Microbial (CFU) counts vary with the vegetable chosen, ambient temperature, organisms present on the food at the start, and how long fermentation is allowed to proceed. Counts are typically in the hundreds of millions, but can reach billions, just as in probiotic supplements. Species that proliferate include several lactobacillus, leuconostoc, and other species, although typically only one to four species are found (unlike the wider species diversity found in commercial probiotic products that we use to "seed" a greater number of species at the start of bowel flora cultivation efforts). Foods other than vegetables can be fermented, too, such as fruits and mushrooms, but vegetables are the easiest and most versatile for the beginner.

Make sure to use water free of chlorine, chloramine (resistant to being removed by boiling, unlike chlorine), and fluoride and salt free of iodine. This means using filtered water (filtered via reverse osmosis, charcoal filtration, or distillation or obtained from a "clean source" such as a fresh spring) and sea salt, kosher salt, or other noniodized salt.

Veggies should be sliced or chopped to encourage the fermentation reaction. For vegetables like onions with an outer layer, remove the woody outermost layer but maintain all the inner softer layers, even if discolored, as they are richer in microbes. A white residue can form along the edges during the fermentation process, representing fungal growth; simply wipe this off but don't consume it.

You will need a fermentation setup that allows you to completely submerge your sliced/chopped veggies in a brine solution. For instance, you can use a clean large, widemouthed jar, weighing the veggies down with a plate with a heavy (clean) stone on top. I have a heavy drinking glass that fits perfectly in the mouth of a widemouthed jar; the glass easily pushes the veggies below the surface. You can also purchase fermentation setups online. The brine solution is created using water with around 1 tablespoon noniodized salt per quart or liter, more if desired.

You will witness the process of fermentation starting at about 48 to 72 hours, with bubbles forming and rising to the surface. Most veggies are fermented after 72 hours and can be kept in the container for around 2 weeks before they start to get stale due to excessive fermentation. Refrigeration can extend shelf life, as it slows fermentation.

Combining vegetables, such as sliced onions and garlic cloves, and/or adding fresh or dried spices and herbs (caraway seeds, fresh dill, or oregano) add even more variety. Below are two simple fermentation recipes to get you started. Anyone wishing to further explore this fascinating health practice can find a much more detailed discussion in *The Art of Fermentation* by Sandor Ellix Katz. For the sake of simplicity, I present these two easy recipes as if you are using a 1-quart vessel for fermentation. Alter the amounts, of course, to suit the size of your fermentation vessel.

Fill a clean vessel with water. Add 1 tablespoon noniodized salt per quart of water to make the brine. Add more salt to taste.

To make red onions and garlic: Remove the outer woody layer from the onions but maintain all fleshy inner layers. Slice both the onions and garlic, add several sprigs of fresh dill, and submerge in the brine. Store in a cool place out of direct sunlight.

To make asparagus with white onions and dill: Asparagus can be fermented either whole or chopped into 1-inch pieces. Remove the outer woody layer from the onions but maintain all fleshy inner layers and slice. Add two or three sprigs of fresh dill. Submerge the vegetables and store in a cool place out of direct sunlight.

Appendix D

Additional Resources

Reliable Secondary Sources for Further Information

Recall that, whenever possible, rely on primary sources of information (i.e., the original source). The National Library of Medicine makes such studies available to anyone on its PubMed site: pubmed.gov.

However, for the sake of saving time and effort, identifying trusted secondary sources of information can be very helpful; these are sources that you have come to trust as reliable and unbiased. Some judgment will be required here. There are many sources of nutritional information, for example, that are blatantly untrustworthy, nothing more than authors who "repackage" conventional advice. You are looking for sources that consistently use sound logic, do not misrepresent or misinterpret information, and are not in the business of selling you a product for hair growth, for instance, in the midst of a conversation about hair loss.

Of course, the Undoctored site (undoctoredhealth.com) can serve as a secondary source that will also, over time, report back the results of the Undoctored experience.

Here are some other trusted secondary sources.

AUTOIMMUNE DISEASES

Dr. Terry Wahls

terrywahls.com

Dr. Wahls personally reversed her incapacitating multiple sclerosis and now makes it her mission to help people navigate all the issues surrounding autoimmune conditions.

BOWEL FLORA/MICROBIOME

Human Food Project: Anthropology of Microbes

humanfoodproject.com

Jeff D. Leach incisively analyzes many facets of human bowel flora, and many of his observations are the result of time spent in Tanzania with the Hadza.

Human Microbiome Project

hmpdacc.org

This Web site provides the unfolding scientific findings of the National Institutes of Health–funded project exploring the human microbiome, including the many studies this effort has generated.

NUTRITION

From Undoctored discussions, you know that we do not rely on agencies such as the American Heart Association, the American Diabetes Association, or the Academy of Nutrition and Dietetics for nutritional advice due to bias and involvement of commercial interests. For unbiased interpretations of the science, the following sites provide comprehensive, scientifically backed information on various facets of nutritional health.

Wheat Belly Blog

wheatbellyblog.com

This blog, which accompanies the discussions provided in the Wheat Belly book series, explores various facets of grain-free living with concepts consistent with the Undoctored lifestyle.

Undoctored

undoctoredhealth.com

In addition to being the place to go to contribute health information that will be tracked and reported back over time, this site will also be a place to obtain new developments in nutritional insights relevant to health and the Undoctored experience.

Undoctored U

undoctoredu.com

Undoctored U is the official training and certification program that trains doctors, nurses, chiropractors, naturopaths, integrative health practitioners, personal trainers, and others interested in delivering the Undoctored program to their clientele.

Art and Science of Low Carb/Jeff S. Volek, PhD, RD, and Stephen D. Phinney, MD, PhD

artandscienceoflowcarb.com

Drs. Volek and Phinney originate considerable original research that explains why carb limitation and ketogenesis are healthy processes. While much of their discussions are geared toward the general public, they also cover a lot of ground helpful to athletes.

Livin' La Vida Low-Carb/Jimmy Moore

livinlavidalowcarb.com

Jimmy is not just a friend but also a terrific connector of people and ideas. He provides an impressive amount of information via podcasts, videos, and even an annual Caribbean cruise.

Dietitians for Professional Integrity

integritydietitians.org

I do not trust the majority of dietitians to provide unbiased information. But there is a growing movement from within the profession to stand apart and help provide information untainted by commercial interests.

The Eating Academy blog/Peter Attia, MD

eatingacademy.com

Dr. Attia has championed the cause of performing and funding real, unbiased science in nutrition to replace the flawed and poorly constructed studies that led to such blunders as cutting fat and consuming high quantities of carbohydrates.

Chris Kresser

chriskresser.com

Chris Kresser is a nutritionist who is committed to the idea that continual learning is the key to health. You can be sure that his ideas and responses are carefully considered.

ORGANIC FOODS

The Organic Center

organic-center.org

The Organic Center is a nonprofit research and consumer advocacy group focused on generating responsible science for organic farming and foods.

Rodale Institute

rodaleinstitute.org

The Rodale Institute (founded by the same J.I. Rodale who founded this book's publisher and the magazine *Organic Gardening*) conducts research on organic farming methods, educating students, scientists, and farmers through webinars, online courses, and on-site programs.

SPECIFIC NUTRIENTS

In general, hospital/health systems, nutritional supplement manufacturers, and even "official" sources such as the USDA MyPlate Web site post nutritional information that is unreliable, based on outdated science, or biased in favor of selling you something and should not serve as sources of information. Here are some sources that have proven to be helpful and unbiased.

Linus Pauling Institute of Oregon State University
lpi.oregonstate.edu/mic
This site provides scientifically responsible discussions about various micronutrients with extensive reviews of the science. Despite being attached to a scientist (Linus Pauling) who had some extreme ideas, this site has consistently maintained objectivity without extreme views.

National Institutes of Health, Office of Dietary Supplements
ods.od.nih.gov
Use this site only for the most basic nutrient information, such as the RDA for iron or zinc, but not for extensive reviews of the science or discussions about ideal, as opposed to just enough, intake of nutrients.

The Vitamin D Council/John J. Cannell, MD
vitamindcouncil.org
For over a decade, Dr. Cannell has championed the vitamin D issue, providing insightful and responsible discussions about the importance of this nutrient.

THYROID HEALTH

Stop the Thyroid Madness/Janie A. Bowthorpe, MEd
stopthethyroidmadness.com
Ms. Bowthorpe is a terrific example of how a person who isn't in health care can develop a high level of sophistication and expertise in a health issue, in this case thyroid health. She has proven to be a reliable and insightful information source for thyroid issues, far better than most doctors I know.

TOXIC EXPOSURES AND SAFE PERSONAL CARE AND CLEANING PRODUCTS

The Environmental Working Group

ewg.org

The Environmental Working Group is the nonprofit, nonpartisan source for information on issues such as the value of organic foods and strategies to avoid pesticides and herbicides, problem ingredients in cosmetics and toiletries (see EWG's Skin Deep database of products), and healthy cleaning products. The group's smartphone apps are available here: ewg.org/apps.

WOMEN'S HEALTH

Our Bodies Ourselves

ourbodiesourselves.org

Discussions focus primarily on reproductive health, contraception, and global advocacy for women's rights.

Womens-Health.com

womens-health.com/boards/forum

This is a busy forum allowing women to discuss a wide variety of life and health issues.

Direct-to-Consumer Lab Testing

The following labs make just about any test available direct to the consumer, except in New York, New Jersey, California, and Rhode Island. (Blame the hospital lobbies for this, as they try to protect hospital profits in those states; they want you to rely on their labs only.) In every other state, it means that nearly any lab test you desire can be obtained without a doctor's order with results delivered directly to you.

ZRT Laboratory

zrtlab.com

ZRT Laboratory is the premiere finger-stick blood, saliva, and urine direct-to-consumer lab, providing access to an impressive array of testing: cortisol, sex hormones, lipids, HbA1c, heavy metals, thyroid, and others.

Direct Labs

directlabs.com

HealthCheckUSA

healthcheckusa.com

Lab Tests Online
labtestsonline.org

GENETIC TESTING

23andme
23andme.com
A saliva sample is all that is needed to obtain an analysis of over 60 (and growing) genetic variants.

Futura Genetics
futuragenetics.com
Through a saliva sample, 28 genetic variants are assessed.

BOWEL FLORA TESTING

uBiome
ubiome.com
A stool swab will yield an extraordinarily detailed bowel flora analysis.

uBiota
ubiota.com

LIPOPROTEIN TESTING

These are the labs that offer advanced lipoprotein testing, which is superior to outdated cholesterol testing. Your doctor can contact the lab, or you can contact one yourself to identify a blood-draw center in your area for the specimen to be obtained. The list is provided in the order of preference, most preferable at the top.

NMR LipoProfile: Now provided through LabCorp
labcorp.com

True Health Diagnostics (which acquired Health Diagnostic Laboratory)
truehealthdiag.com

Quest Diagnostics (which acquired Berkeley HeartLab)
questdiagnostics.com/home/patients/tests-a-z/heart-disease.html

Lab Values to Consider Tracking through Your Undoctored Program

While you can track easy measures such as body weight, blood pressure, and waist circumference at the beginning and along the way in the Undoctored process, you can also track some important lab values. These lab values will reflect reemerging health in blood sugar levels, triglycerides, and factors that reflect risk for heart disease, stroke, and other conditions.

Note that blood work should generally not be obtained during the Undoctored 6-week process because weight loss occurs in the majority during this period, which will temporarily disrupt lab values, making, for instance, blood sugar and triglycerides high (due to the flood of fatty acids into the bloodstream that is a natural part of weight loss). Ideally, blood should be drawn no sooner than 4 weeks after weight loss has plateaued.

Here are lab values to consider tracking.

Fasting glucose, hemoglobin A1c, fasting insulin—all reflecting blood-sugar and insulin-resistance status

NMR lipoproteins (NMR LipoProfile) or other advanced lipoprotein testing service (see above)

25-hydroxy vitamin D—an assessment of your vitamin D status

Thyroid-stimulating hormone (TSH), free T_3, free T_4, reverse T_3, thyroid antibodies—all measures of thyroid status

Other measures specific to your individual health concerns can be tracked also, such as a complete blood count (CBC) and ferritin if iron deficiency is suspected.

Preferred Probiotic Products

These probiotics contain among the highest CFUs (colony-forming units, a count of bacteria), making it easier to obtain the desired dosage of at least 50 billion CFUs per day. Each also provides a minimum of 10 species and has been assessed by independent labs as delivering the stated amount of CFUs of viable organisms at the time of purchase.

Renew Life Ultimate Flora
renewlife.com

Garden of Life RAW
gardenoflife.com

VSL#3
vsl3.com

NOW Foods Probiotic-10
nowfoods.com

Dr. Mercola Complete Probiotics
probiotics.mercola.com

Preferred Fish Oil Sources

The quality of fish oil has improved over the past decade. Some companies that sold fish oil containing excessive oxidative breakdown products have cleaned up their acts, and the old excessively fishy, belch-provoking low-quality products are increasingly uncommon. I advise avoiding cod liver oil sources, however, as they have been shown to contain excessive polychlorinated biphenyls, PCBs. Nonetheless, there are superior brands of fish oil that have been shown by independent analyses to contain negligible quantities of contaminants, such as mercury and PCBs, as well as oxidative breakdown products.

The triglyceride form that mimics the natural form of EPA and DHA found in fish is the best absorbed and tends to be the most concentrated, while the more common ethyl ester form is somewhat less well absorbed and less concentrated. Triglyceride forms come as liquids that are minimally fishy and flavored with citrus or berry and must be refrigerated, also available in capsules. Ethyl ester forms come in capsules and do not have to be refrigerated, though are best stored in a cool, dark place. All brands listed below are obtained from sustainable and/or low-food-chain sources (e.g., sardines, anchovies, menhaden) to minimize environmental impact and contaminants.

As with several other Undoctored strategies, ignore the dose recommendations on the label and follow the target dose found in Chapter 12. Remember: We aim for ideal health, not average or acceptable health.

Ascenta NutraSea
ascentahealth.com
NutraSea is a high-quality triglyceride form of fish oil in both liquid and capsules. They also offer a unique vegetarian product containing EPA and DHA. This brand is widely available in Canadian stores, less available in the

United States and elsewhere, but it can be obtained through the company's Web site or other online retailers.

Kirkland Signature Natural Fish Oil

This is the Costco brand available at a low cost in a medium-potency ethyl ester capsule with 684 milligrams EPA and DHA per enteric-coated capsule.

Natural Factors Maximum Triple Strength RxOmega-3

A high-potency ethyl ester preparation with 900 milligrams EPA and DHA per capsule. Less potent preparations are also available.

Nordic Naturals

nordicnaturals.com

Nordic Naturals offers some of the most concentrated fish oil products available, allowing you to take less liquid or fewer capsules to obtain the desired intake of EPA and DHA. The company also makes a vegetarian source of EPA and DHA available.

NutriGold Triple Strength Omega-3 Gold

A high-potency triglyceride-form capsule providing 1,000 milligrams EPA and DHA.

Simply Right (Sam's Club) Triple-Strength Fish Oil

This is a low-cost, high-potency ethyl ester form with 900 milligrams EPA and DHA per capsule.

Trader Joe's Omega-3

This is a medium-potency ethyl ester form of fish oil, each capsule providing 600 milligrams EPA and DHA.

Endnotes

INTRODUCTION

1   Centers for Medicare & Medicaid Services, *National Health Expenditures 2014 Highlights,* accessed September 9, 2016, cms.gov/Research-Statistics-Data-and-Systems /Statistics-Trends-and-Reports/NationalHealthExpendData/Downloads/highlights.pdf.

2   P. Densen, "Challenges and Opportunities Facing Medical Education," *Transactions of the American Clinical and Climatological Association* 122 (2011): 48–58.

3   A. Kadish and J. Goldberger, "Selecting Patients for ICD Implantation: Are Clinicians Choosing Appropriately?" *JAMA* 305, no. 1 (2011): 91–92.

CHAPTER 1

1   M. A. Huffman, "Forest Pharmacy," *Healthy Options,* March 2000, www.pri .kyoto-u.ac.jp/shakai-seitai/shakai-shinka/huffman/CHIPP/3.-5%20CHIMPP.pdf.

2   W. Davis, S. Rockway, and M. Kwasny, "Effect of a Combined Therapeutic Approach of Intensive Lipid Management, Omega-3 Fatty Acid Supplementation, and Increased Serum 25 (OH) Vitamin D on Coronary Calcium Scores in Asymptomatic Adults," *American Journal of Therapeutics* 16, no. 4 (2009): 326–32.

3   "PatientsLikeMe Survey Shows Vast Majority of People with Health Conditions Are Willing to Share Their Health Data," PatientsLikeMe, January 23, 2014, news.patientslikeme.com/press-release/patientslikeme-survey-shows-vast-majority-people -health-conditions-are-willing-share-t.

4   C. Marzuillo, C. De Vito, S. Boccia, et al., "Knowledge, Attitudes and Behavior of Physicians regarding Predictive Genetic Tests for Breast and Colorectal Cancer," *Preventive Medicine* 57, no. 5 (2013): 477–82.

CHAPTER 2

1   K. E. Joynt, S. T. Le , E. J. Orav, and A. K. Jha, "Compensation of Chief Executive Officers at Nonprofit US Hospitals," *JAMA Internal Medicine* 174, no. 1 (January 2014): 61–67.

2   A. Hill, S. Khoo, J. Fortunak, B. Simmons, and N. Ford, "Minimum Costs for Producing Hepatitis C Direct-Acting Antivirals for Use in Large-Scale Treatment Access Programs in Developing Countries," *Clinical Infectious Diseases* 58, no. 7 (April 2014): 928–36.

3   A. Palumbo, L. Giaccone, A. Bertola, et al., "Low-Dose Thalidomide plus Dexamethasone Is an Effective Salvage Therapy for Advanced Myeloma," *Haematologica* 86, no. 4 (2001): 399–403.

4   Geeta Anand, "How Drug's Rebirth as Treatment for Cancer Fueled Price Rises," *Wall Street Journal,* November 15, 2004, wsj.com/articles/SB110047032850873523.

5   L. P. Garrison, S. Wang, H. Huan, et al., "The Cost-Effectiveness of Initial Treatment of Multiple Myeloma in the U.S. with Bortezomib plus Melphalan and Prednisone versus Thalidomide plus Melphalan and Prednisone or Lenalidomide plus Melphalan and Prednisone with Continuous Lenalidomide Maintenance Treatment," *Oncologist* 18, no. 1 (2013): 27–36.

6   Infectious Diseases Society of America and HIV Medicine Association, letter to Tom Evegan and Kevin Bernier of Turing Pharmaceuticals, September 8, 2015, hivma .org/uploadedFiles/HIVMA/HomePageContent/PyrimethamineLetterFINAL.pdf.

7   Writing group for the WHI investigators, "Risks and Benefits of Estrogen plus Progestin in Healthy Postmenopausal Women: Principal Results of the Women's Health Initiative Randomized, Controlled Trial," *JAMA* 288, no. 3 (2002): 3231–33.

8   A. A. Ciociola, L. B. Cohen, and P. Kulkami, "How Drugs Are Developed and Approved by the FDA: Current Process and Future Directions," *American Journal of Gastroenterology* 109 (May 2014): 620–23.

9   Global Business Intelligence (GBI) Research, *Rheumatoid Arthritis Market to 2020: A Crowded Market Characterized by Modest Growth,* January 2015, gbiresearch.com/report-store/market-reports/therapy-analysis/rheumatoid-arthritis -market-to-2020-a-crowded-market-characterized-by-modest-growth?companyid =rs-gbijune15pr&utm_source=pr&utm_medium=pr&utm_campaign=gbihcpr150608a &utm_nooveride=1.

10   S. M. Al-Khatib, A. Hellkamp, J. Curtis, et al., "Non–Evidence-Based ICD Implantations in the United States," *JAMA* 305, no. 1 (January 5, 2011): 43–49.

11   Biotronik, *2014 Medicare Payment and Coding Book for Physicians, Hospitals and Ambulatory Surgery Centers,* accessed September 5, 2016, biotronik.com/files/41EBF3 01387FC1B2C1257CFA00262842/$FILE/RF153r3sc.pdf.

12   J. Skinner, E. S. Fisher, and J. E. Wennberg, "The Efficiency of Medicare," in *Analyses in the Economics of Aging,* ed. D. A. Wise (Chicago: University of Chicago Press, 2005), 129–60.

13   K. Baicker and A. Chandra, "Medicare Spending, the Physician Workforce, and Beneficiaries' Quality of Care," supplement, *Health Affairs* (April 7, 2004): W4-184– W4-97, doi:10.1377/hlthaff.w4.184.

14   Boston Scientific, *2015 Procedural Reimbursement Guide: Select Percutaneous Coronary Interventions,* accessed September 5, 2016, bostonscientific.com/content /dam/bostonscientific/Reimbursement/IC/IC%202015%20PPG_Nov2014_Final.pdf.

15   Reed Abelson and Julie Creswell, "Hospital Chain Inquiry Cited Unnecessary Cardiac Work," *New York Times,* August 6, 2012, nytimes.com/2012/08/07/business /hospital-chain-internal-reports-found-dubious-cardiac-work.html?_r=0.

16   K. Davis, K. Stremikis, D. Squires, and C. Schoen, *Mirror, Mirror on the Wall, 2014 Update: How the U.S. Health Care System Compares Internationally,* The Commonwealth Fund, June 16, 2014, commonwealthfund.org/publications/fund -reports/2014/jun/mirror-mirror.

17   A. Carr, "Arthroscopic Surgery for Degenerative Knee: Overused, Ineffective, and Potentially Harmful," *British Journal of Sports Medicine* 49 (2015): 1223–24.

18   L. S. Lohmander, J. B. Thorlund, and E. M. Roos, "Routine Knee Arthroscopic Surgery for the Painful Knee in Middle-Aged and Old Patients—Time to Abandon Ship," *Acta Orthopaedica* 87, no. 1 (2016): 2–4.

19 "Total Abdominal Hysterectomy," Healthcare Bluebook, accessed September 5, 2016, healthcarebluebook.com/page_ProcedureDetails.aspx?id=102&dataset=md&g=Total+Hysterectomy+%28no+cancer%29.

20 J. T. James, "A New, Evidence-Based Estimate of Patient Harms Associated with Hospital Care," *Journal of Patient Safety* 9, no. 3 (September 2013): 122–28.

CHAPTER 3

1 Centers for Disease Control and Prevention, *National Diabetes Statistics Report: Estimates of Diabetes and Its Burden in the United States, 2014* (Atlanta: US Department of Health and Human Services, 2014).

2 American Diabetes Association, "Economic Costs of Diabetes in the U.S. in 2012," *Diabetes Care* 36 (2013): 1033–46.

3 Centers for Disease Control and Prevention, "Trends in Intake of Energy and Macronutrients—United States, 1971–2000," *Morbidity and Mortality Weekly Report* 53, no. 4 (February 6, 2004): 80–82.

4 Ibid.

5 American Diabetes Association, "Revenues Received from Pharmaceutical Companies/Device Makers, 2014," accessed September 5, 2015, main.diabetes.org/dorg/PDFs/2014-pharma-financial-revenues.pdf.

6 R. D. Feinman and J. S. Volek, "Carbohydrate Restriction as the Default Treatment for Type 2 Diabetes and Metabolic Syndrome," *Scandinavian Cardiovascular Journal* 42, no. 4 (August 2008): 256–63.

7 N. F. Sheard, N. G. Clark, J. C. Brand-Miller, et al., "Dietary Carbohydrate (Amount and Type) in the Prevention and Management of Diabetes: A Statement by the American Diabetes Association," *Diabetes Care* 27, no. 9 (September 2004): 2266–71.

8 Institute of Medicine, Food and Nutrition Board, *Dietary Reference Intakes for Energy, Carbohydrate, Fiber, Fat, Fatty Acids, Cholesterol, Protein, and Amino Acids* (Washington, DC: National Academies Press, 2005).

9 A. B. Evert, J. L. Boucher, M. Cypress, et al., "Nutrition Therapy Recommendations for the Management of Adults with Diabetes," *Diabetes Care* 36, no. 11 (November 2013): 3821–42.

10 American Diabetes Association. "Revenues Received from Pharmaceutical Companies, 2014," http://main.diabetes.org/dorg/PDFs/2014-pharma-financial-revenues.pdf.

11 "Cadbury Schweppes Americas Beverages Joins American Diabetes Association in the Fight against Diabetes, Obesity," PR Newswire, April 21, 2005, prnewswire.com/news-releases/cadbury-schweppes-americas-beverages-joins-american-diabetes-association-in-the-fight-against-diabetes-obesity-54372597.html.

12 J. H. Freeland-Graves and S. Nitzke, "Position of the Academy of Nutrition and Dietetics: Total Diet Approach to Healthy Eating," *Journal of the Academy of Nutrition and Dietetics* 113, no. 2 (February 2013): 307–17.

13 "Meet Our Sponsors," Academy of Nutrition and Dietetics, accessed September 5, 2016, eatrightpro.org/resources/about-us/advertising-and-sponsorship/meet-our-sponsors.

14 M. Kaplan, "The National Academy of Sugar," *The Blog*, Huffington Post, August 24, 2015, huffingtonpost.com/marty-kaplan/the-national-academy-of-sugar_b_8018066.html.

15 M. Simon, *And Now a Word from Our Sponsors: Are America's Nutrition Professionals in the Pocket of Big Food?* Eat Drink Politics, January 2013, eatdrinkpolitics.com/wp-content/uploads/AND_Corporate_Sponsorship_Report.pdf.

16 K. D. Brownel and K. E. Warner, "The Perils of Ignoring History: Big Tobacco Played Dirty and Millions Died. How Similar Is Big Food?," *Milbank Quarterly* 87, no. 1 (March 2009): 259–94.

17 American Heart Association, 2014–2015 Annual Report: heart.org/HEARTORG /General/2014-2015-Annual-Report_UCM_448427_Article.jsp#.WE7v5pI-a8U

18 American Heart Association, National Supporters and Sponsors: heart.org /HEARTORG/HealthyLiving/National-Supporters-and-Sponsors_UCM_436493 _Article.jsp#

19 J. Lenzer, "Alteplase for Stroke: Money and Optimistic Claims Buttress the 'Brain' Attack Campaign," *BMJ* 324 (2002): 723–29.

20 N. J. Stone, J. Robinson, A. H. Lichtenstein, et al., "2013 ACC/AHA Guideline on the Treatment of Blood Cholesterol to Reduce Atherosclerotic Cardiovascular Risk in Adults," *Circulation* 129, no. 25, supplement 2 (June 24, 2014): S1–S45.

21 J. Kung, R. R. Miller, and P. A. Mackowiak, "Failure of Clinical Practice Guidelines to Meet Institute of Medicine Standards: Two More Decades of Little, if Any, Progress," *Archives of Internal Medicine* 172, no. 21 (November 26, 2012): 1628–33.

22 American Heart Association, "Get with the Guidelines" (2015), heart.org/idc /groups/heart-public/@wcm/@gwtg/documents/downloadable/ucm_476918.pdf.

23 J. E. Bekelman, Y. Li, and C. P. Gross, "Scope and Impact of Financial Conflicts of Interest in Biomedical Research," *JAMA* 289, no. 4 (2003): 454–65.

24 E. G. Campbell, J. S. Weiss, S. Ehringhaus, et al., "Institutional Academic-Industry Relationships," *JAMA* 298, no. 15 (2007): 1779–86.

25 Marcia Angell, "Drug Companies & Doctors: A Story of Corruption," *New York Review of Books,* January 15, 2009, nybooks.com/articles/2009/01/15/ drug-companies-doctorsa-story-of-corruption/#fn-7.

26 E. H. Turner, A. M. Matthews, E. Linardatos, et al., "Selective Publication of Antidepressant Trials and Its Influence on Apparent Efficacy," *New England Journal of Medicine* 358, no. 3 (2008): 252–60.

27 B. M. Psaty and R. A. Kronmal, "Reporting Mortality Findings in Trials of Rofecoxib for Alzheimer Disease or Cognitive Impairment: A Case Study Based on Documents from Rofecoxib Litigation," *JAMA* 299, no. 15 (April 16, 2008): 1813–17.

28 A. Lundh, S. Sismondo, J. Lexchin, O. A. Busuioc, and L. Bero, "Industry Sponsorship and Research Outcome," *Cochrane Database of Systematic Reviews* 12 (December 12, 2012): MR000033, doi:10.1002/14651858.MR000033.pub2.

29 R. Smith, "The Trouble with Medical Journals," *Journal of the Royal Society of Medicine* 99, no. 3 (March 2006): 115–19.

30 United States General Accounting Office, *Briefing Report to the Honorable Howard Metzenbaum, United States Senate: Six Former HHS Employees' Involvement In Aspartame's Approval,* July 22, 1986, archive.gao.gov/d4t4/130780.pdf.

31 "Conflict of Interest," Duke Clinical Research Institute, accessed September 5, 2016, dcri.org/about-us/conflict-of-interest.

32 "Senate Should Reject President's Nominee to Be the Next FDA Commissioner," Public Citizen, September 16, 2015, citizen.org/documents/2276.pdf.

33 Anna Wilde Mathews, "In Debate over Antidepressants, FDA Weighed Risk of False Alarm: Doubting Data on Suicide and Kids, Officials Stopped Presentation by Staffer," *Wall Street Journal,* May 25, 2004, wsj.com/articles/SB108542623318719773.

34 D. J. Graham, D. Campen, R. Hui, et al., "Risk of Acute Myocardial Infarction and Sudden Cardiac Death in Patients Treated with Cyclo-Oxygenase 2 Selective and Non-Selective Non-Steroidal Anti-Inflammatory Drugs: Nested Case-Control Study," *Lancet* 365, no. 9458 (February 5–11, 2005): 475–81.

35 "Statement of Policy—Foods Derived from New Plant Varieties; Guidance to Industry for Foods Derived from New Plant Varieties; Policy Statement, 22984," *Federal Register* 57, no. 104 (May 29, 1992): 22984, fda.gov/Food/GuidanceRegulation/Guidance DocumentsRegulatoryInformation/Biotechnology/ucm096095.htm.

36 J. Spiroux de Vendomois, F. Roullier, D. Cellier, and G. E. Seralini, "A Comparison of the Effects of Three GM Corn Varieties on Mammalian Health," *International Journal of Biological Sciences* 5, no. 7 (2009): 706–26.

37 G. E. Séralini, E. Clair, R. Mesnage, et al., "Long-Term Toxicity of a Roundup Herbicide and a Roundup-Tolerant Genetically Modified Maize," *Environmental Sciences Europe* 26 (2014): 14.

38 S. Thongprakaisang, A. Thiantanawat, N. Rangkadilok, T. Suriyoc, and J. Satayavivad, "Glyphosate Induces Human Breast Cancer Cells Growth via Estrogen Receptors," *Food and Chemical Toxicology* 59 (September 2013): 129–36.

39 V. L. De Liz Oliveira Cavalli, D. Cattani, C. E. Heinz Rieg, et al., "Roundup Disrupts Male Reproductive Functions by Triggering Calcium-Mediated Cell Death in Rat Testis and Sertoli Cells," *Free Radical Biology & Medicine* 65 (December 2013): 335–46.

40 C. Gasnier, C. Dumont, N. Benachour, et al., "Glyphosate-Based Herbicides Are Toxic and Endocrine Disruptors in Human Cell Lines," *Toxicology* 262, no. 3 (August 21, 2009): 184–91.

41 Food and Agriculture Organization of the United Nations and World Health Organization, *Joint FAO/WO Meeting on Pesticide Residues: Summary Report, October 2015,* who.int/foodsafety/areas_work/chemical-risks/summary_report _JMPR_2015_Final.pdf?ua=1.

42 L. Schinasi and M. E. Leon, "Non-Hodgkin Lymphoma and Occupational Exposure to Agricultural Pesticide Chemical Groups and Active Ingredients: A Systematic Review and Meta-Analysis," *International Journal of Environmental Research and Public Health* 11, no. 4 (April 23, 2014): 4449–527.

43 "About The Heart Truth," National Heart, Lung, and Blood Institute, last modified March 17, 2016, nhlbi.nih.gov/health/educational/hearttruth/about/index.htm.

44 N. J. Stone, J. Robinson, A. H. Lichtenstein, et al., "2013 ACC/AHA Guideline on the Treatment of Blood Cholesterol to Reduce Atherosclerotic Cardiovascular Risk in Adults," *Circulation* 129, no. 25, supplement 2 (June 24, 2014): S1–S45.

CHAPTER 4

1 D. Oken, "What to Tell Cancer Patients: A Study of Medical Attitudes," *JAMA* 175 (April 1, 1961): 1120–28.

2   J. McIntosh, "Patients' Awareness and Desire for Information about Diagnosed but Undisclosed Malignant Disease," *Lancet* 2, no. 7980 (August 7, 1976): 300–303.

3   D. Hiroto and M. Seligman, "Generality of Learned Helplessness in Man," *Journal of Personality and Social Psychology* 31, no. 2 (1975): 311–27.

4   J. B. Lemaire and J. E. Wallace, "How Physicians Identify with Predetermined Personalities and Links to Perceived Performance and Wellness Outcomes: A Cross-Sectional Study," *BMC Health Services Research* 14 (November 29, 2014): 616.

5   "HHS Finalizes Patients' Right to Access Report of Clinical Laboratory Test Results," Centers for Medicare & Medicaid Services, February 3, 2014, cms.gov/Newsroom /MediaReleaseDatabase/Fact-sheets/2014-Fact-sheets-items/2014-02-03.html.

CHAPTER 5

1   H. C. Muldoon, *Lessons in Pharmaceutical Latin and Prescription Writing and Interpretation* (New York: Wiley, 1916).

2   C. Wagner and A. Suh, "The Wisdom of Crowds: Impact of Collective Size and Expertise Transfer on Collective Performance," in *47th Hawaii International Conference on System Science* (2014): 594–603, doi:10.1109/HICSS.2014.80.

3   A. W. Woolley, C. F. Chabris, A. Pentland, et al., "Evidence for a Collective Intelligence Factor in the Performance of Human Groups," *Science* 330, no. 6004 (October 29, 2010): 686–88.

4   B. G. Druss and S. C. Marcus, "Growth and Decentralization of the Medical Literature: Implications for Evidence-Based Medicine," *Journal of the Medical Library Association* 93, no. 4 (2005): 499–501.

5   P. Wicks, T. Vaughan, and J. Heywood, "Subjects No More: What Happens When Trial Participants Realize They Hold the Power?," *BMJ* 348 (2014): g368.

6   J. D. Hixson, K. Parko, T. Durgin, et al., "Patients Optimizing Epilepsy Management via an Online Community: The POEM Study," *Neurology* 85 (2015): 1–8.

CHAPTER 6

1   S. L. Schnorr, M. Candela, S. Rampelli, et al., "Gut Microbiome of the Hadza Hunter-Gatherers," *Nature Communications* 5 (April 15, 2014): 3654.

2   P. Carrera-Bastos, M. Fontes-Villalba, J. O'Keefe, et al., "The Western Diet and Lifestyle and Diseases of Civilization," *Research Reports in Clinical Cardiology* 2 (2011): 15–35.

3   G. P. Murdock, "The Current Status of the World's Hunting and Gathering Peoples," in *Man the Hunter,* eds. R. B. Lee and I. DeVore (Piscataway, NJ: Aldine Transaction, 2009), 13–29.

4   J. Day, A. Bailey, and D. Robinson, "Biological Variations Associated with Change in Lifestyle among the Pastoral and Nomadic Tribes of East Africa," *Annals of Human Biology* 6, no. 1 (January–February 1979): 29–39.

5   D. L. Christensen, J. Eis, A. W. Hansen, et al., "Obesity and Regional Fat Distribution in Kenyan Populations: Impact of Ethnicity and Urbanization," *Annals of Human Biology* 35, no. 2 (March–April, 2008): 232–49.

6   F. J. Fernandes-Costa, J. Marshall, and C. Ritchie, "Transition from a Hunter-Gatherer to a Settled Lifestyle in the !Kung San: Effect on Iron, Folate, and Vitamin B_{12}

Nutrition," *American Journal of Clinical Nutrition* 40, no. 6 (December 1984): 1295–303.

7 S. G. Gimeno, D. Rodrigues, E. N. Canó, et al., "Cardiovascular Risk Factors among Brazilian Karib Indigenous Peoples: Upper Xingu, Central Brazil, 2000–3," *Journal of Epidemiology & Community Health* 63, no. 4 (April 2009): 299–304.

8 S. G. Agostinho Gimeno, D. Rodrigues, H. Pagliaro, et al., "Metabolic and Anthropometric Profile of Aruák Indians· Mehináku, Waurá and Yawalapití in the Upper Xingu, Central Brazil, 2000–2002," *Escola Nacional de Saúde Pública* 23, no. 8 (August 2007): 1946–54.

9 K. O'Dea, "Marked Improvement in Carbohydrate and Lipid Metabolism in Diabetic Australian Aborigines after Temporary Reversion to Traditional Lifestyle," *Diabetes* 33, no. 6 (June 1984): 596–603.

10 H. Kruse, A. M. Kirkemo, and K. Handeland, "Wildlife as Source of Zoonotic Infections," *Emerging Infectious Diseases* 10, no. 12 (December 2004): 2067–72, wwwnc.cdc.gov/eid/article/10/12/04-0707.

11 Food and Agriculture Organization of the United Nations, Agricultural Commodities: Profiles and Relevant WTO Negotiating Issues, accessed September 5, 2016, fao.org/docrep/006/y4343e/y4343e00.htm#Contents.

12 M. N. Cohen and G. M. M. Crane-Kramer, eds., "Editors' Summation," in *Ancient Health: Skeletal Indicators of Agricultural and Economic Intensification* (Gainesville: University Press of Florida, 2007), 320–43.

13 L. Cordain, "Cereal Grains: Humanity's Double-Edged Sword," *World Review of Nutrition and Dietetics* 84 (1999): 19–73.

14 C. Roberts and K. Manchester, "Dental Disease," in *The Archaeology of Disease* (Ithaca, NY: Cornell University Press, 2005), 63–83.

15 C. J. Adler, K. Dobney, L. S. Weyrich, et al., "Sequencing Ancient Calcified Dental Plaque Shows Changes in Oral Microbiota with Dietary Shifts of the Neolithic and Industrial Revolutions," *Nature Genetics* 45, no. 4 (April 2013): 450–55.

16 R. Y. Tito, D. Knights, J. Metcalf, et al., "Insights from Characterizing Extinct Human Gut Microbiomes," *PLOS ONE* 7, no. 12 (2012): e51146, doi:10.1371/journal.pone.0051146.

17 S. Pearce, R. Savlle, S. Vaughan, et al., "Molecular Characterization of Rht-1 Dwarfing Genes in Hexaploid Wheat," *Plant Physiology* 157 (December 2011): 1820–31.

18 R. Batista, N. Saibo, T. Lourenço, and M. M. Oliveira, "Microarray Analyses Reveal That Plant Mutagenesis May Induce More Transcriptomic Changes Than Transgene Insertion," *Proceedings of the National Academy of Sciences of the United States of America* 105, no. 9 (2008): 3640–45.

19 P. Sabelli and P. M. Shewry, "Characterization and Organization of Gene Families at the Gli-1 Loci of Bread and Durum Wheat by Restriction Fragment Analysis," *Theoretical and Applied Genetics* 83 (1991): 209–16.

20 H. C. Van den Broeck, H. C. de Jong, E. M. J. Salentijn, et al., "Presence of Celiac Disease Epitopes in Modern and Old Hexaploid Wheat Varieties: Wheat Breeding May Have Contributed to Increased Prevalence of Celiac Disease," *Theoretical and Applied Genetics* 121 (2010): 1527–39.

21 A. Rubio-Tapia, R. A. Kyle, E. Kaplan, et al., "Increased Prevalence and Mortality in Undiagnosed Celiac Disease," *Gastroenterology* 137, no. 1 (July 2009): 88–93.

22 C. Zioudrou, R. A. Streaty, and W. A. Klee, "Opioid Peptides Derived from Food Proteins. The Exorphins," *Journal of Biological Chemistry* 254, no. 7 (April 1979): 2446–49.

23 D. D. Kitts and K. Weiler, "Bioactive Proteins and Peptides from Food Sources. Applications of Bioprocesses Used in Isolation and Recovery," *Current Pharmaceutical Design* 9, no. 16 (2003): 1309–23.

24 M. Takahashi, H. Fukunaga, H. Kaneto, et al., "Behavioral and Pharmacological Studies on Gluten Exorphin A5, a Newly Isolated Bioactive Food Protein Fragment, in Mice," *Japanese Journal of Pharmacology* 84, no. 3 (November 2000): 259–65.

25 F. C. Dohan and J. C. Grasberger, "Relapsed Schizophrenics: Earlier Discharge from the Hospital After Cereal-Free, Milk-Free Diet," *American Journal of Psychiatry* 130, no. 6 (June 1973): 685–88.

26 M. R. Cohen, R. M. Cohen, D. Pickar, and D. L. Murphy, "Naloxone Reduces Food Intake in Humans," *Psychosomatic Medicine* 47, no. 2 (March–April 1985): 132–38.

27 A. Drewnowski, D. D. Krahn, M. A. Demitrack, et al., "Naloxone, an Opiate Blocker, Reduces the Consumption of Sweet High-Fat Foods in Obese and Lean Female Binge Eaters," *American Journal of Clinical Nutrition* 61 (1995): 1206–12.

28 X. Gao, S. W. Liu, Q. Sun, and G. M. Xia, "High Frequency of HMW-GS Sequence Variation through Somatic Hybridization between Agropyron Elongatum and Common Wheat," *Planta* 23, no. 2 (January 2010): 245–50.

29 X. L. Zhao, X. C. Xia, Z. H. He, et al., "Characterization of Three Low-Molecular-Weight Glu-D3 Subunit Genes in Common Wheat," *Theoretical and Applied Genetics* 113, no. 7 (November 2006): 1247–59.

30 W. J. Peumans, H. M. Stinissen, and A. R. Carlier, "Isolation and Partial Characterization of Wheat-Germ-Agglutinin-Like Lectins from Rye (Secale Cereale) and Barley (Hordeum Vulgare) Embryos," *Biochemical Journal* 203, no. 1 (April 1982): 39–43.

31 V. Lorenzsonn and W. A. Olsen, "In Vivo Responses of Rat Intestinal Epithelium to Intraluminal Dietary Lectins," *Gastroenterology* 82, no. 5, part 1 (May 1982): 838–48.

32 R. Gibson, "Zinc Nutrition in Developing Countries," *Nutrition Research Reviews* 7 (1994): 151–73.

33 L. H. Allen, "The Nutrition CRSP: What Is Marginal Malnutrition and Does It Affect Human Function?," *Nutrition Reviews* 51 (1993): 255–67.

34 P. B. Holm, K. N. Kristiansen, and H. B. Pedersen, "Transgenic Approaches in Commonly Consumed Cereals to Improve Iron and Zinc Content and Bioavailability," *Journal of Nutrition* 132, no. 3 (March 2002): 514S–16S.

35 C. Larré, R. Lupi, G. Gombaud, et al., "Assessment of Allergenicity of Diploid and Hexaploid Wheat Genotypes: Identification of Allergens in the Albumin/Globulin Fraction," *Journal of Proteomics* 74, no. 8 (August 12, 2011): 1279–89.

36 E. A. Pastorello, L. Farioli, A. Conti, et al., "Wheat IgE-Mediated Food Allergy in European Patients: Alpha-Amylase Inhibitors, Lipid Transfer Proteins and Low-Molecular-Weight Glutenins. Allergenic Molecules Recognized by Double-Blind, Placebo-Controlled Food Challenge," *International Archives of Allergy and Immunology* 144, no. 1 (2007): 10–22.

37 K. Foster-Powell, S. H. A. Holt, and J. C. Brand-Miller, "International Table of Glycemic Index and Glycemic Load Values: 2002," *American Journal of Clinical Nutrition* 76 (2002): 5–56.

38 S. Liu, W. C. Willett, J. E. Manson, et al., "Relation between Changes in Intakes of Dietary Fiber and Grain Products and Changes in Weight and Development of Obesity among Middle-Aged Women," *American Journal of Clinical Nutrition* 78, no. 5 (November 2003): 920–27.

39 K. Foster-Powell, S. H. A. Holt, and J. C. Brand-Miller, "International Table of Glycemic Index and Glycemic Load Values: 2002," *American Journal of Clinical Nutrition* 76 (2002): 5–56.

40 A. Fasano, "Zonulin, Regulation of Tight Junctions, and Autoimmune Diseases," *Annals of the New York Academy of Sciences* 1258, no. 1 (July 2012): 25–33.

41 E. Vainio and E. Varionen, "Antibody Response against Wheat, Rye, Barley, Oats, and Corn: Comparison between Gluten-Sensitive Patients and Monoclonal Antigliadin Antibodies," *International Archives of Allergy and Immunology* 106, no. 2 (February 1995): 134–38.

42 J. P. Ortiz-Sanchez, F. Cabrera-Chavez, and A. M. de la Barca, "Maize Prolamins Could Induce a Gluten-Like Cellular Immune Response in Some Celiac Disease Patients," *Nutrients* 5, no. 10 (October 21, 2013): 4174–83.

43 M. P. Valencia Zavala, G. B. Vega Robledo, M. A. Sanchez Olivas, et al., "Maize (Zea Mays): Allergen or Toleragen? Participation of the Cereal in Allergic Disease and Positivity Incidence in Cutaneous Tests," *Revista Alergia México* 53, no. 6 (November–December 2006): 207–11.

44 A. Ramachandran, C. Snehalatha, A. S. Shetty, and A. Nanditha, "Trends in Prevalence of Diabetes in Asian Countries," *World Journal of Diabetes* 3, no. 6 (June 15, 2012): 110–117.

45 F. Faita, L. Cori, F. Bianchi, and M. G. Andreassi, "Arsenic-Induced Genotoxicity and Genetic Susceptibility to Arsenic-Related Pathologies," *International Journal of Environmental Research and Public Health* 10, no. 4 (April 12, 2013): 1527–46.

46 Y. Chen, F. Parvez, M. Gamble, et al., "Arsenic Exposure at Low-to-Moderate Levels and Skin Lesions, Arsenic Metabolism, Neurological Functions, and Biomarkers for Respiratory and Cardiovascular Diseases: Review of Recent Findings from the Health Effects of Arsenic Longitudinal Study (HEALS) In Bangladesh," *Toxicology and Applied Pharmacology* 239, no. 2 (September 1, 2009): 184–92.

CHAPTER 7

1 P. S. Ungar, "Dental Evidence for the Diets of Plio-Pleistocene Hominins," supplement, *American Journal of Physical Anthropology* 146, no. S53 (2011): 47–62.

2 L. Aiello and P. Wheeler, "Energetics and the Evolution of the Genus Homo," *Annual Review of Anthropology* 31 (2002): 323–38.

3 R. W. Wrangham and L. Conklin-Brittain, "The Biological Significance of Cooking in Human Evolution, Part A," *Comparative Biochemistry and Physiology* 136 (2003): 35–46.

4 R. N. Carmody and R. W. Wrangham, "Cooking and the Human Commitment to a High-Quality Diet," *Cold Spring Harbor Symposia on Quantitative Biology* 74 (2009): 427–34.

5   K. Milton, "Diet and Primate Evolution," *Scientific American* 269 (1993): 86–93.

6   M. Hession, C. Rolland, U. Kulkami, et al., "Systematic Review of Randomized Controlled Trials of Low-Carbohydrate vs. Low-Fat/Low-Calorie Diets in the Management of Obesity and Its Comorbidities," *Obesity Reviews* 10, no. 1 (January 2009): 36–50.

7   P. W. Siri-Tarino, Q. Sun, F. B. Hu, and F. M. Krauss, "Meta-Analysis of Prospective Cohort Studies Evaluating the Association of Saturated Fat with Cardiovascular Disease," *American Journal of Clinical Nutrition* 91, no. 3 (March 2010): 535–46.

8   R. Micha, S. K. Wallace, and D. Mozaffarian, "Red and Processed Meat Consumption and Risk of Incident Coronary Heart Disease, Stroke, and Diabetes Mellitus: A Systematic Review and Meta-Analysis," *Circulation* 121 (2010): 2271–83.

9   US Department of Health and Human Services and US Department of Agriculture, *2015–2020 Dietary Guidelines for Americans,* 8th ed., December 2015, health.gov /dietaryguidelines/2015/resources/2015-2020_Dietary_Guidelines.pdf.

10   S. O'Keefe, S. Gaskins-Wright, V. Wiley, and I. Chen, "Levels of Trans Geometrical Isomers of Essential Fatty Acids in Some Unhydrogenated U.S. Vegetable Oils," *Journal of Food Lipids* 1, no. 3 (September 1994): 165–76.

11   D. M. Klurfeld, "What Do Government Agencies Consider in the Debate over Added Sugars?" *Advances in Nutrition* 4, no. 2 (March 1, 2013): 257–61.

12   K. L. Stanhope, J. M. Schwarz, and P. J. Havel, "Adverse Metabolic Effects of Dietary Fructose: Results from the Recent Epidemiological, Clinical, and Mechanistic Studies," *Current Opinion in Lipidology* 24, no. 3 (June 2013): 198–206.

13   C. S. Kwok, S. Umar, P. K. Myint, et al., "Vegetarian Diet, Seventh Day Adventists and Risk of Cardiovascular Mortality: A Systematic Review and Meta-Analysis," *International Journal of Cardiology* 176, no. 3 (October 20, 2014): 680–86.

14   P. Appleby, F. L. Crowe, K. E. Bradbury, et al., "Mortality in Vegetarians and Comparable Nonvegetarians in the United Kingdom," *American Journal of Clinical Nutrition* 103 (2016): 218–30.

15   W. Herrmann, H. Schorr, R. Obeid, and J. Geisel, "Vitamin B-12 Status, Particularly Holotranscobalamin II and Methylmalonic Acid Concentrations, and Hyperhomocysteinemia in Vegetarians," *American Journal of Clinical Nutrition* 78 (2003): 131–36.

16   R. Pawlak, S. J. Parrott, S. Raj, et al., "How Prevalent Is Vitamin B(12) Deficiency among Vegetarians?," *Nutrition Reviews* 71, no. 2 (February 2013): 110–17.

17   A. L. Wilson and M. J. Ball, "Nutrient Intake and Iron Status of Australian Male Vegetarians," *European Journal of Clinical Nutrition* 53, no. 3 (March 1999): 189–94.

18   B. C. Davis and P. M. Kris-Etherton, "Achieving Optimal Essential Fatty Acid Status in Vegetarians: Current Knowledge and Practical Implications," supplement, *American Journal of Clinical Nutrition* 78, no. S3 (September 2003): 640S–46S.

19   B. Burns-Whitmore, E. Haddad, J. Sabaté, and S. Rajaram, "Effects of Supplementing N-3 Fatty Acid Enriched Eggs and Walnuts on Cardiovascular Disease Risk Markers in Healthy Free-Living Lacto-Ovo-Vegetarians: A Randomized, Crossover, Free-Living Intervention Study," *Nutrition Journal* 13 (March 27, 2014): 29.

20   R. C. Block, W. S. Harris, and J. V. Pottala, "Clinical Investigation: Determinants of Blood Cell Omega-3 Fatty Acid Content," *Open Biomarkers Journal* 1 (2008): 1–6.

21 J. V. Pottala, K. Yaffe, and J. G. Robinson, "Higher RBC EPA + DHA Corresponds with Larger Total Brain and Hippocampal Volumes: WHIMS-MRI Study," *Neurology* 82, no. 5 (February 4, 2014): 435–42.

22 T. A. Sanders, "DHA Status of Vegetarians," *Prostaglandins, Leukotrienes and Essential Fatty Acids* 81, no. 2–3 (August–September 2009): 137–41.

23 G. K. Davey, E. A. Spencer, P. N. Appleby, et al., "EPIC-Oxford: Lifestyle Characteristics and Nutrient Intakes in a Cohort of 33,883 Meat-Eaters and 31,546 Non Meat-Eaters in the UK," *Public Health Nutrition* 6 (2003): 259–69.

24 F. L. Crowe, M. Steur, N. E. Allen, et al., "Plasma Concentrations of 25-Hydroxyvitamin D in Meat Eaters, Fish Eaters, Vegetarians and Vegans: Results from the EPIC-Oxford Study," *Public Health Nutrition* 14, no. 2 (February 2011): 340–46.

25 J. W. Beulens, S. L. Booth, E. G. van den Heuvel, et al., "The Role of Menaquinones (Vitamin K_2) in Human Health," *British Journal of Nutrition* 110, no. 8 (October 2013): 1357–68.

26 S. J. Elder, D. B. Haytowitz, J. Howe, et al., "Vitamin K Contents of Meat, Dairy, and Fast Food in the U.S. Diet," *Journal of Agricultural and Food Chemistry* 54, no. 2 (January 25, 2006): 463–67.

27 N. N. Haroon, R. K. Marwaha, M. M. Godbole, and S. K. Gupta, "Role of B_{12} and Homocysteine Status in Determining BMD and Bone Turnover in Young Indians," *Journal of Clinical Densitometry* 15, no. 3 (July–September 2012): 366–73.

28 U. Kapil and A. S. Bhadoria, "Prevalence of Folate, Ferritin and Cobalamin Deficiencies amongst Adolescent in India," *Journal of Family Medicine and Primary Care* 3, no. 3 (July–September 2014): 247–49.

29 M. Glick-Bauer and M. Yeh, "The Health Advantage of a Vegan Diet: Exploring The Gut Microbiota Connection," *Nutrients* 6, no. 11 (November 2014): 4822–38.

30 R. Nagai, J. Shirakawa, Y. Fujiwara, et al., "Detection of AGEs as Markers for Carbohydrate Metabolism and Protein Denaturation," *Journal of Clinical Biochemistry and Nutrition* 55, no. 1 (July 2014): 1–6.

31 C. Prasad, V. Imrhan, F. Marotta, et al., "Lifestyle and Advanced Glycation End Products (AGEs)," *Aging and Disease* 5, no. 3 (June 1, 2014): 212–17.

32 N. Miyazawa, Y. Kawasaki, J. Fuji, et al., "Immunological Detection of Fructated Proteins In Vitro and In Vivo," *Biochemical Journal* 336, part 1, (November 15, 1998): 101–7.

33 E. Bonora, "Postprandial Peaks as a Risk Factor for Cardiovascular Disease: Epidemiological Perspectives," supplement, *International Journal of Clinical Practice* 129 (July 2002): 5–11.

34 J. C. de Beer and L. Liebenberg, "Does Cancer Risk Increase with HbA1c, Independent of Diabetes?," *British Journal of Cancer* 110, no. 9 (April 29, 2014): 2361–68.

35 K. L. Stanhope, J. M. Schwarz, P. J. Havel, "Adverse Metabolic Effects of Dietary Fructose: Results from the Recent Epidemiological, Clinical, and Mechanistic Studies," *Current Opinion in Lipidology* 24, no. 3 (June 2013): 198–206.

36 G. Marek, V. Pannu, P. Shanmugham, et al., "Adiponectin Resistance and Pro-Inflammatory Changes in the Visceral Adipose Tissue Induced by Fructose Consumption via Ketohexokinase-Dependent Pathway," *Diabetes* 64, no. 2 (February 2015): 508–18.

37 T. Goldberg, W. Cai, M. Peppa, et al., "Advanced Glycoxidation End Products in Commonly Consumed Foods," *Journal of the American Dietetic Association* 104 (2004): 1287–91.

38 D. M. Lyon and D. M. Dunlop, "The Treatment of Obesity: A Comparison of the Effects of Diet and of Thyroid Extract," *QJM* 1, no. 2 (1932): 331–52.

39 A. Kekwick and G. L. S. Pawan, "Calorie Intake in Relation to Body-Weight Changes in the Obese," *Lancet* 271 (1956): 155–61.

40 P. Newsholme, V. Cruzat, F. Arfuso, and K. Keane, "Nutrient Regulation of Insulin Secretion and Action," *Journal of Endocrinology* 221, no. 3 (June 2014): R105–20.

41 L. A. Bazzano, T. Hu, K. Reynolds, et al., "Effects of Low-Carbohydrate and Low-Fat Diets: A Randomized Trial," *Annals of Internal Medicine* 161, no. 5 (September 2, 2014): 309–18.

42 W. S. Yancy Jr., M. K. Olsen, J. R. Guyton, et al., "A Low-Carbohydrate, Ketogenic Diet versus a Low-Fat Diet to Treat Obesity and Hyperlipidemia: A Randomized, Controlled Trial," *Annals of Internal Medicine* 140, no. 10 (May 18, 2004): 769–77.

43 G. D. Foster, H. R. Wyatt, J. O. Hill, et al., "Weight and Metabolic Outcomes after 2 Years on a Low-Carbohydrate Versus Low-Fat Diet: A Randomized Trial," *Annals of Internal Medicine* 153, no. 3 (August 3, 2010): 147–57.

44 V. S. Volek, T. Noakes, and S. D. Phinney, "Rethinking Fat as a Fuel for Endurance Exercise," *European Journal of Sport Science* 15, no. 1 (October 2014): 1–8.

45 S. D. Phinney, "Ketogenic Diets and Physical Performance," *Nutrition & Metabolism* 1, no. 1 (August 17, 2004): 2.

46 C. Zioudrou, R. A. Streaty, and W. A. Klee, "Opioid Peptides Derived from Food Proteins. The Exorphins," *Journal of Biological Chemistry* 254, no. 7 (April 1979): 2446–49.

47 M. R. Cohen, R. M. Cohen, D. Pickar, and D. L. Murphy, "Naloxone Reduces Food Intake in Humans," *Psychosomatic Medicine* 47, no. 2 (March–April 1985): 132–38.

48 A. Drewnowski, D. D. Krahn, M. A. Demitrack, et al., "Naloxone, an Opiate Blocker, Reduces the Consumption of Sweet High-Fat Foods in Obese and Lean Female Binge Eaters," *American Journal of Clinical Nutrition* 61 (1995): 1206–12.

49 M. T. Bardella, C. Fredella, L. Prampolini, et al., "Body Composition and Dietary Intakes in Adult Celiac Disease Patients Consuming a Strict Gluten-Free Diet," *American Journal of Clinical Nutrition* 72, no. 4 (October 2000): 937–39.

50 R. B. Elliott, D. P. Harris, J. P. Hill, et al., "Type I (Insulin-Dependent) Diabetes Mellitus and Cow Milk: Casein Variant Consumption," *Diabetologia* 42, no. 3 (March 1999): 292–96.

51 R. P. Evershed, S. Payne, A. G. Sherratt, et al., "Earliest Date for Milk Use in the Near East and Southeastern Europe Linked to Cattle Herding," *Nature* 455 (September 25, 2008): 528–31.

52 A. Ranciaro, M. C. Campbell, J. B. Hirbo, et al., "Genetic Origins of Lactase Persistence and the Spread of Pastoralism in Africa," *Cell* 94, no. 4 (2014): 496–510.

53 M. De Vrese, A. Stegelmann, B. Richter, et al., "Probiotics—Compensation for Lactase Insufficiency," *American Journal of Clinical Nutrition* 73, no. 2 (2001): 421s–29s.

54 S. Mummah, B. Oelrich, J. Hope, et al., "Effect of Raw Milk on Lactose Intolerance: A Randomized Controlled Pilot Study," *Annals of Family Medicine* 12, no. 2 (March–April 2014): 134–41.

55 T. He, M. G. Priebe, Y. Zhong, et al., "Effects of Yogurt and Bifidobacteria Supplementation on the Colonic Microbiota in Lactose-Intolerant Subjects," *Journal of Applied Microbiology* 104, no. 2 (February 2008): 595–604.

56 S. Mummah, B. Oelrich, J. Hope, et al., "Effect of Raw Milk on Lactose Intolerance: A Randomized Controlled Pilot Study," *Annals of Family Medicine* 12, no. 2 (March–April 2014): 134–41.

57 R. B. Elliott, D. P. Harris, J. P. Hill, et al., "Type I (Insulin-Dependent) Diabetes Mellitus and Cow Milk: Casein Variant Consumption," *Diabetologia* 42, no. 3 (March 1999): 292–96.

58 H. Teschemacher, G. Koch, V. Brantl, and P. S. Ungar, "Milk Protein-Derived Opioid Receptor Ligands," *Biopolymers* 43, no. 2 (1997): 99–117.

59 J. Wasilewska, E. Sienkiewicz-Szlapka, E. Kuzbida, et al., "The Exogenous Opioid Peptides and DPPIV Serum Activity in Infants with Apnoea Expressed as Apparent Life Threatening Events (ALTE)," *Neuropeptides* 45, no. 3 (June 2011): 189–95.

60 V. Brantl, H. Teschemacher, J. Bläsig, et al., "Opioid Activities of Beta-Casomorphins," *Life Sciences* 28, no. 17 (April 27, 1981): 1903–9.

61 M. Nilsson, M. Stenberg, A. H. Frid, J. J. Holst, and I. M. Björck, "Glycemia and Insulinemia in Healthy Subjects after Lactose-Equivalent Meals of Milk and Other Food Proteins: The Role of Plasma Amino Acids and Incretins," *American Journal of Clinical Nutrition* 80 (2004): 1246–53.

62 T. Paajanen, T. Tuure, T. Poussa, and R. Korpela, "No Difference in Symptoms during Challenges with Homogenized and Unhomogenized Cow's Milk in Subjects with Subjective Hypersensitivity to Homogenized Milk," *Journal of Dairy Research* 70, no. 2 (May 2003): 175–79.

63 G. Walcher, M. Gonano, J. Kummel, et al., "Staphylococcus Aureus Reservoirs during Traditional Austrian Raw Milk Cheese Production," *Journal of Dairy Research* 81, no. 4 (November 2014): 462–70.

64 "Nonpasteurized Disease Outbreaks, 1993–2006," Centers for Disease Control and Prevention, last modified December 12, 2014, cdc.gov/foodsafety/rawmilk/nonpasteurized-outbreaks.html.

65 T. J. Robinson, J. M. Scheftel, and K. E. Smith, "Raw Milk Consumption among Patients with Non-Outbreak-Related Enteric Infections, Minnesota, USA, 2001–2010," *Emerging Infectious Diseases* 20, no. 1 (January 2014): 38–44.

66 P. L. Ruegg, "Management of Mastitis on Organic and Conventional Dairy Farms," supplement, *Journal of Animal Science* 87, no. S13 (April 2009): 43–55.

67 E. Palupi, A. Jayanegara, A. Ploeger, and J. Kahl, "Comparison of Nutritional Quality between Conventional and Organic Dairy Products: A Meta-Analysis," *Journal of the Science of Food and Agriculture* 92, no. 14 (November 2012): 2774–81.

CHAPTER 8

1 J. Gahche, R. Bailey, V. Burt, et al., "Dietary Supplement Use among U.S. Adults Has Increased Since NHANES III (1988–1994)," *NCHS Data Brief* 61 (April 2011): 1–8.

2   "Dietary Supplements: Background Information," National Institutes of Health, Office of Dietary Supplements, last modified June 24, 2011, ods.od.nih.gov/factsheets /DietarySupplements-HealthProfessional.

3   D. F. Birt, T. Boylston, S. Hendrich, et al., "Resistant Starch: Promise for Improving Human Health," *Advances in Nutrition* 4, no. 6 (November 6, 2013): 587–601.

4   A. M. Leung, L. E. Braverman, and E. N. Pearce, "History of U.S. Iodine Fortification and Supplementation," *Nutrients* 4, no. 11 (November 13, 2012): 1740–46.

5   L. Frank and L. E. Quint, "Chest CT Incidentalomas: Thyroid Lesions, Enlarged Mediastinal Lymph Nodes, and Lung Nodules," *Cancer Imaging* 12 (March 5, 2012): 41–8.

CHAPTER 9

1   B. Hesselmar, A. Hicke-Roberts, and G. Wennergren, "Allergy in Children in Hand versus Machine Dishwashing," *Pediatrics* 135, no. 3 (February 2015): e1–8.

2   S. Lindeberg, "Risks with the Paleolithic Diet," in *Food and Western Disease* (Oxford: Wiley-Blackwell, 2010), 99.

3   T. L. Blasbalg, J. R. Hibbeln, C. E. Ramsden, et al., "Changes in Consumption of Omega-3 and Omega-6 Fatty Acids in the United States during the 20th Century," *American Journal of Clinical Nutrition* 93, no. 5 (May 2011): 950–62.

4   R. Dudley, "Ethanol, Fruit Ripening, and the Historical Origins of Human Alcoholism in Primate Frugivory," *Integrative and Comparative Biology* 44, no. 4 (2004): 315–23.

5   M. A. Carrigan, O. Uryasev, C. B. Frye, et al., "Hominids Adapted to Metabolize Ethanol Long before Human-Directed Fermentation," *Proceedings of the National Academy of Sciences of the United States of America* 112, no. 2 (2015): 458–63.

6   M. H. Ward, "Too Much of a Good Thing? Nitrate from Nitrogen Fertilizers and Cancer: President's Cancer Panel—October 21, 2008," *Reviews on Environmental Health* 24, no. 4 (2009): 357–63.

7   D. C. Paik, D. V. Saborio, R. Oropeza, and H. P. Freeman, "The Epidemiological Enigma of Gastric Cancer Rates in the US: Was Grandmother's Sausage the Cause?," *International Journal of Epidemiology* 30, no. 1 (February 2001): 181–82.

8   R. C. Massey, P. E. Key, R. A. Jones, and G. L. Logan, "Volatile, Non-Volatile and Total N-Nitroso Compounds in Bacon," *Food Additives & Contaminants* 8, no. 5 (1991): 585–98.

9   J. Haorah, L. Zhou, X. Wang, et al., "Determination of Total N-Nitroso Compounds and Their Precursors in Frankfurters, Fresh Meat, Dried Salted Fish, Sauces, Tobacco, and Tobacco Smoke Particulates," *Journal of Agricultural and Food Chemistry* 49, no. 12 (December 2001): 6068–78.

CHAPTER 11

1   M. Burton, E. Cobb, P. Donachie, G. Judah, V. Curtis, and W. P. Schmidt, "The Effect of Handwashing with Water or Soap on Bacterial Contamination of Hands," *International Journal of Environmental Research and Public Health* 8, no. 1 (January 2011): 97–104.

2   A. H. Sachdev and M. Pimeltel, "Gastrointestinal Bacterial Overgrowth: Pathogenesis and Clinical Significance," *Therapeutic Advances in Chronic Disease* 4, no. 5 (September 2013): 223–31.

3   S. L. Schnorr, M. Candela, S. Rampelli, et al., "Gut Microbiome of the Hadza Hunter-Gatherers," *Nature Communications* 5 (April 15, 2014): 3654.

4   A. J. Obregon-Tito, R. Y. Tito, J. Metcalf, et al., "Subsistence Strategies in Traditional Societies Distinguish Gut Microbiomes," *Nature Communications* 6 (March 25, 2015): 6505.

5   J. P. Zackular, N. T. Baxter, K. D. Iverson, et al., "The Gut Microbiome Modulates Colon Tumorigenesis," *mBio* 4, no. 6 (November 5, 2013): e00692-13.

6   A. Horvath, P. Dziechciarz, and H. Szajewska, "Glucomannan for Abdominal Pain-Related Functional Gastrointestinal Disorders in Children: A Randomized Trial," *World Journal of Gastroenterology* 19, no. 20 (2013): 3062-68.

7   S. Lohner, D. Küllenberg, G. Antes, et al., "Prebiotics in Healthy Infants and Children for Prevention of Acute Infectious Diseases: A Systematic Review and Meta-Analysis," *Nutrition Reviews* 72, no. 8 (August 2014): 523-31.

8   M. Giovannini, E. Verduci, D. Gregori, et al., "Prebiotic Effect of an Infant Formula Supplemented with Galacto-Oligosaccharides: Randomized Multicenter Trial," *Journal of the American College of Nutrition* 33, no. 5 (2014): 385-93.

9   N. Foolad and A. W. Armstrong, "Prebiotics and Probiotics: The Prevention and Reduction in Severity of Atopic Dermatitis in Children," *Beneficial Microbes* 5, no. 2 (June 2014): 151-60.

10   J. A. Parnell and R. A. Reimer, "Prebiotic Fiber Modulation of the Gut Microbiota Improves Risk Factors for Obesity and the Metabolic Syndrome," *Gut Microbes* 3, no. 1 (January-February 2012): 29-34.

11   M. D. Robertson, J. M. Currie, L. M. Morgan, et al., "Prior Short-Term Consumption of Resistant Starch Enhances Postprandial Insulin Sensitivity in Healthy Subjects," *Diabetologia* 46, no. 5 (May 2003): 659-65.

12   S. A. Abrams, I. J. Griffin, K. M. Hawthorne, and K. J. Ellis, "Effect of Prebiotic Supplementation and Calcium Intake on Body Mass Index," *Journal of Pediatrics* 151 (2007): 293-98.

13   K. Schmidt, P. J. Cowen, C. J. Harmer, G. Tzortzis, S. Errington, and P. W. Burnet, "Prebiotic Intake Reduces the Waking Cortisol Response and Alters Emotional Bias in Healthy Volunteers," *Psychopharmacology* 232, no. 10 (May 2015): 1793-801.

14   R. Luoto, K. Laitinen, M. Nermes, and E. Isolauri, "Impact of Maternal Probiotic-Supplemented Dietary Counselling on Pregnancy Outcome and Prenatal and Postnatal Growth: A Double-Blind, Placebo-Controlled Study," *British Journal of Nutrition* 103, no. 12 (June 2010): 1792-99.

15   Y. Kadooka, M. Sato, K. Imaizumi, et al., "Regulation of Abdominal Adiposity by Probiotics (Lactobacillus Gasseri SBT2055) in Adults with Obese Tendencies in a Randomized Controlled Trial," *European Journal of Clinical Nutrition* 64 (2010): 636-43.

16   A. S. Andreasen, N. Larsen, T. Pedersen-Skovsgaard, et al, "Effects of Lactobacillus Acidophilus NCFM on Insulin Sensitivity and the Systemic Inflammatory Response in Human Subjects," *British Journal of Nutrition* 104 (2010): 1831-38.

17   H. Bishop, A. C. Frazer, G. B. Robinson, and R. Schneider, "The Nature of the Antiperistaltic Factor from Wheat Gluten," *British Journal of Pharmacology* 21 (1963): 328-43.

18 M. A. Froetschel, "Bioactive Peptides in Digesta That Regulate Gastrointestinal Function and Intake," *Journal of Animal Science* 74 (1996): 2500–2508.

19 J. H. Exon, L. D. Koller, C. A. O'Reilly, and J. P. Bercz, "Immunotoxicologic Evaluation of Chlorine-Based Drinking Water Disinfectants, Sodium Hypochlorite and Monochloramine," *Toxicology* 44, no. 3 (1987): 257–69.

20 L. Lombardo, M. Foti, O. Ruggia, and A. Chiecchio, "Increased Incidence of Small Intestinal Bacterial Overgrowth during Proton Pump Inhibitor Therapy," *Clinical Gastroenterology and Hepatology* 8, no. 6 (June 2010): 504–8.

21 A. Lanas and F. Sopeña, "Nonsteroidal Anti-Inflammatory Drugs and Lower Gastrointestinal Complications," *Gastroenterology Clinics of North America* 38, no. 2 (June 2009): 333–52.

22 B. Chassaing, O. Koren, J. K. Goodrich, et al., "Dietary Emulsifiers Impact the Mouse Gut Microbiota Promoting Colitis and Metabolic Syndrome," *Nature* 519 (March 2015): 92–96.

23 J. Suez, T. Korem, D. Zeevi, et al., "Artificial Sweeteners Induce Glucose Intolerance by Altering the Gut Microbiota," *Nature* 514 (October 2014): 181–86.

24 G. Laden and R. Wrangham, "The Rise of the Hominids as an Adaptive Shift in Fallback Foods: Plant Underground Storage Organs (USOs) and Australopith Origins," *Journal of Human Evolution* 49, no. 4 (October 2005): 482–98.

25 J. G. Muir and K. O'Dea, "Measurement of Resistant Starch: Factors Affecting the Amount of Starch Escaping Digestion In Vitro," *American Journal of Clinical Nutrition* 56, no. 1 (July 1992): 123–27.

26 D. J. Jenkins, D. Cuff, T. M. Wolever, et al., "Digestibility of Carbohydrate Foods in an Ileostomate: Relationship to Dietary Fiber, In Vitro Digestibility, and Glycemic Response," *American Journal of Gastroenterology* 82 (1987): 709–17.

27 M. M. Murphy, J. S. Douglass, and A. Birkett, "Resistant Starch Intakes in the United States," *Journal of the American Dietetic Association* 108, no. 1 (2008): 67–68.

CHAPTER 12

1 R. Vieth, "Vitamin D Supplementation, 25-Hydroxy Vitamin D Concentrations, and Safety," *American Journal of Clinical Nutrition* 69, no. 5 (May 1999): 842–56.

2 M. A. Cabral, C. N. Borges, J. M. Maia, et al., "Prevalence of Vitamin D Deficiency during the Summer and Its Relationship with Sun Exposure and Skin Phototype in Elderly Men Living in the Tropics," *Journal of Clinical Interventions in Aging* 8 (2013): 1347–51.

3 C. C. Sung, M. T. Liao, K. C. Lu, and C. C. Wu, "Role of Vitamin D in Insulin Resistance," *Journal of Biomedicine and Biotechnology* 2012 (2012): 634195.

4 B. Schöttker, U. Haug, L. Schomburg, et al., "Strong Associations of 25-Hydroxyvitamin D Concentrations with All-Cause, Cardiovascular, Cancer, and Respiratory Disease Mortality in a Large Cohort Study," *American Journal of Clinical Nutrition* 97, no. 4 (April 2013): 782–93.

5 M. F. Holick, "Vitamin D: The Underappreciated D-Lightful Hormone That Is Important for Skeletal and Cellular Health," *Current Opinion in Endocrinology, Diabetes and Obesity* 9 (2002): 87–98.

6   I. Karakis, M. P. Pase, A. Beiser, et al., "Association of Serum Vitamin D with the Risk of Incident Dementia and Subclinical Indices of Brain Aging: The Framingham Heart Study," *Journal of Alzheimer's Disease* 51, no. 2 (February 2016): 451–61.

7   G. Tamer, S. Arik, I. Tamer, and D. Coksert, "Relative Vitamin D Insufficiency in Hashimoto's Thyroiditis," *Thyroid* 21, no. 8 (August 2011): 891–96.

8   E. Hypponen, E. Laara, A. Reunanen, et al., "Intake of Vitamin D and Risk of Type 1 Diabetes: A Birth Cohort Study," *Lancet* 358 (2001): 1500–1503.

9   A. Ascherio, "Environmental Factors in Multiple Sclerosis," supplement, *Expert Review of Neurotherapeutics* 13, no. S12 (December 2013): 3–9.

10 S. Gandini, F. Francesco, H. Johanson, B. Bonanni, and A. Testori, "Why Vitamin D for Cancer Patients?," *ecancermedicalscience* 3 (2009): 160.

11 A. Valcour, F. Blocki, D. M. Hawkins, and S. D. Rao, "Effects of Age and Serum 25-OH-Vitamin D on Serum Parathyroid Hormone Levels," *Journal of Clinical Endocrinology & Metabolism* 97, no. 11 (November 2012): 3989–95.

12 A. K. Heath, E. J. Williamson, D. Kvaskoff, et al., "25-Hydroxyvitamin D Concentration and All-Cause Mortality: The Melbourne Collaborative Cohort Study," *Public Health Nutrition* (March 29, 2016): 1–10.

13 U. Lehmann, F. Hirche, G. I. Stangl, et al., "Bioavailability of Vitamin D(2) and D(3) in Healthy Volunteers, A Randomized Placebo-Controlled Trial," *Journal of Clinical Endocrinology & Metabolism* 98, no. 11 (November 2013): 4339–45.

14 E. Hypponen, E. Laara, A. Reunanen, et al., "Intake of Vitamin D and Risk of Type 1 Diabetes: A Birth Cohort Study," *Lancet* 358 (2001): 1500–1503.

15 M. F. Holick, "Vitamin D: The Underappreciated D-Lightful Hormone That Is Important for Skeletal and Cellular Health," *Current Opinion in Endocrinology, Diabetes and Obesity* 9 (2002): 87–98.

16 I. R. Reid, S. M. Bristow, and M. J. Bolland, "Calcium Supplements: Benefits and Risks," *Journal of Internal Medicine* 278, no, 4 (October 2015): 354–68.

17 C. Y. Yang, P. S. Leung, I. E. Adamopoulos, and M. E. Gershwin, "The Implication of Vitamin D and Autoimmunity: A Comprehensive Review," *Clinical Reviews in Allergy & Immunology* 45, no. 2 (October 2013): 217–26.

18 H. A. Bischoff-Ferrari, W. C. Willett, E. J. Orav, et al., "A Pooled Analysis of Vitamin D Dose Requirements for Fracture Prevention," *New England Journal of Medicine* 367 (2012): 40–49.

19 C. Annweiler, Y. Rolland, A. M. Schott, et al., "Higher Vitamin D Dietary Intake Is Associated with Lower Risk of Alzheimer's Disease: A 7-Year Follow-Up," *Journals of Gerontology Series A: Biological Sciences and Medical Sciences* 67, no. 11 (November 2012): 1205–11.

20 A. M. Leung, L. E. Braverman, and E. N. Pearce, "History of U.S. Iodide Fortification and Supplementation," *Nutrients* 4, no. 11 (November 2012): 1740–46.

21 K. L. Caldwell, G. A. Miller, R. Y. Want, et al., "Iodine Status of the U.S. Population, National Health and Nutrition Examination Survey 2003–2004," *Thyroid* 18, no. 11 (November 2008): 1207–14.

22 J. Jiskra, Z. Limanova, Z. Vanickova, and P. Kocna, "IgA and IgG Antigliadin, IgA Anti-Tissue Transglutaminase and Antiendomysial Antibodies in Patients with Autoimmune Thyroid Diseases and Their Relationship to Thyroidal Replacement Therapy," *Physiological Research* 52, no. 1 (2003): 79–88.

23 R. Shimizu, M. Yamaguchi, N. Uramaru, et al., "Structure-Activity Relationships of 44 Halogenated Compounds for Iodotyrosine Deiodinase-Inhibitory Activity," *Toxicology* 314, no. 1 (December 2013): 22–29.

24 A. Elnour, L. Hambraeus, M. Eltom, et al., "Endemic Goiter with Iodine Sufficiency: A Possible Role for the Consumption of Pearl Millet in the Etiology of Endemic Goiter," *American Journal of Clinical Nutrition* 71, no. 1 (January 2000): 59–66.

25 W. R. Ghent, B. A. Eskin, D. A. Low, and L. P. Hill, "Iodine Replacement in Fibrocystic Disease of the Breast," *Canadian Journal of Surgery* 36, no. 5 (October 1993): 453–60.

26 S. Venturi and M. Venturi, "Iodine in Evolution of Salivary Glands and in Oral Health," *Nutrition and Health* 20, no. 2 (2009): 119–34.

27 K. L. Caldwell, G. A. Miller, R. Y. Want, et al., "Iodine Status of the U.S. Population, National Health and Nutrition Examination Survey 2003–2004," *Thyroid* 18, no. 11 (November 2008): 1207–14.

28 B. O. Asvold, T. Bjøro, T. I. Nilsen, et al., "Thyrotropin Levels and Risk of Fatal Coronary Heart Disease: The HUNT Study," *Archives of Internal Medicine* 168, no. 8 (April 2008): 855–60.

29 A. G. Juby, M. G. Hanly, and D. Lukaczer, "Clinical Challenges in Thyroid Disease: Time for a New Approach?," *Maturitas* 87 (May 2016): 72–78.

30 S. De Coster and N. van Larebeke, "Endocrine-Disrupting Chemicals: Associated Disorders and Mechanisms of Action," *Journal of Environmental and Public Health* 2012 (2012): 713696.

31 National Research Council Committee on the Toxicological Effects of Methylmercury, *Toxicological Effects of Methylmercury* (Washington, DC: National Academies Press, 2000).

32 "Product Review: Fish Oil and Omega-3 Fatty Acid Supplements Review (Including Krill, Algae, Calamari, Green-Lipped Mussel Oil)," ConsumerLab.com, April 5, 2014, consumerlab.com/reviews/fish_oil_supplements_review/omega3.

33 S. K. Raatz, J. T. Silverstein, L. Jahns, and M. J. Picklo, "Issues of Fish Consumption for Cardiovascular Disease Risk Reduction," *Nutrients* 5, no. 4 (March 2013): 1081–97.

34 J. Mariani, H. C. Doval, D. Nul, et al., "N-3 Polyunsaturated Fatty Acids to Prevent Atrial Fibrillation: Updated Systematic Review and Meta-Analysis of Randomized Controlled Trials," *Journal of the American Heart Association* 2, no. 1 (February 2013): e005033.

35 E. A. Miles and P. C. Calder, "Influence of Marine N-3 Polyunsaturated Fatty Acids on Immune Function and a Systematic Review of Their Effects on Clinical Outcomes in Rheumatoid Arthritis," supplement, *British Journal of Nutrition* 107, no. S2 (June 2012): S171–S84.

36 A. Laviano, S. Rianda, A. Molfino, et al., "Omega-3 Fatty Acids in Cancer," *Current Opinion in Clinical Nutrition & Metabolic Care* 16, no. 2 (March 2013): 156–61.

37 M. De Lorgeril, P. Salen, P. Defaye, and M. Rabaeus, "Recent Findings on the Health Effects of Omega-3 Fatty Acids and Statins, and Their Interactions: Do Statins Inhibit Omega-3?," *BMC Medicine* 11 (2013): 5.

38 E. M. Balk, A. H. Lichtenstein, M. Chung, et al., "Effects of Omega-3 Fatty Acids on Serum Markers of Cardiovascular Disease Risk: A Systematic Review," *Atherosclerosis* 189, no. 1 (2006): 19–30.

39 P. E. Miller, M. Van Elswyk, and D. D. Alexander, "Long-Chain Omega-3 Fatty Acids Eicosapentaenoic Acid and Docosahexaenoic Acid and Blood Pressure: A Meta-Analysis of Randomized Controlled Trials," *American Journal of Hypertension* 27, no. 7 (July 2014): 885–96.

40 P. Xun, B. Qin, Y. Song, et al., "Fish Consumption and Risk of Stroke and Its Subtypes: Accumulative Evidence from a Meta-Analysis of Prospective Cohort Studies," *European Journal of Clinical Nutrition* 66, no. 11 (2012): 1199–1207.

41 E. A. Miles and P. C. Calder, "Influence of Marine N-3 Polyunsaturated Fatty Acids on Immune Function and a Systematic Review of Their Effects on Clinical Outcomes in Rheumatoid Arthritis," supplement, *British Journal of Nutrition* 107, no. S2 (June 2012): S171–S84.

42 E. Cabre, M. Manosa, and M. A. Gassull, "Omega-3 Fatty Acids and Inflammatory Bowel Diseases—A Systematic Review," supplement, *British Journal of Nutrition* 107, no. S2 (2012): S240–S52.

43 R. M. Ortega, E. Rodriguez-Rodriguez, and A. M. Lopez-Sobaler, "Effects of Omega 3 Fatty Acids Supplementation in Behavior and Non-Neurodegenerative Neuropsychiatric Disorders," supplement, *British Journal of Nutrition* 107, no. S2 (2012): S261–S70.

44 M. W. Hess, J. G. Hoenderop, R. J. Bindels, and J. P. Drenth, "Systematic Review: Hypomagnesaemia Induced by Proton Pump Inhibition," *Alimentary Pharmacology & Therapeutics* 36, no. 5 (September 2012): 405–13.

45 L. Tosiello, "Hypomagnesemia and Diabetes Mellitus. A Review of Clinical Implications," *Archives of Internal Medicine* 156 (1996): 1143–48.

46 D. Thomas, "A Study on the Mineral Depletion of the Foods Available to Us as a Nation over the Period 1940 to 1991," *Nutrition and Health* 17, no. 2 (2003): 85–115.

47 A. W. Hoes, D. E. Grobbee, J. Lubsen, et al., "Diuretics, Beta-Blockers, and the Risk for Sudden Cardiac Death in Hypertensive Patients," *Annals of Internal Medicine* 123 (1995): 481–87.

48 S. C. Larsson and A. Wolk, "Magnesium Intake and Risk of Type 2 Diabetes: A Meta-Analysis," *Journal of Internal Medicine* 262 (2007): 208–14.

49 J. M. Peacock, T. Ohira, W. Post, N. Sotoodehnia, W. Rosamond, and A. R. Folsom, "Serum Magnesium and Risk of Sudden Cardiac Death in the Atherosclerosis Risk In Communities (ARIC) Study," *American Heart Journal* 160 (2010): 464–70.

50 U. Gröber, J. Schmidt, and K. Kisters, "Magnesium in Prevention and Therapy," *Nutrients* 7, no. 9 (September 23, 2015): 8199–226.

51 R. Hoffman, E. Benz, S. Shattil, et al., "Disorders of Iron Metabolism: Iron Deficiency and Overload," chap. 26 in *Hematology: Basic Principles and Practice,* 3rd ed. (London: Churchill Livingstone, 1999).

52 M. Foster and S. Samman, "Vegetarian Diets across the Lifecycle: Impact on Zinc Intake and Status," *Advances in Food and Nutrition Research* 74 (2015): 93–131.

53 P. Bonaventura, G. Benedetti, F. Albarède, and P. Miossec, "Zinc and Its Role in Immunity and Inflammation," *Autoimmunity Reviews* 14, no. 4 (April 2015): 277–85.

54 B. S. Oberlin, C. C. Tangney, K. A. Gastashaw, and H. E. Rasmussen, "Vitamin B12 Deficiency in Relation to Functional Disabilities," *Nutrients* 5, no. 11 (November 12, 2013): 4462–75.

55 S. J. Eussen, L. C. de Groot, R. Clarke, et al., "Oral Cyanocobalamin Supplementation in Older People with Vitamin B12 Deficiency: A Dose-Finding Trial," *Archives of Internal Medicine* 165, no. 10 (May 23, 2005): 1167–72.

56 K. Okuda, K. Yashima, T. Kitazaki, and I. Takara, "Intestinal Absorption and Concurrent Chemical Changes of Methylcobalamin," *Journal of Laboratory and Clinical Medicine* 81 (1973): 557–67.

57 "USDA Food Composition Databases," US Department of Agriculture, Agricultural Research Service, accessed September 9, 2016, ndb.nal.usda.gov/ndb/foods.

58 R. Green, "Indicators for Assessing Folate and Vitamin B-12 Status and for Monitoring the Efficacy of Intervention Strategies," *American Journal of Clinical Nutrition* 94, no. 2 (August 2011): 666S–72S.

59 M. Ebbing, K. H. Bønaa, O. Nygård, et al., "Cancer Incidence and Mortality after Treatment with Folic Acid and Vitamin B12," *JAMA* 302, no. 19 (2009): 2119–26.

60 J. B. Mason, A. Dickstein, P. F. Jacques, et al., "A Temporal Association between Folic Acid Fortification and an Increase in Colorectal Cancer Rates May Be Illuminating Important Biological Principles: A Hypothesis," *Cancer Epidemiology, Biomarkers & Prevention* 16, no. 7 (July 2007): 1325–29.

61 A. E. Czeizel, I. Dudás, L. Paput, and F. Bánhidy, "Prevention of Neural-Tube Defects with Periconceptional Folic Acid, Methylfolate, or Multivitamins?" *Annals of Nutrition and Metabolism* 58, no. 4 (October 2011): 263–71.

62 M. Fava and D. Mischoulon, "Folate in Depression: Efficacy, Safety, Differences in Formulations, and Clinical Issues," supplement, *Journal of Clinical Psychiatry* 70, no. S5 (2009): 12.

CHAPTER 13

1 S. R. Patel and F. B. Hu, "Short Sleep Duration and Weight Gain: A Systematic Review," *Obesity* 16, no. 3 (March 2008): 643–53.

2 P. Branger, E. M. Arenaza-Urquijo, C. Tomadesso, et al., "Relationships between Sleep Quality and Brain Volume, Metabolism, and Amyloid Deposition in Late Adulthood," *Neurobiology of Aging* 41 (May 2016): 107–14.

3 N. H. Rod, M. Kumari, T. Lange, et al., "The Joint Effect of Sleep Duration and Disturbed Sleep on Cause-Specific Mortality: Results from the Whitehall II Cohort Study," *PLOS ONE* 9, no. 4 (April 3, 2014): e91965, doi:10.1371/journal.pone.0091965.

4 G. Tosini, N. Pozdeyev, K. Sakamoto, and P. M. Iuvone, "The Circadian Clock System in the Mammalian Retina," *BioEssays* 30, no. 7 (July 2008): 624–33.

5 A. M. Chang, D. Aeschbach, J. F. Duffy, and C. A. Czeisler, "Evening Use of Light-Emitting Readers Negatively Affects Sleep, Circadian Timing, and Next-Morning Alertness," *Proceedings of the National Academy of Sciences of the United States of America* 112, no. 4 (January 2015): 1232–37.

6 R. G. Stevens, D. E. Blask, G. C. Brainard, et al., "Meeting Report: The Role of Environmental Lighting and Circadian Disruption in Cancer and Other Diseases," *Environmental Health Perspectives* 115, no. 9 (September 2007): 1357–62.

7   W. Zhang, W. Y. Chen, S. W. Su, et al., "Exogenous Melatonin for Sleep Disorders in Neurodegenerative Diseases: A Meta-Analysis of Randomized Clinical Trials," *Neurological Sciences* 37, no. 1 (January 2016): 57–65.

8   M. M. Heitkemper, C. J. Han, M. E. Jarrett, et al., "Serum Tryptophan Metabolite Levels during Sleep in Patients with and without Irritable Bowel Syndrome (IBS)," *Biological Research for Nursing* 18, no. 2 (March 2016): 193–98.

9   A. Bougea, N. Spanbideas, V. Lyras, et al., "Melatonin 4 mg as Prophylactic Therapy for Primary Headaches: A Pilot Study," *Functional Neurology* 31, no. 1 (January–March 2016): 33–37.

10 G. H. Song, P. H. Leng, K. A. Gwee, et al., "Melatonin Improves Abdominal Pain in Irritable Bowel Syndrome Patients Who Have Sleep Disturbances: A Randomised, Double Blind, Placebo Controlled Study," *Gut* 54, no. 10 (October 2005): 1402–7.

11 D. J. Kim, K. I. Cho, E. A. Cho, et al., "Association among Epicardial Fat, Heart Rate Recovery and Circadian Blood Pressure Variability in Patients with Hypertension," *Clinical Hypertension* 21 (November 22, 2015): 24.

12 A. Goyal, P. D. Terry, H. M. Superak, et al., "Melatonin Supplementation to Treat the Metabolic Syndrome: A Randomized Controlled Trial," *Diabetology & Metabolic Syndrome* 6 (November 18, 2014): 124.

13 E. Walecka-Kapica, G. Klupińska, J. Chojnacki, et al., "The effect of Melatonin Supplementation on the Quality of Sleep and Weight Status in Postmenopausal Women," *Przegląd Menopauzalny* 13, no. 6 (December 2014): 334–38.

14 M. Yurcheshen, M. Seehuus, W. Pigeon, et al., "Updates on Nutraceutical Sleep Therapeutics and Investigational Research," *Evidence-Based Complementary and Alternative Medicine* 2015 (2015): 105256.

15 G. Mazzoccoli, S. Carughi, M. Sperandeo, et al., "Neuro-Endocrine Correlations of Hypothalamic-Pituitary-Thyroid Axis in Healthy Humans," *Journal of Biological Regulators & Homeostatic Agents* 25, no. 2 (April–June, 2011): 249–57.

16 Y. H. Wu and D. F. Swaab, "The Human Pineal Gland and Melatonin in Aging and Alzheimer's Disease," *Journal of Pineal Research* 38, no. 3 (April 2005): 145–52.

17 W. C. Miller, "Effective Diet and Exercise Treatments for Overweight and Recommendations for Intervention," *Sports Medicine* 31, no. 10 (2001): 717–24.

18 M. Fogelholm, "Physical Activity, Fitness and Fatness: Relations to Mortality, Morbidity and Disease Risk Factors. A Systematic Review," *Obesity Reviews* 11 (2010): 202–21.

19 M. N. Silverman and P. A. Deuster, "Biological Mechanisms Underlying the Role of Physical Fitness in Health and Resilience," *Interface Focus* 4 (2014): 20140040.

20 S. M. Ryan and Y. M. Nolan, "Neuroinflammation Negatively Affects Adult Hippocampal Neurogenesis and Cognition: Can Exercise Compensate?," *Neuroscience & Biobehavioral Reviews* 61 (February 2016): 121–31.

21 B. Cerdá and J. D. Pérez-Santiago, "Gut Microbiota Modification: Another Piece in the Puzzle of the Benefits of Physical Exercise In Health?," *Frontiers in Physiology* 7 (February 18, 2016): 51.

22 H. J. Foulds, S. S. Bredin, S. A. Charlesworth, et al., "Exercise Volume and Intensity: A Dose-Response Relationship with Health Benefits," *European Journal of Applied Physiology* 114, no. 8 (August 2014): 1563–71.

23 S. S. Ho, S. S. Dhaliwal, A. P. Hills, and S. Pal, "The Effect of 12 Weeks of Aerobic, Resistance or Combination Exercise Training on Cardiovascular Risk Factors in the Overweight and Obese in a Randomized Trial," *BMC Public Health* 12 (August 28, 2012): 704.

24 K. Gebel, D. Ding, T. Chey, et al., "Effect of Moderate to Vigorous Physical Activity on All-Cause Mortality in Middle-Aged and Older Australians," *JAMA Internal Medicine* 175, no. 6 (June 2015): 970–77.

25 J. B. Gillen, B. J. Martin, M. J. MacInnis, et al., "Twelve Weeks of Sprint Interval Training Improves Indices of Cardiometabolic Health Similar to Traditional Endurance Training Despite a Five-Fold Lower Exercise Volume and Time Commitment," *PLOS ONE* 11, no. 4 (2016): e0154075, doi:10.1371/journal.pone.0154075.

26 S. S. Ho, S. S. Dhaliwal, A. P. Hills, and S. Pal, "The Effect of 12 Weeks of Aerobic, Resistance or Combination Exercise Training on Cardiovascular Risk Factors in the Overweight and Obese in a Randomized Trial," *BMC Public Health* 12 (August 28, 2012): 704.

27 E. J. Bassey and S. J. Ramsdale, "Increase in Femoral Bone Density in Young Women Following High-Impact Exercise," *Osteoporosis International* 4, no. 2 (March 1994): 72–75.

28 L. A. Tucker, J. E. Strong, J. D. LeCheminant, and B. W. Bailey, "Effect of Two Jumping Programs on Hip Bone Mineral Density in Premenopausal Women: A Randomized Controlled Trial," *American Journal of Health Promotion* 29, no. 3 (January–February 2015): 158–64.

29 E. G. Wilmot, C. L. Edwardson, and F. A. Achana, et al., "Sedentary Time in Adults and the Association with Diabetes, Cardiovascular Disease and Death: Systematic Review and Meta-Analysis," *Diabetologia* 55, no. 11 (November 2012): 2895–905.

30 E. B. Fortescue, A. Y. Shin, D. S. Greenes, et al., "Cardiac Troponin Increases among Runners in the Boston Marathon," *Annals of Emergency Medicine* 49, no. 2 (2007): 137–43.

31 L. Mont, R. Elosua, and J. Brugada, "Endurance Sport Practice as a Risk Factor for Atrial Fibrillation and Atrial Flutter," *EP Europace* 11, no. 1 (January 2009): 11–17.

32 C. J. Lavie, J. H. O'Keefe, and R. E. Sallis, "Exercise and the Heart—The Harm of Too Little and Too Much," *Current Sports Medicine Reports* 14, no. 2 (March–April 2015): 104–9.

33 J. D. Pillay, T. L. Kolbe-Alexander, W. van Mechelen, and E. V. Lambert, "Steps That Count: The Association between the Number and Intensity of Steps Accumulated and Fitness and Health Measures," *Journal of Physical Activity and Health* 11, no. 1 (January 2014): 10–17.

34 N. B. Hopf, A. M. Ruder, and P. Succop, "Background Levels of Polychlorinated Biphenyls in the U.S. Population," *Science of the Total Environment* 407, no. 24 (December 2009): 6109–19.

35 US Environmental Protection Agency, *An Exploratory Study: Assessment of Modeled Dioxin Exposure in Ceramic Art Studios* (Washington, DC: US Environmental Protection Agency, 2008).

36 F. Xin, M. Susiarjo, M. S. Bartolomei, et al., "Multigenerational and Transgenerational Effects of Endocrine Disrupting Chemicals: A Role for Altered Epigenetic Regulation?," *Seminars in Cell & Developmental Biology* 43 (July 2015): 66–75.

37 M. Barański, D. Srednicka-Tober, N. Volakakis, et al., "Higher Antioxidant and Lower Cadmium Concentrations and Lower Incidence of Pesticide Residues in Organically Grown Crops: A Systematic Literature Review and Meta-Analyses," *British Journal of Nutrition* 112, no. 5 (September 14, 2014): 794–811.

38 M. Kruger, P. Schledorn, W. Schrödl, H. W. Hoppe, W. Lutz, and A. A. Shehat, "Detection of Glyphosate Residues in Animals and Humans," *Journal of Environmental & Analytical Toxicology* 4 (2014): 2.

39 B. S. Rubin, "Bisphenol A: An Endocrine Disruptor with Widespread Exposure and Multiple Effects," *Journal of Steroid Biochemistry and Molecular Biology* 127, no. 1–2 (October 2011): 27–34.

40 P. D. Darbre and P. W. Harvey, "Paraben Esters: Review of Recent Studies of Endocrine Toxicity, Absorption, Esterase and Human Exposure, and Discussion of Potential Human Health Risks," *Journal of Applied Toxicology* 28, no. 5 (July 2008): 561–78.

41 P. A. Thompson, M. Khatami, C. J. Baglole, et al., "Environmental Immune Disruptors, Inflammation and Cancer Risk," supplement, *Carcinogenesis* 36, no. S1 (June 2015): S232–S53.

42 R. Verkerk, M. Schreiner, A. Krumbein, et al., "Glucosinolates in Brassica Vegetables: The Influence of the Food Supply Chain on Intake, Bioavailability and Human Health," supplement, *Molecular Nutrition & Food Research* 53, no. S2 (September 2009): S219.

43 M. L. Pall and S. Levine, "Nrf2, a Master Regulator of Detoxification and Also Antioxidant, Anti-Inflammatory and Other Cytoprotective Mechanisms, Is Raised by Health Promoting Factors," *Sheng Li Xue Bao* 67, no. 1 (February 25, 2015): 1–18.

44 M. E. Sears, K. J. Kerr, and R. I. Bray, "Arsenic, Cadmium, Lead, and Mercury in Sweat: A Systematic Review," *Journal of Environmental and Public Health* 2012 (2012): 184745.

Index

Underscored page references indicate boxed text.

H